REPORT:

Commission for the Control of
HUNTINGTON'S DISEASE
and Its Consequences

Volume IV, Part 5 — Public Testimony
New Orleans, New York, Seattle

October, 1977

U.S. Department of Health, Education, and Welfare
Public Health Service   National Institutes of Health

New Orleans, Louisiana

December 17, 1976

TABLE OF CONTENTS

Chronological List of Witnesses
New Orleans, Louisiana

December 17, 1976

Page

FERRIS, Robert M., Ph.D.
Burroughs Wellcome and Company   5-5

DORSEY, Richard F., M.D.
Merrell-National Laboratories   5-10

BAYNE, Gilbert M., M.D.
Merck Sharp & Dohme and Company   5-19

SLATER, Irwin H., M.D.
Eli Lilly and Company   5-24

KOPIN, Irwin, M.D.
National Institute of Mental Health   5-58

CARLSSON, Arvid, M.D.
Goteborg, Sweden   5-59

UDENFRIEND, Sidney, Ph.D.
Hoffman-LaRoche, Inc.   5-60

FREEDMAN, Daniel X., M.D.
University of Chicago   5-61

HOLLISTER, Leo E., M.D.
Stanford University   5-62

BUNNEY, William E., Jr., M.D.
National Institute of Mental Health   5-63

BENNETT, Ivan F., M.D.
Eli Lilly and Company   5-83

P R O C E E D I N G S

GUTHRIE: I see that one of our guests has walked into the room, at the end of the table. Since we asked all of you to come, those who are coming at your convenience, would you tell us who you are, and perhaps we could take some time out to speak with you.

FERRIS: Yes. I'm Robert Ferris, and I'm from Wellcome Research Labs with Burroughs Wellcome and Company.

CHASE: I understand that you're developing a GABA mimetic or a GABA inhibitor which might have some use in treating Huntington's chorea patients.

FERRIS: We are interested in GABA mechanisms in general. For the last five or six years, we've utilized the crayfish neuro-muscular junction preparation in our studies. Very recently we've set up the GABA binding assay, and we also have methods for studying the transport systems for GABA in flial cells and synaptosomes. In the neuropharmacology laboratories we are evaluating animal models for Huntington's disease. We also have set up the procedures for measuring GABA-T and GAD activity and would be interested in finding active compounds. Progress has been slow, and we don't really have anything suitable for treating Huntington's disease at the present time.

We have, for a number of years, been interested in the rela-tionship of GABA to the dopaminergic tracts. We feel such studies have the potential to lead to the development of drugs for the treatment of several disease states. So, we're looking at GABA systems in a much broader sense than simply the development of drugs for Huntington's disease; but that certainly would be one of our interests.

MC KHANN: Where are your labs?

FERRIS: In Research Triangle Park, North Carolina.

MC KHANN: Is Pedro Cuatrecasas with your group?

FERRIS: He's our Vice President of Research, Development and Medicine.

CHASE: That may explain the interest in GABA. We were just discussing when you came in what motivates drug companies to try to develop drugs for relatively rare diseases where the markets may not be that great. Can you speak to that issue at all?

FERRIS: I can tell you how we started with ours. I think you might have to look at Wellcome Research Laboratories in a little bit different light from many other industrial groups. Individual scientists are given a large prerogative to go into the type of research and development which interests them, if it fits within a framework of potential therapeutic applications. GABA was an interest of a former member of our staff in the CNS Section, Dr. Gerald McKenzie. He started our current program. So a general interest in the study of GABA systems was generated in our laboratories, rather than simply a desire to study Huntington's disease. While Huntington's disease certainly is something that we are concerned with, there's much more to the clinical implications of GABA systems than simply Huntington's disease. I think our research management appreciates this concept. We have reasonable freedom to do basic research, and we are encouraged to develop drugs from basic research ideas.

Really, when one looks at muscimol (and there's a real problem now in getting a hold of enough of it for everybody), one wonders if you can develop a more potent agent. Muscimol is an extremely potent agonist, at least in the receptor binding assay and other data that we've seen. It turns out to be a very difficult problem to synthesize muscimol-type compounds.

CHASE: Let's say you can develop a GABA mimetic, a GABA receptor agonist. Do you see any difficulties with bringing these drugs to clinical trial that this Commission should know about? Are there any problems you foresee that a commission of this type might deal with?

FERRIS: You're asking me questions that I don't really have the experience to answer. We certainly would recommend it to our Research Committee who makes the final decisions. I, personally, feel that they probably would develop the drug but at what level of priority, I don't know.

MC KHANN: Maybe it would be helpful to us if you could outline how things work through a company such as yours. Supposing you come up with a GABA agonist, for example, where do you go from there, in terms of taking it beyond your model systems?

FERRIS: Once we get the drug to this point, a complete
pharmacological profile in vivo is obtained by our general screening laboratories, as well as additional information in more
sophisticated secondary screening procedures. If the agent looks
like it's going to be a good agonist and has a reasonable therapeutic ratio, we would take it out of the research and screening
status into what we call program status. At this stage (and
there's some overlap between these various stages), we would try
to optimize activity by studying related compounds to see if we
have obtained the best one.

When the best compound is selected, we would recommend to
our Research Committee that this compound be developed for
clinical trial. If agreed to by the Research Committee, it would
be given project status. The Toxicology Department would get it
and take it through the necessary studies. If cleared by the
toxicologist, the compound would proceed on through to the filing
of an IND and into a phase 1 study. Our Medical Department would
be responsible for the clinical development of the drug.

N. WEXLER: How long would such a project take, approximately?

FERRIS: I can tell you for one drug, a new antipsychotic
agent that we have. We started the program in 1971-72, and the
projected date for marketing (with nothing going wrong) is approximately 1984.

N. WEXLER: For an antipsychotic, that's very good.

MC KHANN: Let me ask you a question about that. In this
13-year period, at what point along that 13 years was the basic
work completed, and how much of that 13 years is now being taken
up with the subsequent steps toward the human?

FERRIS: Actually, the basic research was started in about
1970 and was finished in '73, '74, somewhere in there. Then it
was recommended to project status.

MC KHANN: So we're saying 10 years?

FERRIS: It's at least 10 years.

N. WEXLER: Can you see any place along that way where the
process could be speeded up?

FERRIS: That's difficult to say. Yes, I think with a maximal effort and a change of priorities among competing projects,
some steps might be eliminated which would probably cut a year
off of development. But outside of that, no. It seems to me
that compliance to FDA regulations necessitates these extended
periods of time for drug testing before it can be marketed.

We're also faced now with the "Good Laboratory Practices"
proposals as printed in the Federal Register recently. I've
looked this over as it relates to efficacy for nonclinical laboratory studies, and I see problems.

CHASE: Do you want to specify some of those problems, because this is brand new for everyone. I'm just sort of curious
what your first impressions are.

FERRIS: This is exactly what it is, a first impression.
I've simply read the proposed regulations over very rapidly coming down here on the plane. It looks like we may have to hire
a few more people and have a quality assurance unit for research
practices, which would check out our laboratory instrumentation,
standardizations, records, et cetera. I think, in general, most
reputable scientists, such as those at Wellcome, do this without
regulation from the FDA. I'm not familiar with the problems that
the FDA has with other industrial laboratories. I know in Wellcome
if you fail to practice good fundamental research you would have
difficulties in maintaining your position. Regulation of what I
consider to be ordinary fundamental procedures for research is
going to take considerable time and money and effort, and I think
actually add more time on to getting a drug to the final stages
of development. That certainly is one of the problems.

CHASE: What you're saying is that you think it's going to
increase the overhead for new drug development and not necessarily
improve the safety of the new drug?

FERRIS: It is possible, certainly. I looked over the regulations, and I really think Wellcome would not gain anything in
terms of the quality of its research. The regulations might
simply be creating more time-consuming utilization of investigators' time in meeting bureaucratic requirements.

CHASE: More record keeping.

FERRIS: More record keeping, yes.

MC KHANN: Can you take advantage of the fact that you're a somewhat international company and move drugs along outside the United States more quickly than inside?

FERRIS: I think this is possible, but how successful this is, I'm really not qualified to answer.

MC KHANN: I want to ask you a more basic question relating, perhaps, to your own work. It seems to me that in the transmitter field (in the potential application to movement disorders) one of the key issues is which systems use which transmitters. Do you see being able to get at that with the use of the GABA binding assay, being able to localize, do you think, for example, which tracts are GABA-minergic a little better than we have already?

FERRIS: There are some problems with the GABA binding assay as it stands now. It's new, and it has to be refined and developed to a further extent, but I think there's a great potential for it. I, personally, would like to see it equated with another response, like cyclic GMP levels, for example; much like what's been done with the alpha receptor binding assay and cAMP levels by Lefkowitz and Snyder, and a number of other investigators. Then one might be able to locate GABA receptors with the assay and in this manner obtain some knowledge of GABA-minergic tracts. I don't think its possible to use the assay to trace the tracts, however, since the axons don't contain receptors.

M. WEXLER: Did you suggest that the initiation of the interest in GABA was because of the interest in the problem of aggression?

FERRIS: Not necessarily aggression, but more with the inter-relationship between the dopaminergic system and the GABA-minergic system and how these systems relate to aggressive and psychotic states.

CHASE: ...academic study, that the scientists are pretty much left to their own devices.

FERRIS: Yes, within the framework of eventually developing therapeutic agents, I think we have great leeway in picking the areas of research with no one really saying to us, "you can" or "you cannot be in this area." So, from that standpoint, yes. We put the emphasis on certain areas of basic research and, as a consequence, influence the further development of drugs within the company. I think we do it very conscientiously and very carefully, trying to consider all developmental aspects. I know in our particular case in the CNS section, we do consult Marketing to see what potential is involved. Marketing considerations are important, but in our company they are not by any means the total motivating force.

CHASE: Do they come to you and say, "We need a drug to do something"?

FERRIS: No. I would imagine that that could happen. It hasn't, as far as I know.

GUTHRIE: I see another guest has joined us. I think it would be nice if we could ask him to introduce himself, too. Maybe he'd like to join our discussion.

DORSEY: I'm Richard Dorsey. I'm a practicing psychiatrist and Director of Psychotherapeutic Research for Merrell National Laboratories, in Cincinnati. As I mentioned to Dr. Wexler yesterday, I did my M.B.A. research on regulation of medical practice and am very much interested in the issues that your Commission is addressing of how regulation can serve or not serve the public interest. I'm delighted to have a chance to join you.

CHASE: Would you care to make a statement, please.

DORSEY: Before making a statement, I'd like to ask (to be sure that I have the correct focus)--your interest is in how Government and the private sector can work together to develop new drugs in the CNS area with Huntington's disease as a model. I gather the particular focus is on what changes in regulation or in operating procedure might serve that goal. Is that a fair statement of what you want to know?

CHASE: Yes.

DORSEY: I'd like to start by talking briefly about regulation, partly as industry researchers perceive it and again from my own perspective of seeing it as a clinician as well. I think industry is probably 10 or 15 years ahead of the practice of medicine in where regulation has gone, for better or worse. With PSROs and a number of other areas that we are facing, I hope that both the medical profession and Government will learn from the experience in industry and adapt somewhat.

Two foci of regulation apply to drug development and to the pharmaceutical industry. The one which concerns us most is documenting and demonstrating the safety and efficacy of new drugs or drugs that are already on the market, because, if safety or efficacy questions come up, drugs can be removed. An example of a group that is about to be removed from the market is the monoamine oxidase inhibitors, a class of antidepressants that simply lack efficacy, proven by 1976 standards, because they are old drugs.

On the other side, questions of safety (e.g., carcinogenecity) will come up with drugs whose efficacy isn't questioned, and then the FDA tends to weigh the public health benefits of a class of drugs, in a therapeutic sense, against safety risks. An example here is the amphetamines for appetite control. There is no question that they're effective for that in the short run. The question that the Congress is asking, the question FDA asks, is: "Is that small degree of efficacy worth the public health hazard of abuse?" That question hasn't been answered.

The other thing FDA does is devote a fair amount of time and energy to monitoring the promotion of drugs to assure that all statements made, whether in advertisements or by the representatives of the companies, are consistent with labeling, which is not quite the same thing as being scientifically correct. They have to be consistent with the labeling; if the labeling is obsolescent, they still must be consistent. Whether that represents 1976 psychopharmacology or not is not the issue. This is a source of some concern to industry and a lot of concern to people who are practicing medicine, because sometimes Government has the view that failure to prescribe in accordance with labeling is somehow unauthorized prescribing or is not practicing medicine right. That's not true. The companies cannot promote outside of the labeling, but physicians can and sometimes should prescribe outside it. A fair amount of FDA time and energy is tied up in what I, personally, think are unproductive hassles over how physicians use drugs, rather than how the companies promote them, which is what FDA's statutory and constitutional mandate is.

If you look at the costs and benefits of regulation generally, which I think you have to do in order to get to the question of what would you change, the costs are pretty clear: First, it costs money; it costs the companies money, which is passed on to the patient and to the general public in tax-supported drug-purchase programs; it costs the FDA money because they've got to hire people to do the regulating and review the material; and it costs the Congress, indirectly, money in the time and effort spent in reviewing the reviewers. So there's a fair amount of money tied up in it.

More of concern, again particularly to the clinician, is the delay; the drug lag that [Wardell] and [Lasagna] have talked about is certainly a fact. What the impact of it is is arguable. But you can go to the meetings in this hotel and hear about drugs that have been used in Europe for a number of years and are not available in the United States. On the other hand, in some countries dubious drugs get on the market. If you look at France, the overall quality of their research is not very high, and some of the things that get on the market there probably shouldn't, by U.S. standards.

There's delay; there's the diversion of resources, and I think there is a decrease in innovation, because the amount of time and effort that we put in as a company (and I know the amount of time and effort I put in personally) to meeting regulatory requirements is not available to test new drugs, to see what the drugs will do. We have a backlog of new compounds we would like to test and will test. But if it's a choice between testing a new drug and keeping an existing drug on the market, there's no question which way we go. If FDA says, "We would like your comments on such and such," whether it's one item or ten pages of items about a drug that's already marketed, that gets first priority. To the extent that regulatory demands or the need to change labeling in order to promote new uses of a drug require a lot of time and effort to prove in effect that the world is round, then that time and effort and money are not available to test new compounds. That's the trade-off that you face.

On the other hand, there is some advantage, as compared with the older system. I think the quality of the pharmaceutical industry research in this country has gone up since 1962, because it has to. If you look at regulatory theory and practice, you see that where something is mandated (that's the price of staying in business), whether you're going to do it or not ceases to be a matter of judgment. If you have to prove efficacy before you

can get a drug on the market, then you have to do more thorough
research than if you have only to establish safety. If you have
to document very carefully that you have done good studies and
that your investigators have complied with your protocols and
have not gone off on tangents, then the scientific quality will
be higher than if you don't have that kind of pressure.

There is the orientation of science as an end in itself
that scientists have. There's an orientation in a commercial
enterprise or in Government (it doesn't make a whole lot of difference, I think) where the larger organization has its own
priorities. Science is, to some extent, a means to an end in
industry. Pharmaceutical companies are not set up exclusively
as scientific, investigatory operations; they're set up as commercial companies that I, personally, believe serve the public
interest very well by doing good science. What regulation does,
I think, is help the commercial managers translate scientific
quality into economic terms by saying that "If you don't have
the scientific quality, you can't go on the market," or "If you
don't have the scientific quality, you can't do the promoting,"
or something like that, in the same sense that regulation does
this in a number of other areas.

Finally, there's the reassurance function that Dr. Crout,
the Director of the Bureau of Drugs of FDA, has spoken to several
times. From that perspective, the amount of money and time you
can put into regulation is infinite, because it depends on how
much reassurance you want. If you want reassurance at a confidence level of only one chance in a million that something could
be wrong, it's going to cost you vastly more than if you'll accept one chance in a hundred. Dr. Crout has made the analogy that
a society can spend as much as it likes on the military, or on
housing, or on highways, depending on what that society values.
For the reassurance function, if you try to reassure some groups
in our society, the spending would approach infinity. If you're
satisfied to reassure the general public, it probably is high
enough now or maybe a little bit too high. How much you want to
spend depends on your target audience.

With that background, let's take a look at what a committee
like this might do to help accelerate the course of drugs going
through industry and through FDA. As you probably know, FDA
already has a kind of special pathway, a priority service, if you
will, for drugs that are genuinely unique, that address disorders

for which there is no good treatment or which are, on the face of
it, qualitatively superior to existing therapy. They'll give top
priority to drugs that will do this. They're doing it now with
an SKF drug for peptic ulcer disease. It seems to have a unique
mechanism of action, level of safety, and level of efficacy.

Even though Huntington's disease is a special disorder, and
if there is an effective drug for it that would get a top priority,
I think it might be worth looking at the broader issues of how
you would improve the whole process. Again, I think that a
commission like this (and hopefully others) could be very helpful
in that regard. If I were on your committee and wanted to do that,
what I would do first is go to the Congress, and I'd take several
messages to them, because I think that the Congress does listen to
testimony, particularly of influential, disinterested citizens or
those who have clear interests but are not parties to the actual
debate going on.

The first message is that you're interested in seeing drugs
that are effective and reasonably safe as a higher priority than
drugs that are safe and reasonably effective. That is the range
of debate today. The sick person wants to get well and usually
will take a fair amount of risk in order to do that, depending on
how sick he is. The person who is well and presuming to speak for
the sick person tends to focus more on wanting things to be safe,
because he's not hurting. The people that come into my office, and
into every physician's office, are there not primarily to debate
abstractions, or to look at the broad public interest; they're
there because they're sick and they want to get well. Somebody
with Huntington's disease, who knows what the prognosis is and
knows what's going to happen to him, is likely to accept a fairly
high risk. I think it's important to make the point on behalf of
the sick people in this country that a higher level of risk to get
the higher benefit is well worthwhile. I think that the medical
profession is starting to make that point and needs to hit it
harder, but I think that you can do that kind of thing particularly
well.

The corollary is that a difference exists between the patient's
interest and the public interest. Again, I think the patient's
interest, or that of the patient's family, is much more focused on
"How do I get well?" and less on concerns about rights, social
costs, or many other things that are reasonable issues, but not

necessarily the central one for medicine, nor the central one for drug development. Somebody needs to speak for the patient and say that this is the patient's concern and the family's concern.

We also need greater focus on another point in the Congressional hearings. This is not by any means uniquely my view, but something that Peter Hutt, Dr. Schmidt, and several Commissioners and Counsel of FDA have said. They would like to see more focus in Congressional hearings on the issue of the risks and benefits of technologic advance rather than on "to what extent has industry corrupted FDA," which, from our perspective, is a bogus issue. I really think that the FDA'ers are conscientious people that are not by any means corrupted by or unduly influenced by industry. I think they listen to industry because industry has a stake in it and does its homework and comes down there with scientific evidence rather than just moral fervor. To say that the central issue is how FDA is in industry's pocket, I think, misses the point, though it's an easy thing to do. It's a lot of fun; it's dramatic. The harder issue is to what extent will society take risks in order to get benefits on the broad technological front. The corollary is to what extent should society stand in the way of the individual patient who wants to take a higher risk than society would like to take. I've got some people in my office who would take a 1-percent risk of mortality, which is a very high risk in terms of drug therapy, if they could stay out of the hospital, or go back to school, or could get out of the home. We generally keep them out of the hospital now, but there are a lot of people who thought they were going to be professionals or were going to go to college, and so on, who are sitting home because, although we can get rid of hallucinations, delusions, and psychotic symptoms, dealing with the social withdrawal is a lot more difficult. They'd take a high risk.

Somebody who'd been in the hospital ten years would probably take a 5-percent risk of mortality to get well. In surgery, nobody thinks anything about 1-percent, 5-percent mortality in terms of the benefit. They don't disregard it, or say, "Well, we don't care about the operative mortality." They do say, "If we can accomplish such and such, we'll take that chance." I think that perspective is an important one to weigh in what we as industry can develop and what we as physicians can prescribe for our patients; there ought to be a broad range. If a doctor and a patient want to take a high risk because that's the way they feel about the issue, then I don't think that society ought to constrain them from doing that.

MC KHANN: May I ask you a question about that?

DORSEY: Yes.

MC KHANN: How do you see, then, limiting the use of a high-risk drug? Say, you have a specific situation. Let's say, for purposes of argument, you had a drug that carried, say, a 5-percent or a 1-percent mortality, but would alter a disease like Huntington's. How do you keep people from trying it (as has occurred with L-dopa) with every other unknown neurological disease?

DORSEY: I think there's something to be said for trying it, particularly if you have olivo cerebeller degeneration, which is a bad disease to have, too. If I had a patient like that, and nothing else worked, I think as a physician--not on a research basis, but simply doing the best I can for a patient that's in a tight situation--I might try it if there's any rationale. If it's something that I know is specific to Huntington's disease, and, on the face of it, it's absurd for anything else, I'm not going to try it.

Much of this kind of therapeutic adventuresomeness comes down again to the question of what else are you going to do? If you've got these people that are going downhill, or are downhill and hope to God they're going to get up, you take some chances. I think several appropriate controls already exist. The best example is the antineoplastic drugs, which have high toxicity and some mortality. Legally, I can prescribe antineoplastic drugs, if I want to. I'd be a fool to because I don't know anything about them. That's one area in which most doctors, I think, exercise self-control over what they do and do some weighing of the risks and benefits. I think there's tighter control in hospitals, via hospital accreditation standards. I think the Government's own program of PSRO is going to make that tighter still on an inpatient and an outpatient basis.

In Ohio, for example, we're planning to monitor prescribing patterns of physicians treating welfare patients, which is Medicaid. We have tentative agreement between the Ohio State Medical Association and the Department of Welfare that where they get physicians prescribing profiles that are three or four standard deviations away from the mean, we'll take a look at them. If they really are unjustified, we will cooperate with the Licensing Board in discouraging that kind of practice. I think that this is the kind of self-regulation on a local basis that is far, far preferable to some Procrustean bed designed in Washington.

What PSRO says, as Senator Wallace Bennett designed it to do (and rightly, I think), is that there are some standards from which deviation is permitted if you've got a good reason. The good reason may be that the patient hasn't responded to any other kind of treatment, or that the doctors in this part of the country, for this kind of population, tend to take a somewhat different view of risks and benefits. Ohio may think differently from Maryland or from Utah. There's a range of opinion in psychiatry, I know. In Utah, the physicians lean very much toward medical psychiatry and prescriptions and short-term psychotherapy. In Maryland, they lean very much toward psychoanalysis. I don't think you can say which is right, but I think you need that kind of diversity, and that you won't get it in a centrally designed and operated system, and you sure won't get it if the drug is not on the market in the first place. If you say, "Well, we'll constrain practice by not making drugs available," then the patient that needs the drug can't get it and is stuck.

M. WEXLER: It seems to me that what limited the extensive and rather careless use of lobotomy was the good judgment of the doctors, not some kind of legislation.

DORSEY: I agree. People find out. A number of procedures never were regulated. When I was a junior medical student, people were excited about freezing ulcers, and every hospital was going to have an ulcer freezing machine. That lasted about two years, and they found out it didn't work. I think that a pure clinician who's not interested in research at all certainly is interested in what works and what doesn't. If it doesn't work in general, and particularly if it has high risk associated, he's likely to give it up.

There's a combination of mechanisms. Another, of course (which we all dislike, but is a fact of life), is malpractice suits. If I have a drug for Huntington's chorea with a 10-percent mortality rate, and I'm giving it to people for transient dizzy spells, and one of them dies, I ought to go to court. I'm going to have a hard time defending myself, and I should have some difficulty like that. I think that's fair enough. But, again, the courts in this context look at what other reasonable physicians under the same circumstances do.

GUTHRIE: I was going to ask you, is there something that we could recommend that would give you that protection, because I happen to agree with what you're saying.

DORSEY: I think there are several things that offer us some
protection. I think what we need the most is protection from the
Washington system that is designed by people who don't know the
practice of medicine throughout the country very well. Malpractice litigation is at the local level, and I think that is not
mainly a Federal concern. Different states are handling it differently. In Ohio, we have reached an agreement with the legislature and have gotten some changes in the law in exchange for our
policing ourselves more tightly by setting up a system, which I had
the pleasure of helping design, that detected the mentally disabled
physician and offered him a choice between voluntarily stopping
practice and getting into treatment or losing his license.

We would like to do more of that. I think in principle,
though not through federal legislation, an increase in the power
of medicine to regulate itself (comparable to that of the Bar to
regulate itself) would serve the public interest well and strike
a responsive chord. I've spent a lot of time traveling in this
quality control area. I've talked to people on the planes, and
they say, "Why don't you doctors take the licenses of these other
people that aren't doing it right?" The answer is, "We can't."
We don't have that power. The state licensing boards are separate
from the medical societies; many people assume that they are like
the Bar, and they are not. You can expel people from medical
societies if they do badly, and they can thumb their noses and say,
"We're going to do it anyway." You can kick them off hospital
staffs, and they can thumb their noses and say, "We're going out to
a county where there isn't a doctor and do as we please."

Finally, where we're catching up to them is with the computerized profiles. You say, "Well, Doctor, here you are doing things
five standard deviations away from what everybody else in the same
situation is doing. If you can't account for that, we're going to
the licensing board with it." That is evolving, and I think it's
better down at the state or local level than through federal legislation. It's a fair question from a Congressman to ask exactly
what you've asked: "If we give wider latitude in drugs getting
on the market, what mechanisms are there?" The answer is the ones
I've mentioned to you. I'd be happy to give you more formal background material, in terms of publications, or something, on that,
if it would help you.

I think the major issue is looking at technology and looking
at public policy, and not engaging in what from the practicing

psychiatrist's viewpoint is kind of a political psychodrama of the virtuous FDA versus the villainous industry. As I say, it gets more headlines, but I don't think it helps the public a lot, and surely it doesn't help the patient.

WILENTZ: Could we get back to the specifics of drugs formulated for these diseases? Is Merrell actively working on GABA mimetics or others?

DORSEY: Not as a major effort, though we do have one compound in this area. In terms of industry, there is a range something like this: Some companies do a lot of basic research, animal pharmacology, early development, as well as clinical testing, and that's where their strength lies. At the other extreme, some companies think, "I don't have to waste the money," and that they will acquire promising compounds. They do not see the reason to maintain a large stable of basic scientists either because overall it's a waste of money, or because that isn't what their strength is, and they don't want to build it. They will go to Europe, particularly, and get promising compounds and develop them then clinically in the U.S. (That we have to go abroad to get the compounds is itself unfortunate, but that's the fact.) Merrell is more toward that end of the spectrum. Burroughs may be more toward developing the compounds themselves. This will vary. I think certainly the regulatory impact on clinical research is the same for both kinds of companies. The weight of good laboratory practices, and so on, falls more heavily on a company that does more of that kind of work.

GUTHRIE: Excuse me, just a minute. We have one guest who told me he had to leave by 11:00 o'clock. I would like to ask him, won't you join our conversation and tell us who you are, please?

BAYNE: I'm Gilbert Bayne, Director of Long-Term Planning for Merck Sharp & Dohme Research Laboratories. I would like to relate to one part of your discussion, the question this gentleman asked, the problem of regulating drugs by restricting distribution. Unfortunately, it does create inequities under certain circumstances. I think you should think a long time before you do it.

For example, the treatment of patients with multiple cancer drugs is a risky procedure and probably best done in a cancer center. On the other hand, if you have a patient who just doesn't

want to go to a cancer center, and you could improve his prognosis
by giving drugs in the home or in the local hospital, I think you
should think awhile before you take away that right to treatment.
We'd prefer, rather, to describe the hazards and the potential
benefits and then rely on the physician and the local controls of
physicians (as you've talked about) to see that the drugs are
properly applied.

MC KHANN: May I ask you, representing a large pharmaceutical
industry which has been quite successful in the neurological area
recently, a question? One of the problems we were discussing before you came in is the problem from the point of view of a drug
manufacturer in relationship to a drug that may be very effective,
but for which the population may be small; in other words, relatively rare diseases in terms of total numbers. How much does
that go into your planning? You mentioned that you're the long-
term planner. How do you see that problem, and, from the point of
view of our Commission, what should we say about it, or what could
we do to change the ideas about this?

BAYNE: There's a potential problem. Most organizations like
our own have many, many projects to work on--more than we have the
capacity to work up for clinical trial at a given point in time.
We are inevitably forced to assign some sort of priorities. However, this does not necessarily exclude from consideration the
drugs that are useful for the treatment of a small population. I
think most of the large companies try to respond to a social need.
For example, we market many such drugs: Actinomycin-D is a limited
use drug. Asparaginase has been supplied for years for the treatment of acute lymphatic leukemia. There are many examples of this,
where you depend on and you usually get a response from the
pharmaceutical industry to provide a service.

It is true that if we're left to our own initiatives, we tend
to attack rather large populations. However, in a company like
Merck, where you have maybe 2,000 scientists (many of them working
on basic mechanisms), you will uncover in a random sort of fashion
drugs for the treatment of diseases you didn't originally seek to
treat. You attack a pharmacological objective, a serotonergic
drug, an antiserotonergic drug, whatever. Once you've found the
drug, it may well have applications more broad than anticipated.
Some of these agents modifying CNS transmitter systems may well
benefit the Huntington's disease patients.

N. WEXLER: I had a related question to that. Given a relatively rare disease, plus Dr. Dorsey's notion (which I think is a
very curious one) that the Government sets itself up to decide
what kinds of risks an ill person should take--I think that's an
interesting concept which I hadn't really thought of before--that
is, given a small population with a high-risk drug that might be
very efficacious, can it possibly be commercially feasible for a
company to really develop that drug? That's really two blows
against you.

BAYNE: As I say, we market many drugs intended for rather
restricted uses. Actinomycin-D is a very toxic drug for a very
specific treatment situation. Asparaginase is the same sort of
thing--many side effects, but, for certain patients, a necessary
treatment.

N. WEXLER: Do you have to be a pretty large company to be
able to do that?

BAYNE: I'm sure that out of the multiple pharmaceutical
companies you'll find somebody who is willing to do that.

DORSEY: I think the answer is, yes, you have to be large.
If you want to expand the pool of companies that might do that,
there was a comment that, in essence, the patients who are buying
other drugs from that company are subsidizing this, something
industry hasn't done much of. But if you want to take a look at
innovation, it's always a nice thing to do.

You can look at the airlines, for example, and see that
Government directly subsidizes service to small communities. In
our part of the country Piedmont Airlines flies into a lot of
places that TWA is not interested in. The reason Piedmont is
interested is that they are getting direct support, taxpayer support, for that, which I think makes some sense.

There are several ways of handling it: One, which I think
theoretically is the most appealing, is that you assure that
there is a market, that the Government (or somebody) will pay
enough for the drug when it's finally developed to make it worthwhile. If you have a small number of patients and somewhat high-
risk kinds of drugs with high legal liability as a consequence,
then the price is going to have to be high to make it worthwhile.

There are many companies, for example, that are serving the renal dialysis market, and that are doing so because they know that Medicare is going to pay for goods and services (or in this case mainly goods) in that area. They know that there's a market if they can find something that will serve it. If everybody were paying out of the pocket for renal dialysis, it'd be a different market.

The other alternative (which I think would require even more change in orientation, but is still worth looking at) is, would the Government be willing to share the cost of development? I think the private sector is still, in general, better at doing applied kinds of development, taking things from the creative stage into a drug that's available for distribution. Would Government, either through direct subsidy or through tax credit (that's another way of doing it and probably preferable, theoretically), be willing to give companies incentives to put some of their money into that kind of venture? Again, I think that would be worth looking at and could serve the public interest even better than having the Government itself do it.

There are other variants that we've been involved with, the swine flu venture, which is not exactly a model for success. That was wholly nonprofit. There are things that you can look at: Will government give a shield from liability? If we're going to test a drug that we know killed 10 percent of animals (and, therefore, the only thing you can guess is that man is going to be at risk), will Government relax its standards or treat something like this as a special case, in terms of its willingness to let it go into patients in the first place? Will Government take the view that the risk is worthwhile and not beat us over the head when the first patient dies, not have a hearing, and not have the president of our corporation up, asking him, "Why are you killing patients and disregarding the public interest?" If we had some kind of assurance that an explicit policy would permit that, I think it would be much more attractive.

MC KHANN: May I ask Dr. Bayne to comment on that, from the point of view of a company like Merck? Do you see this kind of Government subsidization as just a road to more interference that you don't want around, or do you see this as an effective route? We had discussed this issue before you came. That's why I ask.

BAYNE: I have mixed emotions on that. There are such programs now, in the sense that the Cancer Chemotherapy group in the NIH has people make compounds for them and do certain other services. When we have done that, we've generally done it in the public spirit of cooperation more than with the idea that it would be productive for the company. I think you have to look at the situation. If there is a logical approach (you understand the disease, you have a good animal model) and you could persuade yourself that if you just spend enough time screening compounds you will find a cure for this disease, I think maybe then you should consider mobilizing resources to do that.

If you really don't understand it, and there is no satisfactory model, then I don't believe you can make a case for simply increased random activity. You might better invest in a better understanding of the disease. People seeking solutions to other problems may in the meantime devise agents which will modify central transmitters in such a way as to benefit the Huntington's disease patients.

I would not like the company to have a very large investment in so-called directed research for the treatment of Huntington's disease unless we felt confident about the hypothesis and the available technology for seeking a solution. I would rather be seeking new types of pharmacology or biology with the expectation that when we understand more about basic mechanisms we'll be able to manipulate nature's interference with the human mechanism. Is this too confusing, the way I'm putting it?

DORSEY: No.

SLATER: I think there's another way of saying it--you talk about the companies doing research, but the research is done by individual people in the companies and by scientists who are dedicated to learning something. If they're not convinced that the research they're doing has meaning and relevance and that the tools they use are really something, they're not going to work on it. This is not a situation where you have people and you say, "Do this. Do that." These are independent men that you have to deal with.

GUTHRIE: Excuse me. Would you introduce yourself to us, please?

SLATER: I'm Dr. Slater, Director of Pharmacology at Eli Lilly and Company. I should say that my statements represent my personal point of view and should not be considered as representing an expression of the policy of the Lilly Research Laboratories or Eli Lilly and Company.

DORSEY: I think what you're hearing is, to some extent, the difference between the creative, basic science companies (which are much harder to direct) and ours or some others, where if we have a compound that we think is going to work, we certainly can and do say that this is what's going to be studied. It's at that point particularly that tax credits, or whatever, can make the difference in choosing to put time, money, and people into drug A rather than B, C, or D. There is a close tie (in our company, certainly) between commercial management and clinical research in decisions on where we go and which compounds and which projects get the priority. I would agree that you cannot direct people to create; you can certainly direct them to test clinically.

MACKAY: Let me ask you another question. You speak of Government intervention. Several hundred patent licenses on new compounds developed with DHEW funding in university facilities have been taken over by drug companies and are in various stages of development. I have no idea what the commercial value of those is, though it's estimated to be in the hundreds of millions of dollars, potentially. Some of them are very far from being actually on the market; I think only one has come on in the last nine years, when DHEW policy was modified to facilitate industry interest. Lately, there's been some talk of tampering with that area. What is the impact of that on your development of new drugs (because, presumably, those would be coming out of basic research enterprises and then would be recognized for marketability or for therapeutic potential)? Are these helpful in drug development?

DORSEY: I can speak only in a very general way. We don't care particularly what the source is as long as it's patented, whether it's Paul Janssen in Belgium, or one of the French companies, or whatever. The concern, from a commercial viewpoint, is, "Does it work or have some probability of working, is it patented, is it safe, and what will it do?" which are the four things you really need to know.

MACKAY: I mentioned it as a way that Government effort does contribute to the development of therapeutic agents.

SLATER: Precisely what are you talking about?

MACKAY: I'm talking about patenting of---

SLATER: Which patents are you talking about?

MACKAY: I'm talking about patents of some 368 compounds in
the period from 1964 to 1973 that were licensed by universities.
They were developed by university scientists under federal funding.
I'm asking, does that have a measurable impact on drug company
development? That is, they may obtain patent rights to that;
they may buy the license to market it, but I have no estimation,
from the drug companies' point of view, of the amount of commercial
or therapeutic potential. These may all just sit on the shelf because they really can't be developed much further, but, in securing
the license, the company has at least made some initial investment
in an eventual payoff. That's what I'm trying to get an answer to.

BAYNE: I'd like to say that I think that is a good thing.
There are many scientists working independently, and they will
create hypotheses in their minds and test them in their own environments and validate some of them. Of the ones that reach that stage,
many will have potential therapeutic application. The next stage
is the role that the pharmaceutical industry is particularly well
set up to do, to take this potential from the point of hypothesis
validation on to a marketed product. There are many, many things
required to develop a good idea and make a product out of it. We
have built an organization with all the skills to do that last part
of the job.

I would hope that new ideas are continually being generated in
the university setting; and after they've taken them as far as they
logically can, I hope they would take the initiative to seek the
help of industry to assist in development and marketing.

M. WEXLER: I'm not quite sure how to organize this question.
You've mentioned two mechanisms: tax relief or some kind of tax
credit and some kind of protection from liability. Is there any
way in which the Government could operate with other mechanisms
to develop drugs felt to be relevant, let's say, to Huntington's
--by way of grant or contract mechanisms?

DORSEY: I had given the first analogy, direct subsidy. I think one of the problems historically with direct subsidy is a kind of Gresham's law, that good money drives out bad. If you get too much subsidy you lose one of the things that makes private enterprise work fairly efficiently, which is the incentive to conserve its own money. You've got the money, and then you've got to do the job and have something left over. If it's cost-plus, historically such industries (whether they're in defense or hospital care) have not performed as well as those that have gotten tax credits or some other way of getting the money and the targeting without the disadvantages of that kind of compensation. There are many ways it could be done. I am just suggesting to you, in a general way, what experience has shown to be the benefits of one versus another.

CHASE: Historically, whenever the Government has subsidized industry, it has imposed some degree of control over that industry; in other words, money goes along with finding somebody with that money. I am just wondering whether the drug companies in general would support the idea of more direct, obvious subsidization of new drug development, number one; and, number two, whether there's any other way of getting around that issue. Drug companies are in business to make a profit. One of the ways of insuring your profit is to diminish the cost of doing research. Perhaps the Government could serve as an insurer against patient suits, as they are in the swine flu program; or, perhaps another way of approaching this problem is to try to figure out how you can diminish the cost of the regulatory process. This sort of gets back to where we were initially. I wonder whether you have any suggestions about how the regulatory process could be improved.

Criticisms against the FDA as the primary regulatory agency abound. Nobody seems to be happy with the FDA. You painted the FDA as being sort of a white knight here. If you talk to Ralph Nader's group, the FDA is the villain. The point is, do you have any real suggestions for improving the whole process and perhaps making it more efficient to introduce new drugs onto the market?

DORSEY: I would say, first, that to get any organization (whether it's regulatory, business, Government) to work well, you have to have agreement on what it's supposed to be doing. One reason that FDA is getting caught in a cross fire is that different people have their own agendas for what FDA should be doing and are judging its performance against those agendas in the absence

of any specific policy definition. Does the public, in terms of
what it'll allow to move in interstate commerce, basically want
to give first priority to safety and then efficacy in drug development, or to efficacy and then safety? If you don't have the
standard by which the agency is supposed to regulate, you are
forever going to have arguments.

I think Nader's position is clearly "safety first." Safety
first and hamstringing business second are ends in themselves, at
least it's our perception that that is so. Industry and the
medical profession tend to lean the other way. I'm not painting
FDA as a white knight, because I think the level of scientific
competence in FDA is not nearly what it should be to discharge the
legal responsibility it has. I'm saying they are basically fair
people, and they are not persuaded by much of anything that
industry can do, except bring forth scientific evidence and show
interest in its own products. If you hear the speeches that the
top executives of FDA make, that's their perception also.

As an FDA staffer, right now I know that if I say "yes,"
either I or the guy above me will have to go down and tell Senator
Kennedy or Congressman Fountain, or somebody, why he said "yes;"
if I say "no," I might get a medal. It's not hard to imagine
which way I'm going to call the doubtful shots. If the Congress
declared the wish to see drugs move faster through FDA and would
investigate why they're moving slowly rather than saying that they
want safety first, we'd see a marked acceleration in drug development. A group like yours would have high credibility in telling
Congress that.

Maybe you could deal with the "consumerists." We, in industry,
have not had much success in such communication; the medical profession hasn't either because of the intense climate of suspicion
and distrust based on a number of factors. I think having people
who speak for those who have the disease talk to health research
groups and tell them that your genuine feeling is that you need
the new drugs and want the new drugs...maybe you could set up a
forum at which you would try again to get "consumerists," public
officials, and industry people to try to work together. Medicine
is very, very complex; so is the pharmaceutical industry. I don't
see how you can run a system that complex and carry on a guerilla
war at the same time. It's a basic principle of management that if
you want a smooth-running organization, you've got to have the
organization set up and going in the same direction. You can't have
a lot of infighting simultaneously. We'd certainly like to see that.

Basically (and this is mundane, but important), I think you
could go to the FDA Advisory Committee meetings to ask, "How is
this project coming?" When some people say that you shouldn't
permit things to move as fast as they are, you can say, "We think
you should move them faster." It's unglamorous, it seems rather
pedestrian, and yet this is what industry does, which the
"consumerists" say is undue influence. Anything that comes up
that's going to affect us, we're there. We try to do our homework
and try to have the scientific evidence, but I think you would
have greater credibility.

GUTHRIE: I think that the consumer is sort of caught between
the two (agreeing with what you're saying), and I can call myself
a consumer. I also feel that what Dr. Slater said influences my
thinking in that I realize that there's a creative process going
on, and I cannot, therefore, go and say, "I'm going to give you
all the money. You better do that work." Your interest is vital.
So we're sort of caught between the two.

DORSEY: I think we're talking now at different stages. The
creativity is harder to regulate or deregulate. It's much more,
as he pointed out, that industry does best. Creativity can occur
in industry, or academia, or wherever. Industry's unique skill,
in the general scheme of things, is taking the original creation
and moving it step by step until it's a drug on the market. You
can have profound influence on that process, and regulation most
clearly can accelerate or retard it. One exception to that has
been in psychopharmacology, where most of the advances have been
by serendipity; new drugs have been tested for one thing, and it
was found they did something else. That, again, comes back to the
trade-off. Would you, as a public official, or an advisor to a
public official, allow more drugs to go into humans earlier with
less safety data on the chance that one of them will turn out to
do something that either wasn't expected, or only a little bit
suspected, rather than having them well proven before they went
into humans?

LI: We are all consumers, of course. We like to see effective drugs moving into use faster. On the other hand, if the
Government does move faster, aren't we going to get another
thalidomide?

DORSEY: That's the risk. It's precisely that.

SLATER: Getting that assurance, from the present techniques, just isn't going to happen no matter how careful you are. No drug goes into clinical trial with more than 5,000 or 10,000 patients. If something has a low incidence, it's going to happen. It's not going to happen right away...and by sitting on the data and waiting and waiting and waiting, you still don't answer the question.

MC KHANN: Could I ask you to make that calculation a little further? That is, in order to substantiate a specific risk, whether it's as striking as [ocamelia] or thalidomide or [toxican-thinitis], what are your numbers?

SLATER: I'm not enough of a statistician to tell you exactly. But if you want to say, at a very high probability, something is not going to occur at the rate of, say, one patient in a thousand, then there are statistical calculations that say it's probably going to take 6,000 or 7,000 patients before you have any idea whether it's going to happen, and you have the assurance it's going to happen once or twice.

MC KHANN: This has particular relevance when you're dealing with a relatively small population of patients, because you may be talking about a significant proportion of those available for testing of the drug.

SLATER: I think that you also have to recognize in this group of patients what the inevitable cost is and what, for some people, a period of benefit means as against the risk of sudden mortality or sudden damage to the patient. This is sort of a hardhearted way of looking at things. One of the things you never know, philosophi-cally, is if you have five patients and two of them are going to die, and you save one patient and only one in five dies, is it the same patient who would have died the other way? Have you killed somebody to save two other people, and are you justified morally in doing this? These are very difficult problems to answer.

DORSEY: One other way of addressing it would be in terms of economic theory--the diminishing marginal utility concept--that if you want to go from 95 percent assurance to 99 percent assurance, it's going to cost you twice as much. If you're going from zero, no assurance at all, to 95, it may cost you, say, $1 million in drug testing. If you want to go from 95 to 99, it's going to cost you another million. If you want to go from 99 to 99.9, it's going to cost you a million on top of that.

This is the risk that we're talking about in industry. It's also the risk that I or any other physician deals with every day. Should we take some chances, including chances of something really bad happening, in order to get the benefit? There isn't any way you can have drugs that are simultaneously highly safe and highly effective in most instances. You've got to go one way or the other.

SCHACHT: I think you also have to recognize individual differences in here, where an individual will react to a drug where no one else might...

DORSEY: That's right. It's partly the response, and the other part is, again, the individual propensity to take risks. One person may say, "Better the devil I know than the one I don't know, and I'm going to stick with my disease." If someone is a psychiatrist, a weakness in the right hand doesn't make a whole lot of difference. If the same person is a surgeon, he's going to take a lot bigger chances to get full strength in his right hand back, which makes a crucial difference to his whole profession.

LI: We all realize the risks we are taking. If we are worried about one type of risk, we take another risk of the second type. We realize all that. My question is, what is the critical thing that helped the United States avoid thalidomide? What is the critical factor?

DORSEY: I think, unfortunately, the answer may be delay, if you sit on it long enough. To some extent, it's an unspoken public policy that we're willing to let Europeans be the clinical screen for our drugs. If it's on the market in Europe for five years, and nobody's died of it, then, "Yeah, all right. We'll expose Americans." The other side of the coin is they don't get the benefit. Frances Kelsey didn't come up with some unique system or divine inspiration; she sat on the thing and got a medal. Everybody knows that.

M. WEXLER: Nobody asked, much more bluntly, how many people died from delay? That problem can't be avoided altogether.

DORSEY: No one died from the delay on thalidomide. It comes back, even at the price of being redundant, to the risk. How many die of delay in marketing an anti-ulcer drug, or an anti-cancer drug? Something that's intensely debated, what about some of the other beta-blocker drugs for hypertension, cardiac arrhythmia, angina? They are diseases that have clear mortality. You get intense argument and, depending on whose statistics you look at, different answers on whether--the fact is that there's only one beta-blocker on the U.S. market and two or three in Europe, including ones that are the drugs of choice there--there are more people dying from untreated hypertension and cardiovascular disease than are being saved by not being exposed to risk. Often, you come down to intangibles.

Personally, I think that public policy would support greater risk for a greater benefit. I don't think that it's always addressed specifically in the Congressional hearings or in the public dialogue where you have something with high morbidity-- and again, if you want to look at Huntington's disease, there you're weighing high morbidity against potential mortality. Nobody's going to die of it next year, but in terms of what it does to the individual, it may be worse than dying.

M. WEXLER: I know the risk-reward problem is much more important than the one I raised before. I'd like to come back to it for a moment. Maybe you could help me. I'd like to make it very concrete. If Burroughs Wellcome is finding it very difficult to synthesize muscimol and is about to give it up because it's a very long-term, expensive, and difficult project, and if Tom Chase were vitally interested in having this kind of GABA analog and felt that it was very important to continue the development of this drug, what types of mechanisms could be used by the Government to insure that they don't drop the synthesis?

DORSEY: Are either of you going to comment on how you would get a particular compound? I think to some extent, again, industry's strength has been partly in making its own decisions based on its perception of what the payoff will be. I think that that is part of private enterprise versus the public sector that tends to look more to the question you're asking of "Who wants it?" rather than "What will the payoff be?"

M. WEXLER: ...indicated their interest and they're excited about the development, but they're really finding that it's problematic because it's difficult to synthesize; so they may want to drop it....But, suppose the Government or NINCDS felt that this was a very important contribution and treatment and wished either

for Burroughs Wellcome or some other drug company to continue the
efforts to synthesize the drug.

DORSEY: Personally, I would not be able to add much more than
what I've suggested already. The economic incentive in one form or
another (whether it's an assured ultimate market, a tax credit, or
a direct subsidy) that says, "We'd like you to stay in this area,
and this is what we'll do for you tangibly," would be what I would
lean toward.

SLATER: I think if you thought it was sufficiently important,
we could do it very easily with grants out in the academic community. You'll find a problem that is of major chemical difficulty
will attract academic people as well as industry people. This type
of problem may be better handled as a study of mechanisms of a
chemical reaction that are in themselves a fulfillment and a source
of provocation to the academician.

CHASE: Maybe the swine flu program is an example of what
Milton is talking about. Here the Government perceived the need,
and the industry was willing to go into it, but was not that
enthusiastic on the basis of market potential. The Government, in
a variety of ways, subsidized the program; yet the whole thing is
collapsing around us. Is it true that when the Government puts its
heavy hand into the private enterprise system, the results may be
less than what one would like to see?

DORSEY: The whole point of contracting out is that somebody
knows how to do it better or has a better track record than you do.
That's one of the main reasons for doing that. If you're going to
contract out and then tell the person every step of the way, it
doesn't make as much sense to contract. The point raised here,
which is an excellent one, is should you go to industry at all, or
should you be going to academia for some of the creative work, or
both? Of all the choices, an assured market tends to be the most
attractive. If you want something short-run, then have the fewest
controls, the most flexibility for industry, because part of what
you're buying, as Government, is industry expertise and fleetness
of foot.

MC KHANN: Let me ask a little different question related to
this. Before you came in we heard that Burroughs Wellcome was
working on a product that was seeded, so to speak, in 1970 or '71,
and it may be as late as 1984 before this is carried through the

entire process. Does this kind of lag interfere with communication and dispersal of new knowledge that could be useful to either academic investigators or people at other pharmaceutical companies who might be looking at it a different way?

I understand the pharmaceutical industry's problem. They've got to know when they can get their money back, plus. On the other hand, we're dealing with a very long period of time where there's information that one group has that others may or may not. I guess the question I'm asking is, during this long delay process, at what point is this public information?

SLATER: It varies enormously with how important and how interesting it is. We can't keep our scientists as creative people who will stay in our company unless we allow them to publish at a reasonable point. So that, by and large, when the patent situation is clearly established, we publish, and we publish before we file foreign patents. Once we have filed an American patent, we will generally publish. So these data are frequently published years before the clinical trials are finished and many years before the FDA accepts the results of these trials. I don't think that this is a serious problem. It is a problem if you have an idea, you work on it for awhile, you have some limited success, but you decide you're not going to get anywhere; then our tendency, probably, is not to publish. But that has nothing to do with the regulatory process.

DORSEY: In the later stages, once you've done clinical trials, the investigator's going to publish the results of the trials, because part of the payoff is direct grant support, and the other part in academia is publications, plus the personal gratification of seeing your own work in print.

FERRIS: I would like to simply substantiate that, too. As a basic research scientist (that really is the level that I'm at at Wellcome), publications are of immediate concern to me and to our company as well. I don't think we really withhold any theoretical information from the scientific community. At the most, there might be a slight delay of a year or so until we get patent coverage before we would publish.

STELLAR: Is Burroughs Wellcome doing any basic research on drugs that may be used or useful for intellectual deterioration as contrasted to antipsychotic drugs?

FERRIS: No.

STELLAR: Is anybody, that you know of?

FERRIS: I don't know.

DORSEY: SKF is moving out of the CNS field as their patents have expired. They had the pioneer breakthrough with chlorpromazine (thorazine), which sort of established modern neuropsychopharmacology, and then the congenor, Stelazine. They are now moving into generics and some other areas. I think, to some extent, you need the perspective that companies tend to play musical chairs every decade or so: they will shuffle around and one will trade, decide that it wants to get into CNS or out of CNS, or somebody else wants to get into cardiovasculars or out of them.

Part of it depends not only on the CNS market, but who you have, if you have good people, or have hired somebody, or something like that. Merrell's interest right now is in getting into CNS. We are moving in that direction and have adopted the view, which has been another problem in industry staffing, that at the clinical level many of the people in the CNS areas are not mainly trained in that area. You have internists, or pediatricians, or some others, who are good generalists, but not knowledgeable in the esoterica of psychopharmacology. My own company has made the commitment that we're going to be staffed with either psychiatrists or neurologists who are at least board-eligible, and we're going to see if that works.

There's a certain amount of experimentation that goes on in the industry, and there's the lure of a very big CNS market, but maybe something like half of it is a couple of drugs which, when their patents expire, will shrink the market. When Valium goes off patent, as Librium has already done, the total dollar volume in the CNS area is going to go down. That's another factor to consider: How much of a particular market depends on a very few highly successful compounds or products? I don't think industry feels, overall, that it's a futile area. Squibb's rationale, as rumor has it in industry, is that they had better things to do with their money. They figure they can do better in cardiovascular or antineoplastic drugs. This is the way businesses (and not just the pharmaceutical industry) operate: Somebody thinks that he can do better in selling fried chicken and wants to get out of hamburgers, or somebody thinks he's got the greatest hamburger man in town and wants to dump chicken.

CHASE: One of the things that I've been wondering about is whether the attitude of the NCI, in terms of trying to develop new antineoplastic drugs, has been helpful, and whether we could consider this as a way that NIMH and NINCDS should go; that is, really step into the drug development business in sort of a peculiar partnership with the industry, to drive it to turn over new ideas and new drugs at a much more rapid rate than we'd probably obtain if the Government was not funding this.

Obviously, there are a lot of pitfalls in this. This has been the program that's probably caused more grief for the NCI than anything else. On the other hand, they are turning the field, and I think there are a lot of outfalls from this. Do you think there's any wisdom in thinking about looking at that model as something which might be extended to the CNS people?

MC KHANN: When we hear that major groups are getting busted up because they don't think they can make any money in this area, and we hear that the time for the people and the top brass of Burroughs Wellcome to figure out whether they're going to make any money on a drug is somewhere around one-third to one-half life of the investigators in the CNS unit--maybe you're younger than I think--obviously, there are some factors here that we ought to look at and see what could be changed.

CHASE: We're really not doing that. Perhaps we're doing it a little bit in the epilepsy field, and perhaps the Psychopharmacology Branch in NIMH is doing some of this, but with quite a different model. Really, NCI has taken a very activist posture, vis-a-vis the drug companies, in trying to screen new molecules for antineoplastic activity.

N. WEXLER: Could you describe that a little more thoroughly, Tom?

CHASE: I don't know the details of how it runs, but the NCI does contract out for an enormous screening program for new molecules. This is a rather unprofitable business, because the chance of any one of these compounds being effective is very low; therefore, there's not a great deal of interest on the part of commercial enterprises to do this. On the other hand, there's a feeling that somebody ought to do it because there may be something there; and that even though private enterprise is not interested in doing it, perhaps the Government should be.

Huntington's chorea may represent an analogous situation. Private enterprise may not be willing to take as big risks for anti-Huntington's chorea drugs as they might for antimyocardial infarction drugs, for example. Is there some way that the Government might look at the NCI model to try to turn over this field at a rate that's faster? I don't know.

GUTHRIE: Tom, I'm just curious to ask you, is there any value, perhaps, in telling the people who are involved in these experiments that there's a whole new market for neurological disorders because you have new technology and you're identifying more and more people who are going to be involved in more and more of these neurological disorders? The numbers are increasing regularly.

CHASE: You mean the patient population?

GUTHRIE: Yes, that's what I'm saying. There's a new market. They may be decreasing the drug but, at the same time, there's a whole new market. Huntington's, by comparison, is actually a very new market. Now we've got a whole slew of new neurological disorders being identified, and they're going to hear about more of them.

CHASE: Certainly, the market factor is going to be important here, because the profit motive is the primary one for drug companies to develop new drugs. On the other hand, I think that the market for most neurologic diseases (Huntington's chorea included) is a drop in the bucket compared with the enormous markets that drug companies usually think about, the markets for cold pills, or vitamins, or something like that.

GUTHRIE: That's what I mean. Maybe we ought to tell them what we're learning, that there is a whole new market that we were not aware of. Huntington's was just the beginning of trying to identify these groups of people who were never identified.

DORSEY: I think what you can do, if you want to stimulate marketing interest--certainly industry can count; you see the numbers of people with all neurologic diseases together compared with all cardiovascular. It is a segment, but it can be a profitable segment. One of the corollary questions I'd mentioned earlier is, will Government (or somebody) pay high prices for drugs for this smaller number of people, or will Government allow private

insurers to pay high prices for small numbers? Another marketing
question is, are you selling to the individual patient through a
drugstore where price is less a constraint, or are you selling to
Government on bid where price is a major factor?

If you wanted to sweeten the pot, saying that price could be
set high by one mechanism or another in acknowledgement of the
relatively small numbers of patients would certainly get the
marketing people and commercial management to look two or three
times. I would be delighted for you to do that. Personally, I
think it's an interesting area to study. Our own company is very
much attuned to marketing potential in deciding where we do
research.

M. WEXLER: Let me ask a question relative to what Tom brought
up. It seems to me that where you have an end point that you can
screen (and that, of course, was the big advantage in the cancer
field--say a child with leukemia, or something like that; but it's
true in neurological disease as well, one of the things we'd like
to get quickly is information about whether a drug is any good at
all, regardless of its theoretical base. That doesn't take very
long, and it doesn't take many patients. The kind of unit, Tom,
that you run over at Bethesda, the kind of thing that has been
done in the clinical research units at universities, is designed
to get that information, if we could find a way to get these
drugs to a very small number of patients who are willing to accept
this risk factor.

CHASE: Interestingly enough, the drug companies often aren't.
For example, one of my major constraints in testing out new drugs
that I know about (and that the drug companies were willing to
talk about) is that the drug companies say, "We will not release
the toxicity information to the FDA to support your IND for the
testing of this drug because we are not satisfied the drug is
clean enough yet. We want to test it in more species for a longer
period of time." Even though the NIH and the FDA are willing to
go ahead with a trial of the drug, the drug companies are taking
a very conservative stance because they're afraid of suits. In
fact, I've faced it on two drugs during this meeting. As a matter
of fact, one was a Merrell drug. They have a GABA-T inhibitor
(coming out of Europe), and they're not convinced that it's clean
enough for clinical trials, and they are not certain that they want
to release it yet.

There is no mechanism now to protect a drug company against suit. If the FDA and the NIH feel as though they want to take the risk, and the patients are willing to take the risk, the drug companies are often not because they feel as though they have a bigger stake. Obviously, a few big suits are a lot more important for a drug company.

WILENTZ: Is there any mechanism that can bypass the American drug company if a drug for a rare disease has been developed in Europe?

CHASE: Yes, we do have that.

WILENTZ: If it has achieved some kind of status as an experimental drug, and if you know the right doctor, you can find it. Otherwise, how is it handled?

MC KHANN: I can tell you quite frankly. We bootleg it. It's so much easier than fooling around with the Government and everybody else. You just go over and get it and bring it home.

CHASE: Fooling around with the drug company. The drug companies are often much more conservative in this regard.

WILENTZ: That's the point. They only handle it for one reason or another; either it's noncommercial or they're afraid of suits.

DORSEY: The other thing you want to look at, though, and this is where you might learn something from NCI--I was talking to one of my counterparts, I guess, at NCI, and they're having the same trouble getting IND (investigational new drug) approval as we are. They're having more trouble because they don't have any lawyers on their staff, and they don't know how to handle the regulatory part. You might talk with the NCI people about their experience in dealing with FDA for IND approval in the absence of any commercial interest, or anything like that. NCI is one agency of Government trying to deal with another. They say they can't get their compounds through as fast as they would like.

Industry has its own conservatism. I think, particularly for Merrell, that it's far too conservative, and I'm trying to change that in the clinical CNS area; but it comes back to the safety-efficacy trade-off. Personally, I would rather test a drug to see

if it's effective, because if it's not effective it doesn't make
any difference whether it's safe or not. There's no use taking
it any further in man, either ethically or commercially. But the
companies are not at that stage. I think if legislation, regulation, and public sentiment say that we want to find out if drugs
work and that's the first priority, we'd be very happy.

MC KHANN: We've taken the following stand (and I don't want
to put it up to a legal test); that is, a physician dealing with
an individual patient can use any licensed compound on an individual basis. That way you can test efficacy. When you set up a
study, then you get into all the other factors that go with it.
But, as a test of efficacy, you can deal with a patient individually.

DORSEY: But it can't move in interstate commerce. That's
where the law comes in. The president of our company was bringing Gerovitol, a procaine hydrochloride CNS solution, back from
Europe for his own interest, to test it, and it was seized by U.S.
Customs. They said, "Sir, you're coming into the country, but
the drugs go back to Europe." That's a problem, unless you're
going to have an intrastate lab that synthesizes material and gives
it to the doctor next door to test on intrastate patients.

The FDA has been wrangling over Laetrile for 5 or 10 years,
and right now they've not done so well in court. It's clear that
wherever Government can prevent something moving in interstate commerce (and certainly, coming into the country in the first place),
it's probably not feasible to study it clinically, unless you want
to get into the smuggling business or bring it in and drop a black
bag in somebody's lap at midnight somewhere. I don't think a lot
of investigators want to take that particular kind of risk.

CHASE: Do you think that the risk of potential suits is one
of the inhibitory factors for drug companies in not allowing
interested investigators to bring new molecules to clinical trials.
Is that a major factor?

DORSEY: You mean, releasing or taking a new compound?

CHASE: Releasing it, yes.

DORSEY: I think suits are one. I think the other is they're
getting scared of going down to Congress.

CHASE: Say this was given to a well-known investigator
operating in a reasonably well-controlled situation.

DORSEY: But the risk is this. Suppose I do those things that you say and the first patient dies. It's a chance. I think it's a reasonable chance, and so on, as a physician. You think so, as an investigator. The publicity is going to say, "Here's one of those moneygrubbing, profit-chasing drug companies compromising the public interest and safety in order to get the drug on the market sooner," and we would be hit over the head with that.

CHASE: I'm sort of thinking of what Guy says. Running clinical trials to test efficacy can be a very quick business, but it has become very ponderous at this point.

MC KHANN: Dr. Bayne, what we were talking about is this-- if you have an end point with a particular disease, it doesn't take very long to find out whether the drug's any good or not, and it takes a relatively small number of patients. The problem is getting the compound to this selected environment of patients. Tom and I both have had significant problems in trying to make that step at all levels: the drug company level, the FDA level, and the local level at times, although that one's the easiest to manage.

BAYNE: You're right. As the regulations get more and more complex, the investment of time to make even that initial drug dosage is a bigger and bigger decision and difficult to do.

PRATT: It would seem to me that there should be some group in the Government that could take the chance and relieve the drug companies of the burden of the suits.

CHASE: That's what I'm getting at.

PRATT: We've got to recommend something.

DORSEY: But the suits are not brought in Federal court, by and large.

PRATT: No, they're not. But there ought to be some way the Government can commandeer this drug, let's say, so you have no choice but to release it to them.

CHASE: What about just simply allowing the Government to act as the insurer for certain compounds during the initial clinical trials by an investigator who is not connected with a drug company?

PRATT: Yes, definitely, just take the insurance over.

CHASE: Would that be a mechanism which might reduce the
conservatism of drug companies in releasing the initial clinical
trials?

DORSEY: I think it would probably do that. You'd run into
a lot of resistance. We had this on swine flu, that there are
many other legal principles---

PRATT: Ways to get at you.

DORSEY: Not just that. From the Congressman's viewpoint,
they're saying, in essence, "If we get Government into the insurance business in this area, are we going to end up insuring all
risks in all businesses, and which drugs are so promising that
it's worth Government taking it on?"

GUTHRIE: But the swine flue is preventative, and we're talking about treatment.

DORSEY: Therapeutics, yes. I'm saying you may be able to
make that case and define it clearly. You're going to have new
legislation and run into some objections of the kind that we
encounter. I regret that I'm going to have to go.

M. WEXLER: Just one little question. May I ask whether
there's a problem of communication? For example, I heard a month
or two ago that Dr. [Perry], of British Columbia, instead of using
a GABA analog, was using an anti-tubercular drug, INH. He found
that this was effective because of another mechanism, an increased
GABA, but felt that perhaps some analog for INH, a more potent
drug along the same lines, might be very useful. Is there any
problem with communication, in getting that information to the
drug houses?

DORSEY: I think what we're paid to do, and what we do do,
is read the scientific literature in our own areas. If we're
basic scientists, we've read the basic science literature. I
certainly read the clinical literature, come to meetings like
this, and so on. I think that whatever has entered the general
scientific arena is well known to the companies. Again, that's
the scientific side of the operation and one of its responsibilities. I think that that kind of communication is no major problem; that we know pretty much what's going on where and try to
inform our colleagues. I wouldn't see that as a particularly
fruitful area to pursue.

BAYNE: I'd like to slip in a minority opinion on that one.
I think if there was something new in this field, and you wanted
people to know it, I'd tell them about it. The scientific literature in toto, I find, is overwhelming. There are certain fields,
depending on the orientation of a company, that may not be monitored very effectively, and others where the company may know essentially all relevant data. I might very well miss the INH
observation referred to by Dr. Wexler, in fact, I have never heard
of it before.

DORSEY: I'm saying that it's not just the scientific literature. I mentioned meetings like this; I spend a fair amount of
time on the phone with people in academia talking about one thing
or another, but finding out what's new. I wouldn't say that I or
any of us would rely exclusively on the published literature. We
usually know what's going to be published before it is. This is
why our companies not only encourage, but insist, that we come
to this kind of meeting, to other meetings, to talk to people.
We're happy to have anything additional called to our attention,
but I don't think there's a wide gap between what's known in
academia and what the companies are aware of. I'd like to thank
you very much for inviting me here. I'd be happy, either individually or on behalf of Merrell, to work with you.

GUTHRIE: Thank you.

MC KHANN: Dr. Bayne, while you were out of the room, Tom
Chase raised the question of whether the role of the Cancer Institute, in generating new drug programs essentially on a contract
basis, had an impact on the drug companies in keeping them in the
cancer field and working with new compounds, either independently
of NCI or very closely with them. Putting that within the context
we've heard, that outfits like Squibb, Abbott, and maybe SKF, have
moved out of the CNS field, one of the questions we're looking at
is what would keep other companies in, or keep them interested, or
keep them active?

BAYNE: I don't know that I can give you a good answer on that.
I would say we have drifted out of the cancer field because we didn't
have any compelling programs, I think. I really don't know what
effect the Cancer Chemotherapy group might have had on that one way
or the other.

I would say that one big problem to combat with mental health drugs, as I'm sure you well know, is that the animal models are so difficult. If you say to yourself, "It's unlikely we're going to make a major breakthrough using the currently available animal models," and consider the problems of selecting compounds and the people to study what they'll do in treatment, it's not as logically explained to management as many other fields (such as the treatment of hypertension) where you feel you have a better grasp of mechanisms. So I can understand some companies getting out of the mental health field just because it's terribly complex.

CHASE: Dr. Bayne, do you feel as though there's any way that the Government can stimulate your company to do more in the CNS field, aside from simply dangling money in front of your face? Are there any subtle mechanisms which might really be effective in trying to reorder your priorities in terms of how you are going to plan your future research efforts?

Dr. Dorsey was talking about assuring markets, tax credits, direct subsidies, and all this. All of these mechanisms are a little frightening to me, because they get the Government further into the business of directing private enterprise. Do you see any other ways of doing this that might really be effective, or is the current system, as you see it, as good as we can get it?

BAYNE: Let me go at it backwards. There's a finite amount of money available to conduct research and development, and it generally comes out of your profits, so that a certain amount is set aside each year. I've been with the company for 28 years. Originally, most of our money was spent on research, and we spent relatively little on development. The increasing regulations have magnified the development costs somewhere between 10 and 100 times, I would say, in the last 10 to 20 years, and a very large amount of money is consumed in handling paper and detail to the extent that you tie up your capacity in doing those things, then you have relatively less time to take new compounds and evaluate them in patients. I think that to the extent the needless detail in research could be reduced, companies would have more money they could apply to investigating new compounds. It's getting overweighted on the development side.

CHASE: Why? Do you mean because of the reporting requirements?

BAYNE: I think the reporting requirements, yes. The NDA
applications are better documented now, and I'm glad; but making
it 100 percent perfect, or trying to approach 100 percent accuracy
in documentation has a logarithmic effect on the cost.

I think it was at this meeting that Dr. Lehman was recalling
that 10 years ago it cost him $60 per patient to study a drug, and
now it's $600--more than that--depending on the study. The cost
of studying a given patient, collecting all of the documentation,
has gone up 10 to 20 times. If that's necessary to protect the
patient, why then we have to do it. But to the extent that it's
unnecessary, it consumes resources and interferes with making these
new probes and looking at low priority projects.

CHASE: Do you think this requirement for documentation is
overweighted in both the efficacy and safety areas, or one more
than the other, or is this sort of across the board?

BAYNE: No, I think it's across the board. Let me be clear
that I am not quarreling with the need for adequate documentation
of the studies from which the efficacy and safety judgments will be
made. The point is that the trend toward increasing regulation
still continues and with it goes the increased cost of development.
This makes it increasingly difficult to allocate resources to low
priority projects of all types. Accordingly, it may well be appropriate for you to devise alternate mechanisms to those used in the
past, if you wish to assure that you maximize the likelihood that
therapies for Huntington's disease will keep up with developing
knowledge.

CHASE: Has your company made any analysis of the impact of
this New Device Act on your operations and what the costs will be
to maintain your company in apparent compliance to this new act?

BAYNE: It is possible that the regulations recently issued
by the FDA under the Medical Device Amendments of 1976 will have an
adverse effect on the availability of investigators if they are en-
forced more broadly to include all clinical investigators. These
regulations further complicate the process and increase risk for
the investigators.

VOICE: Is access to clinical investigators a limiting factor
in bringing along new drugs?

BAYNE: I don't think so, really. We can generally get
qualified people to study the drugs. That's not really a problem.
We have to supply them with more support, because now they have a
battery of data recorders. We have our own people who monitor, in
addition. As far as getting people who are competent, generally
it's no problem. There are occasional problems, like right now I
would say it's difficult to get somebody to study a beta-blocker
because there are four or five of them under study at the same
time, but that's unusual. The new pressures on investigators
defined in the New Device Regulations may change this, however.

GUTHRIE: Would you say that today most or all pharmaceutical
houses are aware of the fact that there is such a disease as
Huntington's and the many disorders that relate to it?

BAYNE: Certainly, I would think they're aware of it.

GUTHRIE: You would say this? Yes?

BAYNE: I would think so. They all have competent physicians
to do the investigations. How well versed they are on the disease,
that's a different story. They're aware of it.

GUTHRIE: No, I didn't mean the physicians. We know the problems of the physicians. What I was concerned with is--as long as
we have pharmaceutical people represented here--there was a time
when we felt you were not aware. I'm happy to hear it.

FERRIS: **Sure**, and I think that even from the basic research
standpoint, if you're halfway conscientious, you can't help but
be aware of it. We were.

GUTHRIE: Today?

FERRIS: Sure.

GUTHRIE: And the increased numbers of people that we're finding? I don't think, though, the significant relevance of the
numbers of people involved with this disorder has yet been eluci-
dated.

FERRIS: Yes, I think we're aware, at least from the research
bench itself. I certainly am aware, and our group is very much
aware, that there are increasing numbers, but I couldn't give you
figures. We know it's a problem.

N. WEXLER: This is a very naive question. It seems that one of the areas that we, as a Commission, would be most concerned with is trying to get rapid turnover and rapid testing of the efficacy of these drugs. My question really is, where would the suit develop? Going back to your example, Tom, if you want to try a certain drug, and the government is willing to allow you to get the IND, et cetera, and you have informed consent, where would this suit originate?

CHASE: The patient. Let's say the patient is injured as a result of taking that drug. He'll sue everybody in sight, including the drug company.

N. WEXLER: It's the best of whatever your knowledge is of the toxicology. I know that legally you can't get a patient to abrogate his or her rights; you can't get the patient to sign something in advance saying, "I promise not to sue in the event of my death," or whatever it is. I guess in some sense it's how powerful a tool informed consent is; if, to the best of the drug company's knowledge and your knowledge as an investigator, you inform that patient.

CHASE: First of all, I have grave reservations about informed consent. I think that's legal fiction or a farce. That has no meaning, as far as I'm concerned.

PRATT: I don't think it stands up.

CHASE: That's something which is a courtroom concept, which, as a practicing physician, I don't understand.

VOICE: This came out in the conference on "Genetics and the Law."

CHASE: Unfortunately, it's become so pivotal in clinical trials.

WEXLER: But the law uses it.

GUTHRIE: I can honestly say that amongst the HD families particularly, at least 90 percent of those who are affected would be willing to risk everything and anything if they have children. I think this is a fact.

CHASE: That's part of the problem in informed consent.

N. WEXLER: It's the same kind of thing, for example, in that there are many patients who would be willing to have a caudate biopsy, which is a risky procedure. It's analogous. Maybe informed consent is fiction (I think in many respects it probably is); but it does have validity in court, or it has been having validity in court.

CHASE: It creates jobs for lawyers.

M. WEXLER: Are the drug companies saying that they wouldn't risk giving the drug for clinical trial because it is such a fiction, that the informed consent of the patient wouldn't stand up?

BAYNE: I'm sorry I wasn't here the whole time, and I've lost the thread of it. But I don't think that is a major problem for us, the idea of suits on investigational compounds.

STELLAR: But it does become a problem when you're talking about things that are ready for use in the patient, such as happened with swine flue. That was a precedent-setting situation, where the drug companies could actually withhold the manufacture and distribution of this drug contrary to the government's recommendation that everybody ought to have it. That, in itself, was disputable anyway. That recommendation was made, but the drug companies had the power to withhold it and, in a sense, the power to make the government accept responsibility. That's very precedent-setting because it could have to do with all kinds of liability suits, not just in medicine, but including the professional malpractice situation, where the threat is much greater against the doctors, and the doctors are much less powerful than the pharmaceutical houses in the sense that they are not in the same position to withhold. They can't, ethically, withhold their services the way a pharmaceutical house could do it, and did do it, and get away with it, for one thing. They're not united; they don't deal in such big numbers. This will have ramifications.

If you talk about protecting the drug houses by the same mechanism as that used in the swine flu situation, there will be a great deal of opposition against it, particularly in the Congress which will legitimately, too, worry about how far that should be extended. Should it be extended to doctors, for example, giving the flu vaccine, or all doctors giving any kind of treatment? There isn't any doubt in my mind that it plays a big role in the thinking of those companies who are involved in the distribution of drugs, because they are very vulnerable. The whole concept in the United States of America is unique as compared with any place else in the world, although, like a lot of other bad ideas of ours, it's spreading. There's no comparison with the situation regarding litigation elsewhere in the world as compared with the United States.

I think that as a Commission we have to take into account the fact that if we want new drugs, and we want them tested and developed, and so on, for the treatment of Huntington's disease and related diseases, something's going to have to be done about suits. It's only part of the problem, of course; it's not the whole thing, but it certainly could grow enough to inhibit the whole program.

I think our Commission also has to be concerned with the fact that there's little or no basic research and certainly no development of drugs for the treatment of the major symptoms of Huntington's disease; namely, the intellectual deterioration. I've checked with some of the large companies (some with whom I've worked, such as Merck, Schering, and also Hoffman-LaRoche) and have gotten the same answer we got here, that nobody is doing any work on this. There is some work being done on memory, and so on, in academic circles, but the drug houses are doing very little on it. There's nothing that you can even begin to test. There's nothing in the basic research. I think we ought to consider recommending support for the basic research, particularly because intellectual deterioration is such a big problem outside Huntington's disease.

STELLAR: I think we should ask for support from them for this kind of thing. I think it's a serious problem. I believe the liability problem is very important. Behind all that, or basic to it, is the fact that there's nothing being done in this field that would lead to testable drugs. There seems to be plenty of evidence, too, that the United States has created such a series of obstacles to the approval of drugs as compared with what is done in other equally civilized and advanced countries (Canada, England, other countries in Europe), that we are lagging seriously in some respects.

In certain drugs and in cardiovascular research, apparently, we
are rather behind. We should do something, if we can, to recommend improvements in that sphere. It's not a simple problem.
We could recommend it.

MC KHANN: I'd like to ask Dr. Bayne which countries he feels
have adequate standards for the testing of new drugs? One of the
questions that comes up is, how do you translate what's going on
in a European country back in the United States after they have
obtained a fair amount of information? The counterargument you
always get is, "Oh, well, they didn't obtain this information in
a way acceptable to us," and so around and around you go. What
are the countries, you feel, in which the relationship between the
pharmaceutical industry and their clinical practice is close enough
so that we should take a close look at it?

BAYNE: I don't quite know how to respond to that. We do
research all over the world. We prepare the protocols within the
company and try to design them in such a fashion that all of the
data we obtain on new drugs will be acceptable to the U.S. and,
of course, acceptable to our internal standards, because, after
all, we want to make decisions based upon valid data. On new
drugs, I would say that anywhere in the world where we do research,
we expect it to be usable data. The only exception to that is
that some countries require a certain amount of experience in their
own country. They may appoint experts whom they designate to treat
a sample of patients, and then they ask them their opinions. These
are not always controlled trials, so there may be a certain small
percentage of the data that's not usable in the U.S.

The countries have different standards, but that doesn't prevent you from doing good research pretty much around the world,
assuming you monitor those studies, and you set them up properly
in the first place. I think it's very difficult to label a
specific country. Generally speaking, Great Britain, Australia,
and New Zealand have good investigators; France, Germany, the
Scandinavian countries, other European countries. We do a lot of
research in South America, and we get useful clinical data.

STELLAR: I think an important case in point really relates
to Sinemet and Parkinson's disease. I happen to have been one of
the clinical investigators studying the drug before it was approved
for Merck. Merck had about 10 or 12 projects out on it. It

happened that we had a large population of patients, and we had
the largest group in the country. But we weren't alone in deciding, rather early, that this had sufficient efficacy and safety
to be approved; and yet there were many people in the United
States who couldn't get the drug, despite the number of centers.
At the same time, the drug was freely available in Switzerland,
I believe, France, and other countries in Europe.

     Perhaps Dr. Bayne could tell us how long it was available
before the United States approved it. I have the impression that
it was at least a couple of years. We investigated it for 3-1/2
years before it was approved; that is, the time from the beginning
of our study till the time it was approved was 3-1/2 years. The
answer, in my opinion (and in the opinion of other investigators),
was available in a year or less. Then, there were the two years
or so, I estimate, that it was available in other countries, and
we couldn't enlarge our program beyond our patients. We had 100
patients on it at all times, and we had another couple of hundred
patients who could have used it, but we couldn't give it to them
ourselves. There were other places where there was no investigator, and the patients in that particular area couldn't get it at
all, unless they wanted to travel. Do you know how long it was,
Dr. Bayne, that they had it in Europe?

     BAYNE: I really don't. Actually, I think the drug lag might
have been even smaller with that than it is with most new agents
just because George Cotzias had done so much of it himself and got
it started in this country. We didn't start it abroad; we started
it sort of worldwide. It did take longer for final approval than
we had hoped, considering it was generally regarded as the drug of
choice.

     STELLAR: There was at least a year just in FDA. But I think
most of the lag was that the FDA requirements are so great that
you can't really present it to them early on. Cotzias's work, the
first report, was published in '67 or '68, and the drug wasn't
approved--no, I'm sorry--I shouldn't say that. That was the initial
work on the L-dopa. Sinemet went for 3-1/2 years in our own group.

     BAYNE: I'm sorry, I just don't know the answer to that, what
the lag was.

STELLAR: I think the Commission should consider making recommendations to improve that situation. I realize that there are arguments against it in some cases, and one can point to other drugs which didn't work out so well and had to be recalled, and so on. You have to have a happy medium somewhere. We don't expect perfection. We're not always going to be able to get drugs out at the earliest possible moment and have the maximum of safety, but we have to have some kind of a reasonable arrangement.

I think, myself, that the arrangement we now have is so cumbersome and so costly that we've passed the point of maximum efficiency. We could certainly bring drugs out faster with equal safety. The drug houses are really being swamped and drowned in paper.

CHASE: Dr. Bayne, a little while ago you said that the threat of litigation wasn't the major constraint, as far as you were concerned, in your company releasing drugs for clinical trials to academic investigators. What do you think the major constraints are, particularly when an investigator comes to you and says, "I hear you have a beta-blocker. We would like to try it out in our university." Often times, these investigators find that the drug company is not quite satisfied with the available data, even though the investigator feels that he can get it through his own review committees and get his own personal IND. What are the constraints towards conservatism that a drug company feels in that situation?

BAYNE: I didn't quite understand the question. This is your beta-blocker or it's my beta-blocker?

CHASE: Your beta-blocker.

BAYNE: Let's go back one step. I think our major problem in getting the drugs out is to get them through all the safety testing and animals that are required before you even give the first dose, get enough data to say, "We can go to man." Then, as you extend this into phase 3, there's a lot of---

CHASE: I'm talking about phases 1 and 2 right now.

BAYNE: Again, it's the priority problem. We have many more compounds we would like to put into animal safety testing than we have the capacity to do. There was a tendency of drug companies to gain some flexibility and farm these out occasionally to outside laboratories. That's getting more and more restricted because the outside laboratories are in trouble.

So we have to make decisions. Sometimes, if someone outside has a compound, and we rate it against our own internal compounds, we don't have any place for it. Actually, that happened with Sinemet. Although we had demonstrated the concept in animals, when we considered putting Sinemet into animal safety trials, we really didn't have a place to put it for a while. Dr. Cotzias was impatient, and he said, "Give me the compound and I'll put it into animals." Fortunately, he had the resources to do that at Brookhaven, so we supplied the material, and he did his own animal safety testing, got his own IND, and demonstrated that it worked in man, too. He had really demonstrated that it worked before we had a place to do the chronic safety testing. We ultimately did the rest of the job to get approval to market.

To the extent that outside institutions are self-sufficient through the point of hypothesis testing, that might speed up the development. In other words, if you could prove that the agent had activity, then people would maybe give it a higher priority.

CHASE: I see this all the time, where we come across a molecule which a drug company has and which, for some reason or other, the drug company is not willing to pursue further because of commercial considerations: "This doesn't look like it's ever going to be profitable," for one reason or another. The drug companies in that situation are often resistant to releasing whatever toxicology they may have to support the IND. I don't understand what the constraints are, as far as the drug companies are concerned.

BAYNE: I don't see a problem with that, myself, but there may be appropriate reasons that do not occur to me at the moment.

CHASE: It's happened with so many companies. There must be some concern that these companies have that is not apparent to the investigators.

BAYNE: Yes, nor to me. Aldomet was an example of that, a compound we had in the laboratory. We gave it to the investigators at the NIH, and it had a very happy ending for us. They validated its utility in hypertension.

CHASE: MK-485 was another example, I suppose, where it was really investigated outside of the Merck confines, as has been pointed out.

Are you concerned about the order of phase 1 and phase 2 testing at all? Does that bother you, that you have to do phase 1 first before you deal with the issue of efficacy; the question of payoff first?

BAYNE: Actually, I don't think we distinguish much in our minds between phase 1 and phase 2. You can do phase 1 on patients. If a drug company is going to do it, we do have monitoring responsibilities that are quite strict. There's a finite limit to how many things we can monitor effectively at a given point in time. I, personally, would be delighted with the opportunity to have somebody else test a compound, assuming they could do it adequately. That's great. You extend your capacity in seeking new activities, and then you can always pick up the development part if somebody finds out it's useful. To me, that's no problem. So I can't really tell you what's worrying other people.

To my knowledge, we have never really had a great problem with a suit on investigational compounds. On marketed products, when you get them out in broad samples--and all sorts of miscellaneous things happen to people while they're taking a drug--then you have many strange suits. On investigational drugs, I can't even remember any.

PRATT: Apart from Merck's protocol that you've set up in other countries, is there any one country that you think had good standards?

BAYNE: Sure. Why?

PRATT: You said U.K. Do you think that that---

BAYNE: By "good standards," you mean---

PRATT: Yes. They're not the standards set up in the U.S., but acceptable standards.

BAYNE: Sure. I think there are many countries, and some of them more difficult than the U.S., only a few.

PRATT: You think, then, that they would be worth investigating as models of requirements?

BAYNE: I think they all work on the same sort of a general principle. It revolves, to some extent, on the personnel in the regulatory agency. Everybody has to make this risk-benefit decision. Some people need more reassurance than others before they say yes. In this country I think there's a lot of hesitation in taking an affirmative stance on things, but the basic problem is there for everyone: What does the drug offer versus what does it cost in the way of side effects? I think every country has a responsibility to do this. I hope you don't get the idea that pharmaceutical companies are against the idea of a regulatory agency.

PRATT: Oh, heavens, no.

VOICE: Alice, you're trying to get at the possible differences, where we could modify our own system.

PRATT: Correct.

STELLAR: I really think it doesn't lie in that sphere, as Dr. Bayne is really implying. If you compare England's system with ours, they are very much the same; but the English do it better. They actually do.

PRATT: They've got a lot of drugs over there that we don't have.

STELLAR: Yes. They're much more sensible, I believe, in their judgments. But I think the real problem is in the differences in basic philosophies between us: We're very strong on the final perfection of the individual rights, and we're rather cumbersome in the way we do it. The English have a similar philosophy, but they seem to handle it much more sensibly. So they'll end up, say, approving a drug in a much shorter time than we will. Of course, their system's not perfect, nor is ours.

I believe it's really the underlying philosophy, what do we have to do? We have a tendency in this country to encumber ourselves with government regulations and other regulations. If you consider hospitals, for example, there was an article published

recently about the hospital system in New York State where I think
164 regulatory agencies have something to say about a patient's
care; in many instances there'd be as many as 20 or 30 or 35
agencies covering the same thing (for example, records or pharma-
ceuticals), all having something to say to the poor, benighted
hospital administrators and others who have to run the place.
The survey I read about covered a period of several years, during
which the number of new personnel added to the rolls in New York
State was about 550 or so; at the same time, the number of
physicians in these agencies went down from 69 to 60. They've got
nine fewer physicians and added 550 new people dealing only with
regulation, recordkeeping, and so on. We have a great tendency
to do too much of that. I think the same thing has happened, to
a great extent, in the regulation of the pharmaceutical industry.
It's become difficult.

GUTHRIE: First of all, I'd like to thank Dr. Bayne. We're
going to have lunch, and perhaps you'd like to join us, if you
have the opportunity, because I'm sure there are others who still
might want to talk to you.

BAYNE: I think I may have to go. I should get a plane. I
appreciate the invitation, though.

GUTHRIE: We appreciate your coming here and joining us. I
think we've learned a lot. We've provoked more questions, haven't
we? We're going to go to lunch because we're due back again at
1:30, and we should be on time.

[Recess.]

MC KHANN: I think we might get started. We have some pressure of time. People want to get back to the meetings. I'm
going to act as temporary chairman for a little bit. I'm Guy
McKhann, a member of the Commission. We're very grateful to you
for coming for a short period of time.

Dr. Bloom and Mr. Melnechuk had gotten together ahead of
time to review some of the basic areas that might relate to
Huntington's. Mr. Melnechuk, maybe you could show us your outline
very briefly; that would give us a focus from which to work.

MELNECHUK: As a believer in the epitomization of ongoing
research, to save everybody time and to make things clear, I've
tried to give an instance of that in charting (no doubt overcrudely)

the outline that Floyd Bloom developed for his subcommittee, which is concerned with many of the molecular sciences that would be researching Huntington's disease.

I've put some claims and some expansions of those on two charts here. The first claim that the subcommittee is making is that Huntington's disease is prototypic of inheritable, degenerative, neurobehavioral disorders. We know that there's a dominant gene involved, the expression of which somehow leads to pathology and comes out in HD, the aspects of which are cognitive, emotional, and motor. That puts that disease in a set of diseases, including such things as PKU, mongolism, demyelinating diseases, and others that are organic, brain, behavioral disorders.

We now know from the twin studies and from the drug psychoses that schizophrenia can be thought to have a genetic component (at least for vulnerability); and that manic depressives, through their susceptibility in some cases to lithium carbonate, a small ion, must have some molecular biological defect that may well be expressive genes, too.

Therefore, we feel that this disease is prototypic, as I say, of a set. This argues the possibility of wider support from representatives of concerns for other diseases, and suggests the possibility of a mechanism that would not serve only HD, but the associated diseases.

Let's take a look at this sequence here, from gene to brain to HD. By the way, these are all tentative. It's precisely your modifications, both of the claims and of the schemes, and contributions to filling out and revising the scheme that we beseech. Our second claim is that Huntington's disease is susceptible to research now, at least in the sense (claim 3) that 50 to 100 researchable questions can be made explicit now with regard to knowledge needed now at a variety of levels. (You have before you something you can look at later.)

As a reductionist, my own feeling is to build up this way, but we could go down that way. Let me follow the arrow sequence. We need to know about the inheritance rules at the genetics level. We need to know about the dominant gene and if viruses (perhaps slow) are somehow amongst them. We need to know what the abnormal

gene product is, whether it affects nuclear processes in the affected cells and/or cytoplasmic processes and/or membrane processes in cell recognition or receptorology , what have you. We
need to know about affected cells, not only at the level of the
individual cell, but the regions and tracts.

The affected cells, of course, give rise to pathophysiology.
We need some psychomotor profiles. We need to know about abnormalities in the endocrine, immuno-, and neurochemistry. We need
to know more about the neuropathology. That all gives rise to the
clinical picture, which could be better depicted. We need to know
more about the natural history of that clinical picture, and post-
mortem studies and the provision of material therefor.

For all of this we need animal models. I'd say that's the
scope that this subcommittee sees as its domain. There are other
subcommittees that overlap with specific concerns from some of the
disciplines represented here. I'm sure that in the ultimate
report some synthesis will be made, but we did it this way at this
time.

We make a fourth claim, that this is in a sociopolitical
matrix, and that issues there must be addressed, too, concerning
at least the training of people and research facilitation (either
by the better dissemination of information or by the ways of
getting people to become interested in this or to perceive that
they are members of the relevant community), and some analysis of
the forces pro and against the selection of this disease as
deserving special treatment. That led to that prior chart showing
that it's prototypical.

This, done by Dr. Bloom (with a little help from me) under
great pressure, is our provisional draft of an outline of the
report our committee will make. We have solicited contributions
as to the researchable questions from the people that have already
expressed some--we want them updated--and we solicit from our
guests now ideas for the revision of this outline and the plugging
in of researchable questions to this.

MC KHANN: Thank you very much. Our time is short. If
nothing else, if we can get some of you to think about these problems and communicate back with us, that would be very helpful. Let
me just emphasize what we'd like to get out of this. If we could,

we would like to get specific ideas in terms of areas of research.
We'd like to get some ideas about how to facilitate these particular areas of research, in terms of getting people interested in
these areas, what kind of support is needed here, and how we can
move this whole field along. Before turning to people specifically, we have a number of guests who've joined us. Maybe we could
have you introduce yourselves very briefly. I'll start here.

HOLLISTER: Leo Hollister, Palo Alto, California.

KOPIN: Irv Kopin, Bethesda, Maryland.

CARLSSON: Arvid Carlsson, Goteborg, Sweden.

BUNNEY: William Bunney, Bethesda, Maryland, NIMH.

FREEDMAN: Dan Freedman, Chicago.

BLOOM: I'm Floyd Bloom, from Salk.

WALTERS: Judy Walters, Bethesda.

YAMAMURA: Hank Yamamura, Arizona.

PRODEN: [Eszem Proden], Howard University, Washington, D. C.

MC KHANN: Irv, I've known you the longest. I'll start with
you. What do you think, in terms of any of these, particularly
the areas of---?

KOPIN: I think they're all important areas, clearly. The
more information one has over a broad spectrum, the greater chance
there is of finding something that's going to be relevant to a
particular disease. I think that one of the main objectives
should be to make this disorder one that comes to mind quickly
amongst those people that are doing research in these various areas,
both in terms of training people and having patients available for
research.

I think the philosophy at the NIH has been (at least in the
Intramural Program at NIMH) to choose good people to work in good
fields. The investigator sort of has a nose for what he wants to
study. He'll try to study those things that are most relevant.
As he comes across something, he will test the relevance on the
various important areas. His knowledge that this area exists is
important, because then he begins to think, "Is my finding relevant to this?"

I don't think it's easy to target research. We continually have this problem. By the time you can target the research, the investigator who has made the initial findings is already targeting it if he is aware, or is made aware of areas of potential importance. As soon as an observation is made in the laboratory that can become relevant (if you have a good group of people, and you have a good interaction between your basic and your clinical scientists), that observation, at a basic level, becomes clinically relevant very rapidly; the right questions are asked.

I think that the important thing is to get broad support for many of these areas not only through your own funding (which is necessarily limited), but through popularization of the disorder and supporting more basic research in a whole lot of areas. There are lots of examples that one can look to in the past (even in relation to this disorder in terms of relatively recent things that have come up) that did not start as part of an investigation of Huntington's disease, such as making antibodies into enzymes. If you can make an antibody to glutamic acid decarboxylase, you're interested in looking for the neuronal pathways involving GABA. If GABA is involved in this disorder, you'll be able to pick this up in post mortem specimens.

Of course, there are a lot of studies that have to be done. I don't want to take too much time, but it's important, in my view, to emphasize the need for a nontargeted, investigator-initiated program, with a program of popularization and information availability about the disease; so that as soon as an investigator makes a finding that could be relevant, either he or one of his clinical associates is able to pick this up and use the information rapidly.

MC KHANN: Dr. Carlsson, you might tell us how you approach this problem in Sweden, or any other aspect you want to talk about.

CARLSSON: I don't know too much about Sweden. I'm not sure whether there is any organized activity in this area. So my point of view would be, rather, the pharmacologist's point of view in this context. First of all, maybe one should take into account that there are some related motor disturbances that might be interesting to remember in this context. We have the tardive dyskinesias observed during the chronic treatment with neuroleptic drugs. We have L-dopa treatment of Parkinson's disease. In both these cases there are motor disturbances that are apparently related to the present one. It's possible that one could join forces with those people who are involved in those kinds of problems.

As a pharmacologist, of course, I also try to ask myself whether there are any new principles of treatment that one could try to support or promote. I think that in the basic research in this area there are some very interesting things coming up. We have the dopa receptor agonists. There are data showing that one of these agonists, apomorphine is indeed active in inhibiting some of these movements. There is a development going on, finding better drugs equally selective as apomorphine, but with better pharmacokinetics. Such drugs have actually been synthesized. There is some research going on along that line. To promote this development, I think, would be really very urgent.

Another thing would be to promote the development of GABA-like drugs, and maybe one should even look at GABA itself because there are some new observations suggesting that GABA may have central actions on its own. These would be the suggestions that I have offhand.

MC KHANN: Dr. Udenfriend?

UDENFRIEND: I'd like to make suggestions as to what not to do, first. Whenever I see a group like this, the first thing that worries me is that someone may try to set up a new Institute of Huntington's Disease, which I think is the first thing not to do.

Second, if that isn't done, a special fund is set aside and earmarked in an institute to study a specific disease, which I think is just as bad. The NIH has had some very traumatic experiences. Even specific drugs have been targeted and money earmarked for them, like for atramid. I think this is a very dangerous move.

The third is not to think that those scientists who are specifically working on a disease will be the ones that will solve the problem. The chances are 99 out of 100 that the man who'll solve it will not be supported by a group devoted to the disease.

With that in mind, what can you do? I think there are some things that you can do, in a practical sense. The word "target" is pretty bad, because you've already mentioned drugs like GABA and related compounds. I think there are two things that this group can do. As you probably know, the climate today in the United States for taking any compound, including GABA, into man is very poor. This is true whether you're at a university, at a clinical center, or in the pharmaceutical industry.

Then, even if you get to do some research in man, somewhere along the line, in the Western world, you've got to deal with the pharmaceutical industry if you want to carry out widespread studies. You've got to convince the pharmaceutical industry that this is a worthwhile project. If you do convince them, then they have to get permission to carry out tests. In other words, somebody has to take the risk of being the first one to administer GABA-related drugs. How can this happen easily in today's climate, and what can we expect?

For instance, with our knowledge of genetics, I can foresee the day that you might even be able to diagnose a Huntington's individual prior to the appearance of symptomology. If you do that, conceivably treatment before the symptoms appear would be something that could be instituted. However, at that time you would be treating a so-called normal person. The question is, how do you get a drug into a normal person, specifically some of the kinds of things we're talking about. As we heard today, some of the drugs cause convulsions in dogs, and some of them cause convulsions in rats. The first thing to remember is that to carry out such experiments involves a risk. I think people tend to forget that just like sending an Apollo rocket to the moon, trying to cure disease means that somebody has to take a risk. I think the atmosphere today is that nobody wants to take a risk. In other words, out of the blue one expects to have a magic bullet presented to us which will have no risk and with which nobody will have to take any chances.

To sum it up, we must keep in mind that medical research will always carry a risk. I also think you have to involve the pharmaceutical industry as a pressure group. I would say that almost every major company is in the GABA field to some extent. That's one field I happen to know. However, there are side effects of the neuroleptics. They are there. If you want to bring more pressure to bear in testing this class of drugs, you don't only bring it at NIH, you can also be a powerful group to bring pressure on industry. Industry is concerned in the development of drugs. They, however, are worried about all the things I talked about. That sort of sums up my comments.

MC KHANN: Dr. Freedman? You're nodding. Talk.

FREEDMAN: I was nodding because I thought I really don't have to speak. I think the points made so far are points I would

like to have made. My view is that it would be felicitous to have
something like an "information center" that can serve as an important leverage point. (I guess maybe I'm at claim 4.) I do not
believe an institute, a research center, a targeted program is wise
or will help, because the science base is flourishing in a variety
of areas. It's there.

The question is, how to attend to it? That means to sponsor
conferences occasionally for both scientists and clinicians and
to see that clinicians better understand the course of this disorder and what it's about, that it's there, as a frame of reference
against which the scientist can say, "Hey, maybe what I've got here
is relevant. Maybe there's something that connects." That kind
of facilitating function is far more important than any kind of
specific contract research, because there's a wealth of develop-
ments in the science field.

I think the interface that Dr. Udenfriend spoke of is terribly
important in the advocacy of clinical research. Today, a large
part of our society is making it more and more difficult to apply
science to man: this means, again, that a "facilitating information" center serves many functions. I think you can get more for
all the effort, with information going to various groups in society
but also to the professionals, than through any other device I know.
That may even begin to set the model for how disease-interested
groups can really begin to facilitate something meaningful for what
they're interested in. That's what we're missing. New institutes
and research centers are not a feasible or useful automatic answer.

MC KHANN: Dr. Hollister?

HOLLISTER: I see something of a historical parallel between
the situation with Parkinson's disease of 25 years ago and Huntington's disease today. At that time we really had very little idea
of how to treat the disorder. Had it not been for Charcot's
empirical discovery of stramonium, we really wouldn't have advanced
much further. But once we had a model of Parkinson's, which
fortuitously came about by the side effects of antipsychotic disease
drugs, in a very short time the concept of striatal dopamine deficiency was developed and replenishment with levodopa was developed
as a treatment.

Now we have again, as Arvid points out, two very interesting
iatrogenic models of Huntington's disease, not perfect by any means,
but similar enough to arouse a lot of interest. One is the levodopa-
induced dyskinesia; the other is tardive dyskinesia. As we now have

more chance to explore the pathogenesis and treatment of these iatrogenically induced disorders, we'll probably have a better understanding of Huntington's disease. In fact, the only reason I have for being around this table is that we started out to treat tardive dyskinesia, and we've begun to use the same treatment to treat Huntington's disease, with about equally successful results.

The time is very right for developing new hypotheses that can be tested and can complete the choice among GABA, acetylcholine, dopamine, and several others. But at least it's possible.

Another aspect that's rather intriguing is Klawan's work. If, indeed, one can predict the person at risk and detect the dominant gene, then theoretically in one generation, with proper eugenic control (and, of course, that's much too idealistic to ever envision), one could perhaps eliminate it. I'm not sure that the levodopa provocative test is all that good, but there could be many better ones with the increasing number of dopamine agonists coming along. I'm speaking as a clinician at a very practical level. I don't care how the genes work yet, and I don't know whether I'd understand it. But there are these two practical approaches at the clinical level: the first is the detection of the presence of the gene and the possible prevention of its spread; and the second is the exploration of new avenues of treatment based on postulated disorders in neuro-transmitters.

MC KHANN: Dr. Bunney, do you want to comment?

BUNNEY: Yes. I'd like to just come back to this schema here, because I think this really does represent the scientific approach to it. Maybe not a lot of time, but a lot of knowledge went into developing that schema. I would just really support that 100 percent as a way to approach this.

Just a couple of other points. Obviously, we could all list the number of specific things, like GABA-dopa interactions, as something that would be terribly important; studies of the well state would be another important area. I think also, coming back to Dan Freedman's suggestion, getting clinicians and basic scientists together. Basic scientists and a great many clinicians have no idea what the clinical course or the symptoms of Huntington's chorea are. Maybe they learned them in medical school, or maybe they never learned them. I really think the Neurosciences

Research Program has a model in which they get people together, put out a bulletin and sometimes pick up a disease like this, and get basic scientists and clinicians to interact. I think the support of this kind of thing would be very valuable in the future.

MC KHANN: Hank?

YAMAMURA: I agree with everyone. [Laughter.] I just wanted to say that in Arizona we have a very active group of laymen and scientists working on the control of Huntington's disease. Dr. Stern , who's a neurologist, actually has a free clinic and is actively participating in the control of Huntington's disease.

I've been supported by the Committee to Combat Huntington's Disease the last couple of years, and have been looking at neuro- transmitter receptors, and feel that perhaps this is a way to go. I've been looking at central cerebral spinal fluid and certain neurotransmitter alterations; also, there are neurological receptors which seem to be in vogue. I think it's one way to go.

MC KHANN: Dr. Bloom, you put this together. We didn't give you a chance to talk yet.

BLOOM: Ted summarized it quite effectively. We were looking for a neutral matrix on which to hand knowledge that we have and knowledge that we seem not yet to have. I think we took Dr. Udenfriend's basic approach, that if we targeted it too much we would not achieve the aim that we're looking for (just by calling attention to a specific thing wrong, we're too likely to say, "That's not the one," because we wouldn't have thought of it if it were the one).

We want a way to have general neurobiological research sup- ported. We think that the great advantage of this Commission would be to call attention to the great deficiency that we have in the understanding of brain-related illnesses of genetic origin. There are an awful lot of features that strike me as making this an effective, initial target that will attract a lot of scientists. We're particularly grateful to those who have expressed an opinion--whether pro, con, or supplemental--on what we have to say.

MC KHANN: Could you make one point about this question of animal models--this issue keeps coming up in various forms and ways--what's available and how does the future of that look?

BLOOM: I'm sure everyone in the room knows as much about the animal models of Huntington's disease as I do. There are the iatrogenic drug treatment diseases which in human beings simulate certain elements of the disease, and there are animal models based on the use of [chyenic] acid injections into the caudate nucleus which can simulate some of the neurochemical, but not necessarily the behavioral or motoric, symptoms of Huntington's disease.

Therefore, while one wants to look at the animal models, it's basically to determine what's different about them that would help us determine what's specific about Huntington's disease. We're probably looking at simulations of end-points of the Huntington's disease, rather than simulations of the original genetic defect which seems to be expressed in a lot of organs other than the central nervous system--the endocrinological system, skin fibro-blasts--all express some aspects of the deficient genome which we can't yet identify. Animal models are useful when you see how closely we have simulated that particular model. But none of them, I think--at least in my opinion--so far come close enough to make them models for treatment, or models for etiology or pathogenesis.

MC KHANN: Dr. Carlsson, you and Dr. Udenfriend brought up the issue of GABA and we discussed this and other aspects during our meeting...is it possible that we're looking too closely at the analogy of Parkinson's and the pathological difference being the marked dropout of cells--that what we're seeing here is the effect of death of cells that use GABA, and that this is the secondary effect? It might have, then, very little relationship either to the basis mechanism of the disease or an approach to therapy.

CARLSSON: Well, I think the question you have raised is very difficult to answer. As I look upon it, the Parkinson's disease model has proven very fruitful, and I feel optimistic about ap-proaching it along similar lines in connection with Huntington's disease, so...if I were to do any work in this area, I would invest a lot of effort into the hypothesis that GABA deficiency is impor-tant in the disease and that substitution for this deficiency would be worthwhile to try.

CHASE: One of the questions that Guy is really asking is how generally applicable is the Parkinson model to the study of other diseases. The idea of Parkinson's disease is that if you can identify the missing neurotransmitter, you can alleviate the symptoms produced by that missing neurotransmitter by giving a drug that activates the receptors. Now with the dopamine system, which is a relatively discrete focus system, it may be true, but when you think about the GABA system--which is a very diffuse system--or the coenergic system, similarly, is it really reasonable to think that it's possible that simply manipulating the GABA or coenergic system by drugs can alleviate those particular systems that we associate with Huntington's disease?

UDENFRIEND: Can I answer that in one sentence? No matter what this Commission or you decide, many people are going to do it anyway. There is no point in discussing it.

CARLSSON: I'm sure of it because you're not going to change his mind, or my mind, no matter what you say. It will be done.

MC KHANN: I was asking the question for another reason. By coming down so hard on a current lead, would we give a false impression that we have an answer we don't have?

CARLSSON: Yes, it's true that GABA has a widespread distribution in the central nervous system; it has many different functions. The fact is that when we apply GABA and GABA-like drugs, the effect on the dopaminergic system is very prominent, and it seems reasonable that such an action would be worthwhile. Maybe one could develop this to become even more selective than we see today.

MELNECHUK: It's also possible that supersensitivity develops with an absence of particular nerves--so that a given dose of a drug that's an agonist will act at the site where there has been a deficiency of the substance. These are leads that are going to be followed, and I don't think that you really have to report that because it's such a hot area that everybody's jumping in and it's going to be taken care of. The question is, if this is not the answer, what should be done? I think you're right back to giving broad support for patient research, both at the conceptual level as well as a level of communication.

UDENFRIEND: To back that up, as I heard your question, this will have to be done because it's there to be done. However, for none of the diseases listed on the first chart do we really know the pathogenic sequence. We know the end results and what to do

about them; however, we've got major problems in really understanding Parkinsonism and its cause. This certainly is true of
the other mental illnesses. We may, to some extent, repair
what's gone wrong. However, we really don't know if we're repair-
ing what's gone wrong. We can help a person who is ill, but that
doesn't mean that we understand the primary sequences that made
it happen. So, if you're warning us about that, I think it's a
good warning. To obtain anything that basic would please anyone.
The only way to obtain such information is to keep trying.

CHASE: I detect that it's almost unanimous that many of the
people who are testifying would say no to targeted research programs; they would say no to research centers; they would say yes
to basic research, information exchange, investigator training,
etc. Now how do you square those opinions, which I share, too,
with the mandate of this Commission which is to conquer Huntington's
chorea? How do you put those two things together in a way which
the Commission can understand and get across to Congress and whoever else is saying, "We want a cure for Huntington's chorea as
quickly as possible?"

MELNECHUK: May I ask a question at this point? I asked Dan
Freedman about your comment, Dr. Bunney, that the NRP (Neurosciences Research Program, which is the mechanism for the rapid
detection and clarification of ongoing research) might be a model
for an information service for this set of diseases, with H.D.
perhaps as a keystone. Some of you have been at meetings; Dr.
Carlsson was. Is that a possible model for useful acceleration
of...?

BUNNEY: I think it has to be a continuing thing; it's not
something that you have one meeting on and assume that there will
be answers. What you want to do is say, "We need more information
about how the brain works, we have to be able to disseminate this
information to those people that are concerned with Huntington's
disease, and we have to make more people at the clinical level
concerned with it. In addition, there must be a continuous process
of siphoning the basic information to the people that are interested."

MC KHANN: Do you think an active policy then, a continuous
program doing that, is indicated?

BUNNEY: I think that's the route if you're really interested
in focussing on something and you don't know where to focus. You
want to siphon all the basic information that becomes available to

a group of people--a group of investigators who are equipped to
interpret this information and apply it. One way of doing that
without supporting individuals to do research (particularly on
Huntington's disease, which will probably not give you your
answers, as I think everyone agrees) is to try to use all the
information available and get a wide base of support. Now a
program, perhaps yearly, to do this at various levels--focussing
on some of the more recent important findings in the neurobiology
area, getting people together who are particularly interested in
Huntington's disease--may facilitate it, but to target anything--
it's almost doomed to failure because if you're able to see it,
the guy who found it is also able to see it. And, he's already
targeting on it.

     UDENFRIEND: There is one area beyond the initial findings
of an individual that Dr. Kopin is talking about. An individual,
even though he may think he's targeting his research, may not do
so, or he may not think of the same type of application. I don't
know if any of you have read Dr. Julius Comrose's writings on the
applications of basic research. He points out that there is a very
long time-lag between a basic discovery and its application. Perhaps this Commission can address itself to that problem. What is
the reason for the time-lag? First of all, if a scientist does
find something, he takes quite a bit of time to publish it. So
symposia and short meetings and workshops are in order, but that's
nothing new. Even if you have those, let us suppose I'm interested
in what Dr. Carlsson is doing. I hear his paper, but I don't get
all the details. I still have to wait for his paper. His paper
comes out, and I take a graduate student or technician and ask him
to set up the methods. He, in turn, spends maybe half a year making all the mistakes that Dr. Carlsson made in setting up his procedures, so it takes me about a year to get organized. I think
there is some area in there where one could pay for the training
in an expert's laboratory and really shorten the time it takes to
transfer the expertise from the laboratory where it was born to
another laboratory. I'm sure that many of us would be delighted
if such training were paid for. In other words, somebody would
call me up and say, "Look, I'd like to send somebody to your
laboratory for two weeks to learn your method for so-and-so."
Secondly, there are special pieces of equipment and instrumentation
that are designed from time to time that industry (and when I say
"industry" now, I mean instrument companies) doesn't want to build
because there's not enough profit in it. Maybe they're wrong.

However, maybe you could stimulate them by underwriting their effort. I'm involved in one such instrument project myself. There
are many things which at the beginning don't seem to be profitable for industrial investment.

I would like to re-emphasize that I think that the actual
process of translation can be helped and that such help would go
a long way towards solving the problems we're talking about. We
should be getting more ideas, more directions for those few basic
findings that are made from time to time, but have it done properly
and rapidly.

SCHACHT: I'd like to ask a question. Do you think it would
be a mistake for the Commission to make a recommendation to set up
a network of diagnostic centers--not just for Huntington's but for
this group of hereditary neurological diseases? I ask this because
of the input of the public testimony.

UDENFRIEND: Well, apparently there are some such things occurring. This again is a clinical question. I wouldn't be able to
answer that. What do you think, Irv?

KOPIN: I think perhaps the question should be addressed to
a neurologist because they're the people that deal with the
patients that come in. Usually a patient that has a neurological
disorder is referred to a center, or at least to the local neurologist who in turn will refer him to a center, if it's a relatively
rare disorder--then presumably the patient gets a final diagnosis
or is put into a group of diagnostic categories. I don't know if
there's a real problem. Perhaps there would be for early detection
of some of these disorders. There you'd need the education. But
I don't know if setting up a center would necessarily increase your
early detection unless you had a lot of education of the general
practitioner, the people in the field.

UDENFRIEND: Wouldn't it be a useful device though, enough
for the epidemiology, for the availability of patient materials...?

KOPIN: I guess a neurologist could answer that better than
we can.

UDENFRIEND: It seems to me they should exist now. It sur-
prises me to hear you say that there are no such things. I thought
they existed.

MC KHANN: Well, this is something that we discussed before.
The problem is how to keep from making them too narrow, but
there's no question that if you want to focus on a disease, it's
a very effective way to do it.

BLOOM: I wanted to comment, as a clinical neurologist dealing with patients in this area, I think that most university centers
have evolved quite naturally out of the interests of people, certain
neurologists who deal with these disorders. In San Diego I've
started to see patients with Huntington's disease, Parkinson's
disease, etc., and established a clinic, and now it serves really
as a sort of internal city referral center for questions like, "Is
this Huntington's disease, or could it be? Could I have Huntington's disease? What are the resources for people and families with
this disease?" I think there are two basic problems that still
exist--problems that this Commission is addressing. How do you
establish an early diagnosis with certainty, and what do you do
about it? I think these are the two problems.

If you diagnose somebody but have nothing to offer them in the
way of treatment or alteration of natural history, I'm not sure
you've accomplished a great deal.

HOLLISTER: Well, that's the ethical dilemma imposed by the
provocative tests that unmask the gene before it becomes clinically
manifested. You have nothing to offer the poor devil after you've
found out he's got it.

CHASE: Except genetic counseling.

HOLLISTER: Yes, you can tell him not to have children but you
still have condemned him to...

CHASE: I think there are a lot of neurological centers, perhaps not identified with this group, in which somebody is trying
to work with these patients and perhaps has a little more experience than others. And I think that's very worthwhile. In my case,
having been in San Diego for two and one-half years, after being in
Dr. Kopin's lab, I've been able to identify a large number of
families in the San Diego area and establish contacts with them.
They, in turn, have contacted other families who have been reluctant
to come forward for medical attention. And I think the whole thing
will help to identify the patients, and if there's something that
can be offered at the local level, this is the way to distribute
and disseminate that information.

HOLLISTER: How many cases do you think there are in the U.S.?

N. WEXLER: Do you want a clinical or a political answer?

GUTHRIE: I tell you that nobody knows the answer, and we have thought about it and discussed at great length what we should do about it. For the very reasons that you have heard today, we find it very difficult to give you an honest answer. We do know this-- that there are more people than you ever thought. And, if you don't mind, I'd like to respond to you this way: we already know that because there are families who have not known their family background and history, eugenics will not work. Therefore, the treatment and diagnosis become very important. I also would like to respond to Dr. Udenfriend that many of us around here do agree very seriously with what you have said. Our problem is, how do you get a group of people who were hiding to come forward so that you can work with real people instead of ghosts? The way to get them if you have nothing to offer, is to tell them the truth-- that you will never have anything to offer, unless they come forward. So, this generation of H.D. families is coming forward, and they are saying to you scientists, "We are willing to be the guinea pigs. Do something." So, you don't have to worry about ethical concerns at this time. The families are willing to say: "Do something. We're willing to step forward here and some day you may even get your prevalence."

VOICE: I would like to ask Dr. Udenfriend, before we have a blanket condemnation of the targeted research: Do you consider that...

UDENFRIEND: I said that there's already a lot of targeted research underway, that's the trouble. It also may be the wrong target. However, there's a tremendous amount of such work going on in many pharmaceutical companies. That's all targeted research that's going on. I believe that there's no need to have more targeted research than we now have in these areas.

VOICE: I think--let me give you a complete example--I think some targeted research in this area when so little is known is probably wasted. Let's take, for example, there is some knowl- edge about something on the cell surface that is producing some kind of immune response, and somebody wants to know what's on the cell surface. Would it be valuable to have some kind of targeted research that would attempt to get an answer by electronmicroscopy or other means? That is, to contract out this kind of research and attempt to find out what that molecule is?

KOPIN: I don't know that we would define targeted research in exactly the terms that you have. That target as you've outlined it is sort of a very logical extension of scientific observation. This, to us, is not targeted research. We can set up questions in a laboratory which are really targeted, but what we mean by targeted (and we are so-called anti-target research) is where you have a very nebulous thing; and for instance, say we want to study schizophrenia or we want to study this--what shall we do about it? In these areas there isn't enough basic information to even ask the right questions, and that's what we feel is a waste. When we get down to specifics, as you have, we are very much in agreement. Yes, if you want to call that targeted research, we're all for it because this is the next logical question in a sequence of observations that are going to lead to further information. And it's a logical thing to do. But some of these other things don't appear to be logical.

HOLLISTER: I'm not at all offended by the fact that we can treat people often better than we can understand their illness. That's certainly true in schizophrenia, and it's true in malaria, for instance. It's only been in this century that we have known the epidemiology of malaria, but we were treating it for two centuries before that with the bark of a tree. The logical order would be to, say, know how the gene works and work right up to the clinical side, but very often in real life it goes the other way around. That's certainly been true in most of neurology today.

CHASE: Well, Parkinson's disease is one of the very few disorders where we can say that there was a logical progression from basic knowledge to therapeutics. I think we'd be the first to admit that most of the drugs we use are really empirical and often found through serendipity.

GUTHRIE: What would be your reaction to the possibility of tacking on to some existing facility a so-called neurological center--we're thinking of this to broaden the scope, you see, and not to suggest just a center for Huntington's--that would include a group of disorders that could be the movement neurological, or the genetic neurological? The Commission hasn't yet reached its conclusions, but we are thinking--because of what you have said--

of trying to tell the Congress why this Commission would like to try to take a broader approach. We're trying to find out how we can say it in the right way and be the most meaningful to the Congress and to our constituency, which is what Tom pointed out. We do have a problem in answering to the constituency that worked to get a Commission. We didn't really work for a Commission--I should clarify that. We asked for help and the way the Congress wanted to get rid of us, we believe, is by making a Commission, and we hope to take a broader view and try to help the whole field through our efforts. Do you have any thoughts about a center of this kind being established in an existing facility?

UDENFRIEND: You're talking about one center?

GUTHRIE: Not one. Several centers where there are qualified people and interested people.

UDENFRIEND: Such a center...what you would include in that area--the epidemiology which is necessary; the identification of the patient; the making available of patients to the investigators, with the patients' approval; and the testing of the drugs--to do this in general rather than for just one disease, I think it probably wouldn't be a bad idea at all.

Chances are, many of these things are already partially in existence. I mean, I don't think it's necessary to build new buildings, but I think as we heard from...I think there's essentially one waiting to be supported there.

GUTHRIE: I think that's what we have in mind. There are seeds of centers already existing in this country, and we're trying to see how we can still meet our Commission's responsibility.

KOPIN: I don't think really you need to go too far afield because I think that one could argue that nature reveals her secret often through the rare disorder, and that we find out a great deal about all of neurological and psychiatric disease by finding out about one rare thing. So, one could say that this is one approach to the study of all biological causes of neurological mental disease. I don't think that you need to even remove the name Huntington's disease from your title. You can still be focussed on this, but the understanding would be that this is one route--another window into our understanding of how the brain works. And if it's taken from this standpoint, you've removed it from the target area and yet it's not removed from the target area. So I can see supporting it and providing the...this disorder for study which will give us a great deal of information about the normal human mind. I don't feel it's really necessary to remove your charge from Congress to investigate Huntington's disease. Also, in doing the support for this, one should look at the broad aspects and say, "We are also interested in the abnormal, and we are one example of the abnormal that may provide for you an insight that would not otherwise be available."

HOLLISTER: I'd be willing to broaden it to "movement dis-orders" perhaps, because you might learn something from treating patients with spastic torticollis or other kinds of movement dis-orders rather than just focussing down on Huntington's disease. Another analogy we haven't brought up, and yet clinically some-times it gives you a little trouble in making distinctions, is Wilson's disease. Here, in a very short time, a tremendously ef-fective treatment was developed. Now we still don't know how the Wilson's gene works, but we know that they have too much unbound copper because they generally lack the copper binding globulin fraction in the plasma, and if you simply provide chelation, you can keep them alive. I've followed some patients with this dis-order for over twenty years now, and I'm sure you have too, so you don't have to understand all the mysteries in order to make a great advance.

CHASE: I'm impressed with the chaos of the way science de-velops, as Leo pointed out, because there's not a great deal of logic that we can even apply when we look backwards. Thinking about our Parkinson's centers, now--I think we're funding four or five of them or something--these were all created after the horse was out of the barn. The problem was solved. And now we have these centers going on, researching L-dopa ten years later. They take on a life of their own and they're still doing the same old experiments that were done in the '60's.

UDENFRIEND: Maybe they should be doing movement disorders now. Maybe they should change it.

CHASE: It's very hard to change it. Because the people who run these centers are invested in a certain set of research, and they're not going to change the focus of their research.

FREEDMAN: You don't need to change them at right angles. You can deviate them slowly.

GUTHRIE: Move them over!

CHASE: That's a political no-no.

MC KHANN: Let me ask a question that came up this morning
when we were talking to some representatives of certain drug
companies...other drug companies...the question was how you get
a logical therapeutic candidate into therapeutic trial more
quickly? The three of you deal with this; I'd like to get your
thoughts on it. Let's take Huntington's disease, a defined
entity where one could judge results of pharmacological agents
very quickly. Now the question is, does the damn stuff work at
all? How can you speed up getting it from your lab to Irv Kopin's
lab, if you choose to work on that?

UDENFRIEND: Obviously there are many factors involved in any
kind of drug that's in development. You've got to have some positive data and a model, which you usually have. Suppose it's in
the GABA area, and you're going to search for an active GABA-like
compound. You carry out toxicity studies of a certain type, and
that's where the rub comes in. If you have to spend years to get
a proper carcinogenic profile, then it becomes very costly to pick
out one or two active compounds which are potential drugs. Let us
go back 15 years when one could, with a limited toxicity, give a
few doses of a drug to patients for up to a week. That's how
Aldomet, a widely used anti-hypertensive drug, was discovered.
Merck would never have gotten Aldomet to market if they had been
required to carry out the two years toxicity needed today prior to
human investigation. They didn't have that much faith in the compound. However, the acute toxic effects of Aldomet in animals were
minimal, much lower than those of any other anti-hypertensive drug.
It was only because it was then permissible to give the drug to
hypertensive patients and obtain an answer in three to five days
of treatment that it was possible to demonstrate the efficacy sur-
mised from basic considerations.

KOPIN: The climate has changed.

UDENFRIEND: Yes, the climate has changed so that a company
really has to be almost absolutely certain that a compound is going
to be successful in man...it's almost like a Catch 22 situation.
Before you can give a drug to patients, you must be certain that it
is effective. That is how the situation has changed. You said you
have people who would volunteer. I don't think they would be permitted to volunteer, would they?

VOICE: No, the climate now...

MC KHANN: How do you see that changing? I mean, for example, are there specific areas that a Commission like this could
address and say, "All right, we think in certain circumstances we
ought to have a different mechanism. Let's do it the way we did
it 15 years ago." Is that possible?

VOICE: There might be certain instances where the flexibility
of the FDA might be improved in terms of trials for specific disorders.

UDENFRIEND: They'll do that for cancer drugs. With cancer
drugs, they've gotten away with it.

KOPIN: Right. But there should be some other disorders...
it should be broadened. A serious neurological disorder is one
approach. Now this would help because the benefit would be so
great, and one could argue this for cancer easily. I think this
argument could be extended to many disorders.

UDENFRIEND: Well, let's put it this way. I think the safeguards that you could offer them would be that if a pharmaceutical
company in conjunction with a reputable clinical group feels that
something ought to be investigated, this Commission could perhaps
take a look at it and say, we will offer to support or underwrite
it.

VOICE: If a particular drug comes along that would be relevant, it would be useful for an ad hoc committee to be set up by
the Commission to say, "This is a drug which should be tried in
patients, because of the seriousness of the illness being at the
level of cancer. We should bypass some of the other phases in the
development of drugs, to accelerate the application of this drug
to a clinical situation."

UDENFRIEND: By the way, let us consider Parkinsonism, I
think that many of you may not know the inside story of how dopa
was proved to be effective. When dopa was being investigated in
Parkinsonism, all the experts in the field came to a conclusion at
a meeting at Columbia University in 1965 that it was a wonderful
tool, but that it would never serve any purpose as a drug. At that
point the FDA came to the conclusion that the maximal dosage one

could give a patient was one gram per day. So, this is what
clinicians used. They went up to one gram, but equivocal results
were obtained. Several months later, Dr. George Cotzias, who had
been treating manganese toxicity with large doses of dopa, got a
group of Parkinson patients and put them on doses up to five grams.
He didn't know about the one-dose limitation of the FDA. Now,
after he got his excellent effects, someone told him, "George, you
have broken the law. You've gone up to five grams." At that
point, he went to the FDA, where a friend of his was on the staff,
and he said to him, "Joe, put handcuffs on me. I've just broken
the law." He then explained the whole situation. Had George
Cotzias abided by the one-gram ruling of the FDA, Parkinsonism
would still be untreated today.

     KOPIN: But he tried it out of the country first. His mang-
anese toxicity work was done in South America.

     UDENFRIEND: I know, but the Parkinson patients were treated
in the United States with five grams. What I'm saying is, had the
law as the FDA set it up with a one-gram limit stayed, Parkinsonism
would still be an untreated disease today.

     HOLLISTER: I think the issue we're addressing ourselves to
is one that is very important, and it bothers me constantly. There
is no provision in the current regulations for using any drug for a
pilot study. You know, sometimes two patients treated for three
days can give you an answer.

     UDENFRIEND: At a fraction of the cost!

     HOLLISTER: And I get so discouraged. I have to apply for an
IND, and I have to go through a committee. Then, maybe in two
patients it won't work, so you then forget it. It could be a good
blow, and we do have evidence, that Huntington's disease can be
quickly reversed with some treatment. So if you want to test a new
drug that might be effective, you don't need to wait six months to
get an answer. I'd love to put oxotremorine into some of them.
But, nobody's done the toxicology necessary simply to get a single
dose of oxotremorine in a man by current FDA standards.

     KOPIN: You're talking about the movement part of it.

     HOLLISTER: Yes.

MELNECHUK: But what about the changes?

HOLLISTER: Well, you bite off all you can.

HOLLISTER: It's true.   If anybody's got any ideas about the mental side of it, I'd appreciate hearing about it.

CHASE: Leo, do you have any suggestions about how a pilot IND set-up might work?   There are a lot of forces you have to balance off, and obviously even the pilot investigator may have some constraints on him.   Do you see how that could work in a very simple way?

HOLLISTER: I think perhaps you have to have some idea of what is the toxic versus the effective dose.

CHASE: For example, do you think an independent university investigator, if he and his own local committee want to do it, would be sufficient?   To bypass the FDA?

KOPIN: No.   But I think there should be some mechanism in the FDA to call an ad hoc committee together to be able to give you permission to try this within, say, a three-month period.   It shouldn't have to be delayed for years as it is right now.   You don't want to remove the power of the FDA, but you want to be able to give it flexibility.

CHASE: Irv, I'm not convinced that the FDA gives any meaningful review for most of the drugs...

KOPIN: That's why you need an ad hoc committee--to get a quick answer.

MC KHANN: But how do you face the problem that you may be talking about, giving a compound to humans the first time?

UDENFRIEND: Let's put it this way.   Everything in the world has to be done sometime for the first time, and all you can do is do to the best of your ability.   I know what you should do.   If you have to give a drug for three days and look for short-term effects, there should be one type of toxicity required.   I don't think you need two years of cancer toxicity for such a study because

I'm sure smoking a pack of cigarettes, or eating a broiled steak, which I've read about lately in science, probably is as dangerous as that. I think you need room for flyer type of experiments. There's something else you should think about. You know that frequently a smaller company can undertake the most audacious type of research because its expenditures are lower as a result of a lower overhead. They may, therefore, be more willing to take a risk. But smaller companies find it most difficult to carry out long-term toxicity. They can't afford long-term cancer toxicity. In fact, they'll be driven out of business and you'll be left only with the very large companies. I hate to say it, but that's what is happening. Innovation is discouraged by the cost of assuring no risk.

KOPIN: Do I understand correctly that the exact procedure for a new drug is that it must be given to a normal man first?

UDENFRIEND: But you can't give a drug to a normal man--he has to have a disease.

KOPIN: Your initial studies have to be done on normal individuals? Now for instance with oxotremorine, it would be reasonable from our knowledge of what the drug does, to go directly to the disease stage where it might be useful. Why does it have to go through normal first?

CHASE: It doesn't really have to. It's up to the company. The normal route is that way, but it's violated often.

KOPIN: I think there should be means of doing this quickly and legally, and I think an ad hoc committee through the FDA might be the way to solve it. I'm sure there are other ways.

BUNNEY: Dr. McKhann asked me if I have anything...the only thing I have is perhaps an analogy to the multiple sclerosis scene. Dr. Kopin and I were asked to be on a panel to evaluate drug therapy in multiple sclerosis, and through a Commission that was jointly sponsored by a third party organization, the M.S. Foundation, there were a number of meetings held in Washington. The entire area was broken down into several sections, one of which was the epidemiology, the pathology, and almost everything we've constructed here. From that the third party organization, the Foundation, has carried forward with small ad hoc groups. The group that I'm involved in

is interested in the evaluation of substances that will perhaps
impede the progress of the disease because there's no evidence
that we will, in fact, repair the disease state as it stands.
To that end, we've asked for voluntary supplies of compounds from
all the major pharmaceutical houses and have had a panel evaluate the probability that those drugs may have an effect on the
inflammatory process versus the autoimmune process, and we believe
that perhaps within the next two or three years we may have a compound or compounds which then the Foundation would be willing to
co-sponsor, with the drug house, clinical trials on. We have had
a continuing dialog with the FDA on how to go about this mechanism
to get around exactly the kind of thing that Dr. Hollister, Dr.
Kopin, and Dr. Udenfriend were mentioning. Now, as you know, the
M.S. Foundation is a rather enormous network on the outside and is
well funded by volunteer contributions and the like, but as far as
I can see, this cooperation between Federal and the private sector
has been most useful in being able to do a number of things that
have not previously been possible. There are other panels
sponsored by the Foundation that address other things, such as,
is there a viral etiology for multiple sclerosis? At the same
time, as you know, the National Institute of Neurological Diseases
has continued to sponsor parallel research at both clinical and
basic levels, but the Foundation has seen to it that when things
drop between the cracks, they pick them up. They encourage various
kinds of clinical trials, both in this country and in Canada and
in South America where, perhaps, the degree of flexibility that
is resident in a federal structure, or even in the pharmaceutical
structure, is not possible.

SINGH: I think that the device for the FDA is something that
needs to be worked on because really there could be defined in
this area, and in others, a short toxicity study in animals and
then a limited time period allowed for trying things in man. That
really is the frontier of many other areas. I don't know whether
this Committee could help in that or not.

VOICE: I'd like to raise an issue that I haven't heard discussed here. Perhaps it was discussed earlier, but talk about
parallels--Huntington's disease to other diseases, one of these is
Parkinson's disease. A big difference is the genetic pattern. If
you look at genetic diseases, they are characterized by deficiencies
of something. These are homozygous recessive diseases. Huntington's
is not. Are we looking in the wrong way at a disease that has an

inheritance pattern? Is this likely to be a biochemical defect
or is there some other process? We should be focussing...is the
Commission...is the thrust of the work too narrowly looking at
chemical and pharmacological mechanisms?

HOLLISTER: Are you suggesting that it might be some developmental structural change in the brain...the wiring is different,
or what?

VOICE: I think it has to be considered from a very broad
sample because I don't really know a good precedence for an
inherited disease that has a biochemical defect.

MELNECHUK: What about going to an extreme animal model, the
work of Seymour Benzer on...where he is attempting to correlate
gene defects with morphological changes in the brain and therefore
behavioral mutations.

LI: Most of the discussions are wrong. There are chemicals.
But for Huntington's disease that is really unnecessary. We don't
really need a chemical which can cure the disease. If we only had
some kind of diagnostic test early enough, clinicians could contribute very little because we have nothing to offer. Actually you
have plenty to offer because that's where work constantly begins--
after diagnosis. As a matter of fact, that's the only way to
decrease the incidence of H.D. in the next generation. So I still
think early detection is...well, it suits me better than you
actually. As to the biochemical defect, of course, it has nothing
to do with dominance or recessiveness. Each gene has its own work
to do. Most of the deficiencies we know are recessive in nature,
but a dominant gene can do peculiar things too. So there could be
similar biochemical defects although it is a dominant effect, and
the fact that it is dominant makes the genetic counseling more
effective. They are far more effective than recessive genes, so
all we need now is reliable, early detection methods. Theoretically,
we can wipe out the disease only with early detection without ever
having a cure for it because there is no such disease, therefore
there is no need for the cure, so if our attention is directed
toward this early detection, accurate diagnosis, and genetic
counseling, if we can combine this operation, then probably we
contribute more to the next generation than if we cure patients.

N. WEXLER: I actually would like to disagree with Dr. Li because I think that there are patients who are even early affected

who decide to have children quite early in life when the disease
is just starting so that they can raise the children before they
become too ill.

MC KHANN: May I take a temporary chairman's perogative and
say that these are not mutually exclusive points of view?

N. WEXLER: They're not. But what I really want is to raise
another issue which is varying from this--from the recommendations
that we've been hearing, it sounds like one top priority recommendation for this Commission to make is that we stay light on our
feet. How do you make recommendations without certain kinds of
structures that will enable quick and rapid and perhaps pilot support of certain ideas without getting bogged down with a lot of
ponderous structures that you're stuck with? For example, we don't
know if neurochemistry is the way to go. Dr. Udenfriend was suggesting that maybe we were offering the wrong tack. There are a
lot of promising leads; how do you give it quick and rapid support,
then, if it doesn't look promising, pull back and start in some
other direction? One of the criticisms that we've heard to the
centers concept is that it can get very rigid and can, in fact,
get stuck in one particular track so that it's very hard to pull
back and support some other avenue. Since we're contemplating the
notion of recommending centers, I'm curious to hear what the responses are about whether or not you can maintain some kind of
flexibility in the centers structure? Or if we set up something--
even if it had a broad title, would we get too rigid if we chose
the centers concept? Is that question clear?

MC KHANN: It's clear, but I would like to suggest that we
break for about ten minutes and then come back.

GUTHRIE: I see a guest walked in, and I'm curious to ask, if I may?

BENNETT: My name is Dr. Ivan Bennett. I'm a psychiatrist from Eli Lilly and Company in Indianapolis.

GUTHRIE: We've had some very nice guests this afternoon who have spoken to us about the work that's being done in the various pharmaceutical houses. Dr. Slater was here.

BENNETT: Yes. He's one of my associates.

GUTHRIE: Would you like to say something to us? We'd be very pleased to...

BENNETT: I think that Dr. Slater has mentioned the research at Lilly. I would have nothing more to contribute because this is his particular field.

GUTHRIE: Well, we ask questions too. We might put you through a little bit of questioning, too, perhaps.

MC KHANN: Dr. Bennett, we were told by a number of your colleagues from various companies this morning that a lot of companies have dropped their CNS research teams. Is Lilly staying in this area, do you know?

BENNETT: Yes.

MC KHANN: What are the factors that drive people out? Why are they moving out?

BENNETT: Well, I don't suppose there were many companies in it originally. Most companies get into it either when its patent expires, or they sell the original drug. We are a diversified company with some 1,200 products. Only a small percentage of our total research is involved in the central nervous system, and such research is confined to screening new compounds for antidepressant, tranquilizing, sedative, and analgesic activity rather than in such specific fields as multiple sclerosis and Huntington's chorea.

MC KHANN: Those things that you're screening for are really enormous markets. What's Lilly's attitude for a drug that might have a much smaller population?

BENNETT: I don't think I can answer that directly because
it depends on how much we know about that disease as to whether
research can be productive in terms of a chemical solution. For
example, in Parkinson's disease, there's much research being done
on L-dopa.

So our main interest at the present time is in antidepressants, anti-anxiety drugs, and analgesic drugs.

SCHACHT: Are you doing the basic research to discover compounds for these actions, or are we talking about development?

BENNETT: We are developing new molecules and modifying old
ones. I've been at Lilly for 18 years as a psychiatrist doing
research in mind drugs. For the first 12 years I had a 45-bed
ward at a state hospital. In the last six years I've been doing
Phase 2 studies. My present role is to develop basic protocols,
to obtain outside investigators, help them do the kind of studies
we want and analyze their results. Today it may take at least
six to eight years to get a drug on the market once it has been
developed as being worthwhile for a certain condition. The cost
of this runs from 8 to 10 million dollars for each drug. There
may be over 4,000 compounds that are screened to get one drug that
can be placed on the market. Once on the market, there is a
period of time in which the drug is covered by patent. This
period is eaten up by the time required for research and development, so there may be only a few years of exclusive rights left
before the patent expires. Research has been a difficult and expensive field. One would like to have a high degree of certainty
that a new compound can be shown to show a marked difference from
the other drugs on the market or can be useful in a condition for
which there had been no effective treatment. We are also concerned
about the new problems in clinical evaluation, such as the current
emphasis upon malpractice insurance and implied consent of the
subject. It's certainly getting more and more difficult to
evaluate new drugs. I mention this because I think it pertains
particularly to your current agenda.

GUTHRIE: We have a very interesting problem in that we have
a population of families with Huntington's who would welcome the
opportunity for experimentation, but you have the problem of the
FDA.

BENNETT: My first experience with Huntington's chorea, as a psychiatrist, is based upon treatment of several patients in mental hospitals--I had maybe half a dozen or so and I know them very well. So I've had some clinical experience, but I know nothing, of course, about the new neuropathology, neurochemistry, and things like that. That's not my field.

MC KHANN: We have heard from other people this morning that there appears to be very little research being done in pharmacological approaches to dementia.

BENNETT: Senile dementia?...

MC KHANN: No, not just that, but also the dementia component associated with Huntington's chorea. Why is that; is it too tough a field or no leads or what?

BENNETT: I suppose that these demented conditions --which can be presenile, senile, arteriosclerotic, or related either to Huntington's chorea or Parkinsonism --may be associated with the dropping out of brain cells which cannot be replaced, so it would be difficult to give them a substitute which they need, like a diabetic needs insulin. The cells are no longer there to perform effectively.

M. WEXLER: In diabetes you have a dropping out of cells, but you are replacing the substance.

BENNETT: But you are replacing the insulin which the cell would normally produce. In brain cells, we simply don't know what we can replace to restore brain function without the cells being there themselves. This is the problem.

CHASE: Do you see any virtue in switching around between your Phase 1 and Phase 2 studies? I'm sort of curious to know how inhibitory it is economically for your company to go through the clinical pharmacology before you have any idea of efficacy, because obviously this increases your costs tremendously. Perhaps this has something to do with why most of your research is in the large marketed area of drugs.

BENNETT: We have an ethical responsibility to make sure, first of all, a new drug is safe. We do a lot of animal toxicity

studies, subacute, acute, and chronic, of blood and liver function and the like before we administer the drug to a subject.
What we generally do for the first few patients is to stagger
the dose so that only one patient has a high dose, so if there's
adverse reaction to dose, only one person gets this effect. We
gradually increase the dose over a period of time--single dose
and multiple dose studies. The first thing to determine is, is
the drug safe for human use? What people don't realize, in terms
of toxicology, is that when a drug is then given to humans, its
activity is then studied in the new species. So we start our
study over again using human species for the first time. We must
be very, very cautious in this phase. That's the reason we go
slowly and why we like to use normal subjects that are physically
and mentally healthy.

    N. WEXLER: But if you're trying to test very rapidly if a
drug will have any efficacy for a patient, you're talking really
about some mechanism to speed up that process so that you could
do the initial testing in a sick patient and you could see very
rapidly with a few patients whether or not it's even worth pursuing.

    BENNETT: If a drug is 100 percent effective, this can be
determined using only a few patients. The answer is right there.
Most drugs in psychiatry, however, are effective in 50-75 percent
of the cases, so we may need a minimum of 2,000 patients in a
clinical evaluation to determine the clinical significance of the
new drug for that particular condition.

    N. WEXLER: One-third of the H.D. population...

    BENNETT: This means, we would need a homogenous group of
patients with several hospitals or centers to have this number in
the study.

New York, New York

September 22, 1976

TABLE OF CONTENTS

Chronological List of Witnesses
New York, New York

September 22, 1976

Page

APRIL, Robert, M.D.
City Hospitals' Chronic Disease Center   5-96

AXELROD, David, M.D.
New York State Department of Health   5-107

SHEPARD, Florence
New York, New York   5-110

BUBBA, Ruth
Paterson, New Jersey   5-114

HIRSCHHORN, Kurt, M.D.
Mt. Sinai Hospital   5-117

CASSIDY, Monsignor James, Ph.D.
Archdiocese of New York   5-124

JAEGER, Steven and Peggy
New York, New York   5-128

SMITH, Jane
Connecticut   5-134

PLERHOPLES, Nancy
Wilmington, Delaware   5-137

LEOPOLD, Norman, D.O.
Hahneman Medical College Hospital   5-140

SIEGEL, Florence
Rego Park, New York   5-145

JAFFE, Lewis
Elkins Park, Pennsylvania   5-150

JONES, Margaret
West Hempstead, New York   5-153

BERGER, Florence
Maplewood, New Jersey   5-156

DUNLEAVY, Patrick
Amityville, New York   5-162

Page

LIEBERMAN, Abraham, M.D.
New York University   5-167

YAHR, Melvin, M.D.
Mt. Sinai Hospital   5-174

KEMPSTER, Stephen, M.D.
New York, New York   5-181

ROSSER, Lynnette
Childrens' Hospital   5-184

FEIGENBAUM, Marcy
Westchester County Department of Social Services 5-188

BLOOM, Arthur, M.D.
Columbia University   5-191

DARLINGTON, Gretchen, Ph.D.
Cornell University   5-197

KLASS, Phyllis
New York Hospital-Cornell Medical Center   5-200

AST, Marc, M.D.
Bernard W. Schlesinger Foundation
Institute for Hereditary Research   5-203

RUBIN, Sylvia, M.S.
Columbia University   5-209

OCHS, Fred
Jewish Community Services of Long Island   5-215

STIRLER, Sharon
New York, New York   5-219

SAINBURG, Imogene, R.N.
Hartwyck Nursing Home   5-222

TAUBMAN, Joseph
New York, New York   5-227

HEIMLER, Audrey, M.S.
Long Island Jewish Hillside Medical Center   5-231

HATTER, Dawn
Babylon, New York   5-235

DAVIS, Jessica, M.D.
North Shore Hospital   5-237

BURKE, Vera
(Read by Irene Kelly)
Jewish Family Services

5-242

BURKE, Vera
(Read by Irene Kelly)
Jewish Family Services

Geographical Index

Connecticut
Beacon Falls
Smith, Jane, 5-134
New Haven
Wexler, Henry, M.D., 5-380

New Jersey
Avenel
Murray, Patricia, 5-326
Bayville
DeFilippis, June, 5-283
Chatham
Mistron, Eunice, 5-319
Jersey City
Zurawiecki, Joseph, 5-388
Livingston
Alpert, Roslyn, 5-245
Maplewood
Berger, Florence, 5-156
Merchantville
Schnepp, Mrs. John J., 5-359
Metuchen
Anonymous, 5-413
Newark
Anonymous, 5-405
Nutley
Undenfriend, Sidney, Ph.D., 5-60
Paterson
Anonymous, 5-409
Anonymous, 5-416
Bubba, Ruth, 5-114
Patterson
McKenzie, Vivian, 5-314
Sirota, Anne, 5-364

Pompton Lakes
Maugen, Ronald J., 5-310
Ridgewood
Sainburg, Imogene, R.N., 5-222
Roselle
Fitzpatrick, Mrs. James, 5-289
Scotch Plains
Checchio, Joseph, 5-262
Checchio, Rose, 5-263
Springfield
Anonymous, 5-407
Swedesboro
Hand, Elsie M., 5-294
Teaneck
Harrison, Lillian, 5-297
Wayne
Mura, Maxine, 5-324

New York
Amityville
Dunleavy, Patrick, 5-162
Babylon
Hatter, Dawn, 5-235
Barphace
Marconi, Grace, 5-306
Bronx
Tellez-Nagel, Isabel, M.D., 5-368
Terry, Robert D., M.D., 5-368
Bronxville
Marks, Joan H., 5-308
Brooklyn
Edelson, Mrs. Sam, 5-287
Epifanio, Richard D., 5-274
Horansky, Joan, 5-299

Geneva
  McDowell, Helen, 5-312
Glen Oaks
  Heimler, Audrey, M.S., 5-231
Huntington Station
  Truglia, Lucy, 5-375
Manhasset
  Davis, Jessica, M.D., 5-237
Mount Vernon
  Tompkins, Muriel M., 5-373
New York
  Anonymous, 5-389
  Anonymous, 5-391
  Anonymous, 5-393
  Anonymous, 5-398
  Anonymous, 5-403
  Anonymous, 5-410
  Anonymous, 5-422
  Anonymous, 5-423
  Anonymous, 5-425
  Anonymous, 5-427
  Anonymous, 5-433
  Anonymous, 5-436
  April, Robert S., M.D., 5-96
  Ast, Marc, M.D., 5-203
  Axelrod, David M.D., 5-107
  Bloom, Arthur D., M.D., 5-191
  Burke, Vera M., 5-255
  C.W. 5-410
  Cassidy, M. James, Ph.D., 5-124
  Cofone, Betty, 5-267
  Darlington, Gretchen J., Ph.D., 5-197
  Faden, Robin, 5-279
  Hirschhorn, Kurt, M.D., 5-117
  Jaeger, Peggy, 5-128
  Jaeger, Steven M., 5-128
  Kempster, Stephen, M.D., 5-181
  Klass, Phyllis, 5-200

  Lieberman, Abraham N., M.D., 5-167
  Powers, Robert B., 5-336
  Rubin, Barbara, 5-349
  Rubin, Sylvia P., M.S., 5-209
  Shephard, Florence, 5-110
  Stirler, Sharon, 5-219
  Taubman, Joseph, 5-227
  Wexler, E., 5-379
  Yahr, Melvin, M.D., 5-174
Rego Park
  Ochs, Fred E., 5-215
  Siegel, Florence, 5-145
Rochester
  Dimmick, Joan H., 5-270
  Freeman, Kerry J., 5-291
  Griepp, Janet, 5-292
  Morrow, Martha, 5-321
  Morrow, Martha, 5-321
  Singh, Bruce, M.D., 5-363
Spring Valley
  Kuperman, Mrs. S.C., 5-303
Stonybrook
  Whittier, John R., M.D., 5-384
West Hempstead
  Jones, Margaret, 5-153
Yonkers
  Feigenbaum, Marcy, 5-188

Pennsylvania
Camp Hill
  Bartlett, Robert W., 5-248
Chester
  Wengert, Janet M., 5-376
Elkins Park
  Jaffe, Lewis, 5-150
Erie
  Deutsch, Mrs. William, 5-268
Harrisburg
  Anonymous, 5-430

Havertown
   Casanova, Mary C., 5-260
McAlisterville
   Anonymous, 5-418
Morrisville
   Schutzbank, Merrill, 5-362
Norristown
   Smolens, Regina, 5-366
Philadelphia
   Anonymous, 5-428
   Mills, Mrs. H., 5-316
   Nible, Jacqueline Jordan, 5-327
   Noonan, Patrick J., 5-329
Pipersville
   Ettenhofer, Mary, 5-276
Pittsburgh
   Rosser, Lynnette, 5-184

Radnor
   Tolson, Jay H., 5-370
Roslyn
   Clayton Family, 5-264
Scranton
   Dobrowolski, Marie, 5-271
Southeastern
   Lachenmayer, Anne, 5-304
St. Marys
   Anonymous, 5-432
Upland Chester
   Leopold, Norman A., D.O., 5-140
Waymart
   White, Beatrice, 5-381
West Chester
   Coates, Barbara, 2-833
   Ridolfi, Joan, 2-904
West Point
   Bayne, Gilbert, M.D., 5-19

P R O C E E D I N G S

McKHANN: The hearings of the Commission for the Control of
Huntington's Disease and Its Consequences will come to order. I
would like to welcome you here and the others who will be coming.
The Commission was established under Public Law 94-63 and charged
with the responsibility of developing a national plan which could
lead to the control of Huntington's disease and its consequences.
In addition, the Commission is responsible for delivering to
Congress next year recommendations which will set forth national
goals and priorities and will recommend the necessary resources to
implement the plan. Maybe at this time I might just let the other
people who are representing the Commission introduce themselves.

PRATT: Good morning. I am Alice Pratt, from Houston, Texas,
with the Huntington's Chorea Foundation.

GUTHRIE: I am Marjorie Guthrie, Chairman of the Commission,
from the Committee to Combat Huntington's Disease.

N. WEXLER: I am Nancy Wexler, Executive Director of the
Commission.

McKHANN: For some of you, I am sure this will be the first
time you have been asked to present yourselves or data before a
commission. I would ask you not to worry about it because this
is the first time we've been on a commission. Let me just make a
few comments. First of all, we'd like to thank Dr. Yahr and his
colleagues for making these facilities available to us, and I would
like to say a few words about the scope of this Commission. We
have had two meetings so far and will be meeting at regular intervals through the rest of the year. We're having hearings here and
in other cities on the east coast around now, and in January we
will be doing the same thing in western parts of the country. We
hope to have our completed document in hand by July or August.

I would like to point out that the impetus for this Commission
is Huntington's disease; but the charge to us, or the scope of
what we have to consider, goes considerably beyond that, as we look
at Huntington's disease as a model for many other problems that
affect the same age populations and create the same problems. In
a sense, it's the model of genetically determined disease,

particularly of the adult; it's the model for the problems of the at-risk family; it's a model for the problems of chronic care in the adult; and it's a model for the problems of what best facilities and what best agencies, either local or Federal, should or could be involved. I imagine today we'll be going beyond just Huntington's disease as we get into these broader issues.

Let me just say a few words about how we'd like to function today. We have a number of people who want to talk to us. We have some time restrictions. For those of you who are not on the program, we will have time for brief questions or statements, at least as much as possible. This is all being tape-recorded, so those things which have not been delivered to us in writing will all be typed out and we will have a chance to review them later. We would like to restrict testimony to 5 minutes so that we can have 5 minutes or so for questions about any particular testimony that comes along. I do have a clock I'll keep an eye on as best I can. As I mentioned, we have some gaps in the schedule where we can get testimony from people who have not told us beforehand that they want to appear before us. One final point: When you do testify, please use the center mike and start with your name, home address, and if you're representing an organization, let us know who that is and then just start talking.

TESTIMONY OF
ROBERT S. APRIL, M.D.
CHIEF OF NEUROLOGY SERVICE
CITY HOSPITALS' CHRONIC DISEASE CENTER

APRIL: I am the Chief of the Neurology Service in a large center for chronic diseases in the city of New York, which is part of the Municipal Hospital System of New York City. In this capacity I have devoted special interest to the diagnosis, treatment, long-term management, and study of patients afflicted with a wide variety of chronic diseases of the central nervous system. Many of these diseases cause dementia, or loss of higher intellectual functioning, and are well known to people who are knowledgeable in neurologic diseases. Huntington's disease, which has been called Huntington's chorea, is one of the degenerative diseases of the central nervous system whose exact cause and mechanism are not known.

The institution, New York Medical College Center for Chronic Disease, was built in 1952 as a hospital for incurables and today has a bed capacity of 1,246; of that number, 275 beds are designated "hospital beds" and are reimbursed as acute hospital beds at the current rates. These are rates commensurate with those reimbursements in acute general hospitals. This part of the institution has full general hospital facilities, both material and personnel. The remaining 971 beds are designated "skilled nursing facility beds" and are reimbursed at a lower rate. The services from the 275 hospital beds are available to the other beds as well.

Today's guidelines state that skilled nursing facilities refer to patients who need at least one skilled nursing procedure per day, whether that be maintenance of an intravenous infusion or nasogastric feeding, parenteral injections, or whatever. One of the large reasons that we can bring patients into skilled nursing facilities today is for the dressing of bedsores (decubitus ulcers), which are unfortunate complications of patients who are bedridden for long periods of time. The patients that are referred to us are directly from nursing homes in the area or a variety of other hospitals where they have been for acute treatment of one kind or another or for diagnostic surveys. The patients' stays in our facilities are prolonged because of the nature of the illnesses that they have, and they often unavoidably remain until their natural demise.

We have on our staff in addition to the full complement of medical-clinical personnel three board-certified neuropathologists who with other members of our staff provide incentive for following patients through to post mortem examination, when that is possible. Because of that we have a large number of autopsies expressed as percentage of total deaths. I will talk about the reason why I think this is valuable later.

The organization of the institution is worthy of some comment. The professional staff is hired and managed directly by the medical school of New York Medical College because of an affiliation contract between the municipal health system and the school; therefore, the institution is a direct affiliation of the medical school and its full teaching program. Because of this we have teaching personnel in every department, including fellows and residents and medical students.

For this testimony I have surveyed the medical records of
our institution between the years 1970 and 1975. I have been there
personally only since 1973. I did this to find out what the incidence of Huntington's disease was in our population to determine
whether this incidence reflected a greater or lesser incidence to
the population at large. Of approximately 5,000 admissions during
that period, there were seven identified cases of Huntington's
disease, at least identified by medical records. This is a percentage of .14 percent of the total population. I do not know if
this figure is falsely high or falsely low, and I do not really
know how it relates to general incidence of disease at this time.
We have diagnosed the disease largely on the basis of clinical
signs and symptoms as well as data from ancillary diagnostic
procedures and, in a few cases, from autopsy examinations.

In my own experience with numbers of cases that I have seen,
which has been about three, each of the patients was severely advanced in the course of the disease and had deteriorated in mental
and motor functions, making independent ambulation hazardous or
impossible and producing always the liability of self-injury and
necessitating a great deal of personal care. The deterioration of
mental function made it impossible for the patients to have the
necessary judgment to care for themselves and in many cases (that
is, two out of three at least) to make any coherent verbal
utterance.

The data that I have just reviewed suggests that the
Huntington's disease population is but a very small portion of
the patients that we see in our particular facility. The individual personal and family histories of afflicted individuals that
I have known raised many questions relative to this testimony
and also reflect themselves onto the the general problems relative
to the other 99.86 percent of the population also suffering from
equally disabling chronic diseases I have seen in our institution.
Again, most of those patients suffer from chronic diseases of the
nervous system.

I would like to briefly state at this time a summary of what
is written here which can go into the testimony; namely, the fact
that the treatment of Huntington's disease, as you all know, is
far from adequate. We have a few drugs that allow us to diminish
symptoms for short periods of time, although the drugs themselves

will produce side effects that are often just as difficult as the disease itself. In general, I have been faced with patients who, for the large part, on admission are bedridden or soon become bed-ridden thereafter, and this leads to a variety of other problems common to the general bedridden population in the hospital. These problems are, briefly, the nursing functions of bed hygiene, toilet care, and feeding, which in the case of Huntington's disease victims are all the more difficult because of their wild, uncontrollable, and involuntary movements, which in themselves impede any other kind of individual care. The need to keep these patients scrupulously clean is essential because of the potential lethal complication I have mentioned; namely, that of chronic, infected bedsores. As a point, I should say that the commonest causes of the terminal course of these patients are progressive infection, debilitation, weight loss, anemia, and ultimately they usually succumb to infections of the respiratory tract.

It has become clear to me that we are dealing with patients who have wild, involuntary movements that are self-damaging by trauma. It is necessary to have special bed facilities so that the patients' movements themselves do not harm them. I have often seen patients whose flailing movements or limbs led to bruises and even bone fractures. The only facilities that we have available in a general chronic disease hospital like ours are paddings that we attempt to put on the bedrails, and these are often insufficient. Therefore, there is need for special kinds of nursing staff, including aides. The chronic disease facility must be staffed with specially trained persons who are constantly exposed to educational programs so that they can give the optimum care necessary to patients who represent such difficult daily problems. These problems necessitate extreme patience in nursing, and these kinds of patients do not give back the kinds of professional gratification that are known in acute general hospitals where patients are treated and often get better very quickly. Indeed, the inability of patients to maintain simple conversations with the staff often diminishes the interest of the untrained para-professional worker in such a facility, and they often don't see the human value of the kinds of scrupulous care necessary on a daily basis. The worker often comes away from such a patient thinking that since the situation is hopeless, it should not dictate the kind of extra care that might be dictated in a situation where a cure or remission is clearly possible.

Thus, what we really need in a facility like this is a certain positive and optimistic approach in order to avoid what we should call occupational hazard, which is gloom and hopelessness on the part of the staff as well as the patients. This reaction is compounded today in a situation where budgetary cuts are not only threatened but often implemented, and where personnel is depleted of the quantity of workers necessary to carry out the large number of tedious and often thankless tasks that are described.

Again, another point that I would like to make is the effect of the disease on families of the patients, the members who are themselves not afflicted but who are involved. In the case of Huntington's disease, our patients have often gone through extensive neurological surveys and workups in other institutions. These are costly and often tax to the utmost the financial resources of the family.

I would like to close by simply asking some questions and proposing some thoughts. One question is why we see such a low incidence of Huntington's disease in one of the major chronic disease facilities of this large city. I have no answer to this. Either the cases are not being identified medically or they are going elsewhere, and where they might be going is only conjectural. I have no such data on this, and I think it should be looked into by a commission of this nature.

As for genetic counseling sources at our hospital so that at-risk individuals can be properly identified and counseled, we have none. I would think that this would be a very important avenue of therapy for the families who have to labor continuously under the anxiety of "Will I get the disease?" This is true for any number of diseases which have a heredofamilial basis.

The final concern is how one can develop from a center like ours a model institution for the treatment and management of chronic disease and for research into the causes and ultimate obliteration of the disease. In addition to this, the question is how best to reimburse facilities like ours for the care that we have to give to patients who are specially needy and different from the majority of patients in an acute general hospital. The problems run the gamut of considerations from organization of health care delivery systems in our city to the problems of what

kinds of equipment and material we should have in a hospital of
our kind.

The additional problem that must be brought to the attention
of legislators is the real need for general medical staffing in
any kind of hospital dealing with the chronically ill. There
must be the modern ancillary techniques of clinical pathology,
radiology, and rehabilitation medicine in order to provide
services for constantly changing medical problems that develop in
patients who have diseases of many systems. The disease may begin
in the nervous system, but it seems to run a course which is like
a medical domino situation in which a handicapped individual with
central nervous system disease ultimately develops complications
in other organ systems (the bedsore, the infection, the renal
infections, et cetera).

In addition, the nature of the chronic diseases of our
population tends towards the age group of the geriatric. This
in itself provides a setting for the existence of multisystem
diseases. A center like ours can only give way to loss of
morale and hopelessness if there is no provision made for clinical
research. By their nature we are dealing with diseases that have
no cure, and therefore we are dealing with diseases that have no
effective treatment that will ultimately improve the patient back
to functional capacity. These diseases are the enigmas of modern
medicine. They are to medicine today what bacterial infections
were to medicine 75 years ago. Unless continuous research is
allowed to take place in a free intellectual setting with patients
in hospital institutions like ours, no progress can be made in
the struggle to combat these illnesses. Therefore, the patients
in our hospital must by the nature of their diseases themselves
present stimulating puzzles to the younger generations of medical
investigators.

We need more, not less, research facilities because only
through research can any progress be made in diseases where there
is no treatment. Naturally, we must always remember to respect
the patients' bill of rights and all the recently legislated protection against victimization. However, it is my personal opinion
that it is the highest of human dignity to help people by con-
quering the unknown which handicaps and mutilates them. Therefore,
along these lines of thought, our institution and those like it

should ally themselves closely with major research organizations in this city and elsewhere. I would propose that clinical specimens and post mortem specimens, as well as the patients themselves for behavioral and other kinds of studies, should be made available to capable, ethical researchers in a variety of domains.

The diseases that we are talking about span a number of basic science areas from infectious disease, virology, cellular pathology, speech and communication sciences, psychology, psychiatry, pharmacology, and neurology. An institution like ours would only flourish and the patients' situations could only improve if Federal moneys could be put together into programs that would promote these kinds of researches into both diagnosis, treatment, and nature of the disease, and would ultimately, I think, minimize operating costs on the basis of increased specialized knowledge and management.

I believe that professionals whose interests do not lie in the treatment, management, and research of chronic disease should not be encouraged to work in situations like this. Rather, I think our institutions should become professional environments for dedicated personnel and therapeutic havens for the unfortunate victims of the diseases rather than depositories or repositories of individuals for whom the medical profession has no greater interest. The problem has largely been compounded, as I see it, from the fact that there is a general confusion in the health distribution industries insofar as there is no recognition of chronic disease beds as a special category for reimbursement.

Today we have a dichotomy: the patient is either a candidate for an acute hospital bed at a huge reimbursement, or he is a candidate for a nursing home at an insufficiently low level of reimbursement where general medical facilities are not available. We are constantly fighting the battle in our hospital of having to define the facility in terms of one or the other of these categories: the acute hospital, which is wasteful and really not relevant, or in terms of a nursing home, which traditionally falls well below the needs of our patients under our care.

Therefore, I would strongly suggest that investigation take place at the level of Federal or State or local governments on how to actually legislate a new category of hospital or institutional bed; namely, that of a chronic disease bed. I believe that

demographic studies would show us that the general tendency in
the population at this time is an increase in this kind of
disease due to an increase in longevity and because of the
general conquest of the spectrum of infectious disease which in
the past restricted longevity. Therefore, our kind of patient
represents a greater and greater need. Unfortunately, at least
in New York City, this patient has not had a community behind
him to represent his political needs. For example, at our hospital
there is no community board made up of a citizenry from the community at large because we are on an island--literally an island--
in the middle of the river which is not contiguous with any major
political community. The patients come from all over the city
and therefore represent people from many communities. Because of
the natures of their illnesses, their ages, and their financial
situations, they are often sequestered away from their families
and abandoned on an island in the middle of the river.

A community board has been made up largely of patients
themselves, but as would be clear readily from thinking about it,
these patients do not have an economic and political impact on
the legislative procedure. Essentially our community board has
functioned in token capacity although being able to do some very
important work. Therefore they have had no input directly to
the medical board or to the funding source, which is the most
important source, and which is the municipal corporation running
the entire gamut of health distribution in New York City. This
is an unfortunate situation, because it again confuses the general
needs of acute hospital patients with the special needs of
patients in our kinds of institutions.

GUTHRIE: I'm very interested in the fact that you believe
that there is an in-between stage between the acute and nursing
home, and I'm very appreciative of your comments on the need for
that in-between stage, particularly since I feel that there are
people who might respond very favorably. Can you tell us a little
more about what you think could be done at that in-between stage?
Can you envision something? Can you give me some example of what
can be done in this in-between stage?

APRIL: I don't know what can be done subsequent to the
organization of an in-between stage hospital. I really don't
think that such a hospital would need to duplicate all of the

advanced technological services that one sees in the acute medical
center. For example, it would be unnecessary to have all neuro-
radiological diagnostic procedures available in such a hospital
if it were affiliated in an organized and functional way with
another parent facility where these procedures could take place.

GUTHRIE: What about cost, for instance, for something like
that? Do you envision that it would be different than you're
saying between these two categories?

APRIL: Yes, because the cost for capital investment would
be less, and the cost for maintaining a highly specialized professional staff that would have to be available all the time would
be less. One could, perhaps, on the basis of examining the actual
need of such an institution and where best this could be carried
out in the region with an acute facilities machinery.

GUTHRIE: Can you envision it as part of your chronic care
facility? Does it have to be separate, or can it be a part of
yours?

APRIL: Well, it could be a part of it but physically
separate. I refer really to the model that I've seen that you
presented to me actually from the State of New Hampshire, in which
I understand all regional State chronic care facilities would be
affiliated with a parent major university medical center in that
state; and that it be kept as a central source and physicians
employed through the central source going out to these hospitals,
being on their staffs, and at the same time having a give-and-take
intellectually with physicians back at the main centers. There,
perhaps, the main research laboratory procedures which are rarely
done in acute hospitals could be done and wouldn't have to be
duplicated, say, at five different points around the region, but
could be coordinated in one, both for the purpose of data-keeping
for seminars, for dispersal of information, as well as for treatment plan. The problem, I think, is that if one has to duplicate
the services of both diagnosis and treatment at every particular
hospital center in an area, especially with patients like this,
one loses the kinds of stimulation that you can get from the researcher who may be in a different area and from those specialists
in clinical-medical fields which should be constantly in touch
with these patients whose needs are as great, if not greater,

than those in the acute hospitals. These problems present
challenging medical problems.

   GUTHRIE: Do you think it's possible, if that kind of
facility were available, that maybe we might be able to then
involve the families who are still concerned and maybe do what
you're suggesting about getting involved in the political scene
and the voice for the patient?

   APRIL: You can see that you would be enjoining a greater
number of interested individuals who have a louder voice. For
example, if genetic counseling is a new and challenging field,
and there are only a number of specialists in it who have real
expertise, those specialists could be at the hub of the wheel
which in its periphery extends out to all of the hospitals where
the patients have the needs and where their families are. As an
aside, one could even plan the structure of these hospitals more
humanely and even have facilities where patients' families who
come from long distances--even if one has to go to an island in
the middle of a river--could stay overnight or could have some
kind of temporary housing, and the families themselves could act
as paramedical workers, taking care of the daily needs of the
patients. When that situation has arisen on a number of occasions
which have been emergencies, we have found that the care given
by the family not surprisingly is equally or more dedicated to the
patient than a daily general worker.

   GUTHRIE: There is one other question: In your facility do
you have available for those who can use it physical therapy or
speech therapy?

   APRIL: Yes. We have a very large physical medicine/rehabil-
itation department which has the largest slice of the budgetary
pie for the entire institution and has available services whose
focus has been largely on rehabilitatable diseases such as acute
strokes or subacute strokes, patients who are paraplegic from
trauma who can be rehabilitated with proper bracing, transfer
techniques, activities of daily living, et cetera. Their facilities are also economically limited by the very fact that budgetary
cuts are continual. With an equally large number, or growing
number, of chronically afflicted patients, many of whom are put
into these skilled nursing beds, the facilities for rehabilitation

of the general acute hospital beds are not really readily available in an optimum way. There just isn't enough to go around to those who need it.

GUTHRIE: But you would recommend it if it were available?

APRIL: Absolutely. That would be a critical part of the daily functions of these kinds of patients even if it meant that trained rehabilitation personnel could educate paraprofessional workers on the ward to do daily range-of-motion exercises and the like.

McKHANN: We're going to have to move on. I just want to ask you one more question. You didn't mention the issue of training. To what extent is your facility used either for medical student or house staff training? You mentioned the need for more personnel and younger personnel being brought in. To what extent are you able to participate in that?

APRIL: I meant to include my young medical personnel and those in training. At this time each department has residency programs, all of which have residents who rotate through the institution. We don't have interns in our institution, and we have a very small number of medical students who only come in for physical diagnosis courses but who really should be incorporated in the meaningful fellowships in the study of chronic diseases at all levels.

PRATT: May I ask you one thing? What do you estimate it costs a family to keep someone in your institution?

APRIL: It costs them everything they have. If you're not broke when you come in, we'll be sure you are when you leave.

PRATT: I saw that, but I wondered if you had any figure in mind.

APRIL: I believe that at least one person who will testify will be able to give you these details.

McKHANN: I would like to ask Dr. Axelrod if he would come forward.

TESTIMONY OF
DAVID AXELROD, M.D.
NEW YORK STATE DEPARTMENT OF HEALTH
ON BEHALF OF HON. HUGH L. CAREY
GOVERNOR, STATE OF NEW YORK

AXELROD: The Commissioner of Health, Dr. Robert Whalen,
requested that I appear on behalf of Governor Carey. As the
Governor of New York State, where very likely the greatest population of patients with Huntington's disease has been identified,
Governor Carey has maintained a major personal interest in dealing
with the human problems associated with Huntington's disease. He
has directed the Department of Health to seek additional sources
of funding to enable the Department to bring its full capability
to bear upon a variety of problems, not only the patients with
Huntington's disease but the tens of thousands of lives affected
secondarily. The classic description of this disease just over
100 years ago by the three generations of Huntington's and
members of their family living near their home in Long Isaand
makes it particularly appropriate for New York State to play a
leading role in developing a meaningful program for the control
of Huntington's disease.

The Department of Health, through its Division of Laboratories and Research, Birth Defects Institute, the Helen Hayes
Hospital, and the Bureaus of Professional and Public Education,
is in a position to mobilize resources to deal with a number of
aspects of the problem: early detection and genetic counseling.
The Birth Defects Institute has been providing genetic counseling.
A clear identification of Huntington's disease has made it possible to offer such assistance to affected individuals prior to and
during their reproductive years. Unfortunately, the late onset of
symptoms in most cases has made genetic counseling particularly
difficult. What is required is the development of a means of
detection so that antenatal intervention might be appropriately
considered.

The extensive application of biochemical techniques through
the analysis of cells obtained in persons with a family history of
Huntington's disease may provide some more rational basis for
antenatal intervention. Although chromosomal number and gross
morphology have been reported to be normal in Huntington's disease,

the application of newly developed techniques may permit the identification of subtle changes in affected fetuses. A re-examination of chromosomes of affected individuals may provide clues as to the nature of the genetic abnormality. Because of its potential to control the disease, we believe that a major investment must be made to explore every avenue for antenatal diagnosis.

Morphologic Features of the Disease: Although morphologic features of the disease have offered little immediate hope for the control of Huntington's disease, it may contribute signifi-cantly to our understanding of the nature of Huntington's disease. The possibility of a generalized metabolic disorder is suggested. The high-voltage electron microscope facility at the Division of Laboratories and Research of the Department of Health provides an ideal environment for a study of tissues from the vast cases of Huntington's disease. Ultrastructural studies carried out by the high-voltage electron microscope have the advantage of more efficient image reporting than is usual in conventional electron microscopy, automation of focusing its stigmatic direction and illumination and line to reduce radiation damage, extended dynamic range and contrast of structures reported, et cetera, the capability to reduce instrumental specimen background noise and blurring of detail and to artificially enhance its contrast, and the ability to disentangle the overlap projected information that results in the reporting of thick objects and so provide better three-dimensional cell structure information.

Therapy and Prevention: The Helen Hayes Hospital of the Department of Health provides a setting where efforts of control of movement disorders can be carried out in conjunction with programs for maintaining the delivery of affected care for patients who can remain at home.

Public and Professional Education: The Department has been engaged in efforts in a number of areas to provide information on both the diagnosis and human problems of the disease. The mechan-isms for effectively disseminating information on Huntington's disease are already in existence.

GUTHRIE: I'm very anxious to ask who in the Department is responsible for or interested in disseminating information of this kind?

AXELROD: There are two bureaus within the Department of
Health: one for professional education and one for public
education.   There are in existence bureaus which disseminate
information.

GUTHRIE: I've never seen anything from the Department; that's
why I'm asking.   I'm interested.

AXELROD: We'll be happy to send you information that we are
disseminating.   We do not currently disseminate anything on Huntington's disease.   I believe that we will be doing such, and I
think that you had a very major role in spurring us to do that
kind of dissemination.

GUTHRIE: Thank you.   I'm very happy to hear that you're
going to do it.   I think there is a great need for public
education.

McKHANN: Dr. Axelrod, is your program adequately funded?

AXELROD: No.

GUTHRIE: I'm just wondering if the Department of Health
would be equally interested in not only disseminating information
but perhaps even helping, if it's feasible, families to know
where to go.

AXELROD: Yes.

GUTHRIE: I think this is one of the other problems: not
only to know what your problem is but where do you go when you
have this kind of problem.

AXELROD: Yes.   We currently have a referral system for such
things as sudden death syndrome, and this would be a similar situation where the Department could provide information.   I think
what we would like to have is a roster of people who would be
willing to discuss their own experiences with other members of
the families in a manner which has been adopted by the people in
the Sudden Death Foundation.

GUTHRIE: That is an excellent idea.

AXELROD: We would be happy to do it.

GUTHRIE: Good. Thank you.

TESTIMONY OF
FLORENCE SHEPARD
NEW YORK, NEW YORK

SHEPARD: I was asked by Dr. April to come and testify at
your hearings as a parent who is involved with the neurological
disease of two children. Both of my children are patients at
Bird S. Coler Hospital. There is a lot I can say to back up what
Dr. April has said about the hospital. I was also the first
Chairman of the Community Board at Coler Hospital.

My children's ages--I have three--the two that are hospitalized are 21 and 19, a girl and a boy. My youngest daughter is
fine. Just briefly, the original diagnosis had been cerebral
palsy. As the years went on I questioned that diagnosis, and I
was proven correct but ended up finding out very little because
the children have a disease that has a descriptive name only.
It's called familial progressive spastic paralysis. It's of
genetic origin and nothing is known about it. They become progressively more paralyzed. The children are intelligent; they
are very bright. As a matter of fact, my son, who is wheelchair
bound, goes to college by a telephone system. Our daughter also
graduated from high school and was admitted to college, but
because of bureaucracy she didn't continue with her education.

As far as the hospital is concerned, Mrs. Pratt asked about
the cost. To date, and this is an increasing and ongoing thing,
we owe the city and State of New York $1/2 million. The children
are covered by Medicaid, but because my husband has a responsible
position we have to contribute towards monthly payments. It is
based on his income, and the cost of living is not included. We
cannot claim the two children who are hospitalized as dependents.
We are only considered as a family of three and not five, and we
are requested to live on a very fixed, unrealistic income.

The hospital was at one time a chronic disease facility.
It's only been in recent years that the State of New York has
decided to drop chronic disease, and they have now just decided
that hospitals are either hospitals with skilled nursing

facilities or hospital-related facilities. When I was Chairman of
the Community Board, this was one of the things which we questioned
so strongly of the State. Why did they drop the term "chronic
disease" since, as Dr. April stated, most of the patients in
this facility have chronic disease? There was no real answer for
this. It was Dr. Whelan's office--in fact, I think it was Dr.
Whelan himself in this budget crisis, when they were discussing
the question of trying to close the three chronic disease
facilities--Coler is one and there is a hospital over on Staten
Island named Seaview and another one on Roosevelt Island; those
are the three municipal hospitals who take care of long-term
patients. But it was Dr. Whelan who came up with the suggestion
that one of the two hospitals on Roosevelt Island be turned into
just a skilled nursing facility, and you're going to take away
the medical resources that Coler presently has and turn it into
a complete skilled nursing facility. It's ridiculous! But it
came from the State. When you talk about educating, we have to
educate the people that are making these damned rules. Excuse
me, but I get pretty excited about this.

You mentioned your interest in an older age. As a parent,
I impore you, please consider children. There are many, many
children that are denied any help because they have a genetic
disorder and you can't get help. In the struggle that I had in
my 20 years, I have been going from one source to another where
doctors wouldn't talk to me and patients are shoved from one
place to another. With the children, sadly, because there are
no facilities for children whatsoever, there are no facilities
for young adults whatsoever for the care when they need long-
term care--and it took political pressure in order to have my
child accepted when she was suffering torment from the disease.
It took political pressure in order to have my child accepted
into a facility when she was suffering severe spasms involved in
her care. So I implore you please do not exclude any age group,
from the time you are born until the time you die. If you have a
chronic disorder, you need help.

GUTHRIE: You, I understand, are very active in the hospital.
Isn't there an organization of some kind that speaks for the
patients? To the best of your ability, could you tell us what
you do?

SHEPARD: I was Chairman of the Community Board. As Chairman of the Community Board, I have gone to a number of hearings. We were involved with the corporation, and I'll pronounce this corporation. One thing, where Dr. April mentioned the Community Board being involved with the budgetary problems, we were--but not the way we should be. The Community Board does get to see what the budgets are for the hospital and approves or makes changes. As a matter of fact, believe it or not, Coler Hospital was a chronic disease facility and never had a psychiatrist. The Community Board fought very strongly, and we now have a psychia- trist, which is one of the top achievements that we have.

But I also am involved with an agency, Easter Seals. I chose Easter Seals because it is the one agency that doesn't care what your illness is. I think that what is needed is to try to get all the various agencies, like Cerebral Palsy or Muscular Dystrophy or Cystic Fibrosis, involved and say, "Hey, our patients need a certain type of care," because there is an awful lot of overlapping in all these agencies. We need the same kind of programs, the same kinds of facilities and to stop saying "just this disease" and naming it. This is what I think is needed because the time has come when there's need for money in neuro- logical diseases, such as they did for tuberculosis. Our youngest daughter, right now there is no way she can be tested to find out if she can have normal children or not.

PRATT: Mrs. Shepard, you said that your Community Board had to fight to get a psychiatrist. Does your Community Board have any power other than a lobbying power?

SHEPARD: No. Right now, as Dr. April stated, the Community Board is made up of 51 percent consumers.

PRATT: Is that regulated by the State, that percentage?

SHEPARD: When the community boards are mandated by the State to be established in the hospitals, this is what was mandated by the State. I was a consumer by my children. My seat was as the parent representative of the child who was using the facility. Because I was ambulatory and I wasn't living there, I was able to be the spokesman for the patients. But, sadly, the Community Board has no strength. The patients don't know how to fight the battles

New York, New York

September 22, 1976

that they have to fight. There's no one there to really get them
organized because they are scattered all over and they can't.
Here's a good facility with a lot of potential, but because of the
budgetary problems with this country, they do not have funding to
give to these problems. For instance, not just medical care that
you need; that's not what we need. We're a social animal and
we don't have social programs. We don't have the proper recreational programs in our facility. Yes, they do have rehabilitation
departments, but, sadly, that department only treats the active
rehab candidates. I would say that out of 1,200 patients they
might see 300 patients. There are a lot of patients who should
really get rehabilitation care, therapy care, but right now they
can't get it.

   McKHANN: Thank you very much.

   PRATT: Is there any occupational therapy?

   SHEPARD: Yes, there is.

   PRATT: Is there any help with education, with schooling?

   SHEPARD: No, other than for the children. There's nothing
for adult education. I fought for it for my child.

   PRATT: I wondered about your son in college.

   SHEPARD: It was through my doing. I insisted that he wanted
to go to college, and I insisted on it, and they were able to get
him established through the telephone, but he was the only one.
My daughter was the first one. She started it, but they had problems with the college.

   PRATT: But very little help on the scene.

   SHEPARD: They need it. Another thing that I want to point
out, there is a tremendous language barrier that no one is addressing themselves to in the care of patients that need it.

   McKHANN: Thank you very much, Mrs. Shepard.

TESTIMONY OF
RUTH BUBBA
PATERSON, NEW JERSEY

BUBBA: My name is Ruth Bubba, and I'm from Paterson, New
Jersey. My father has Huntington's disease. It took 10 long
years of going from doctors to psychiatrist to neurologist to
finally diagnose it correctly. The neurologist at Mt. Sinai
Hospital in New York explained the disease to my mother and what
it meant to her husband and two daughters, but she did not tell
us right away because I was pregnant with my third child at the
time. She did give me the name of the disease and I sent away for
a booklet. When I read it, I was in a panic. I called my obste-
trician. He said there was a test they could do on the unborn
child, but he wouldn't advise it. This is how uninformed he was,
because there is no such test.

Three years ago, with Congressman Roe's help, my father was
admitted to the National Institutes of Health. We felt this was
the answer to all our prayers. It wasn't, but not because they
didn't try. He couldn't have been treated better anywhere and
you couldn't have found a more dedicated medical staff. They decided to try a new technique called a family conference. My aunts,
uncles, and cousins were asked to attend to learn about Huntington's disease. The social worker and the doctor spoke to us in a
very blunt manner. They said that Huntington's disease is hereditary, each child has a 50-50 chance of becoming a victim, and
the only way to stamp Huntington's disease out was to stop having
children. Well, it was three children too late for me and two of
my cousins who have five children between them.

My sister, who was getting married, had to face a childless
future. She has since adopted a beautiful little boy from South
America. It was a traumatic experience for all of us, but my
father, who they made sit there through the whole thing, just
broke down and cried. Can you imagine how he felt, knowing that
what was happening to him could happen to his children and grandchildren as well?

The first question I asked was at what age do I tell my
children that their mother, and possibly themselves, are at risk?
The social worker said 9 years old, which I feel is

ridiculous. I will not ruin my children's lives at such a young
age. On the other hand, do you wait and ruin their teenage years
or when they are ready to get married? I have asked this question
of genetic counselors, psychiatrists, and psychologists, and they
all say it depends on the child.

After this horrible event, I joined CCHD and became obsessed
with finding a cure. Day and night that's all I thought about--
raise money to find a cure. It almost broke up our marriage.
Finally, I went to a psychiatrist, and with his help I have learned
to live a normal life and still help raise money for H.D.

The worst experience we had--and the only one that affected
my husband--involved my daughter. She was only 2 at the time.
She started having these movements with her hands and feet. I
took her to my doctor, who is a relative and involved with H.D.,
and he refused to see anything wrong with her. The next morning
we went to a pediatrician from India who knew all about the
disease, and he said she was having chorea-like movements. My
husband ran out of the examining room while my mother and I just
stood there in shock. It was not Huntington's disease and was
gone in a few days, but all we did that whole weekend was stare
at this little girl who was acting like her grandfather. On the
way home, in tears, I said to my husband, "What did I do to her?"

I have learned to live with Huntington's disease because a
tomography test showed that there are no signs present at this
time. This test will show signs of Huntington's only after they
appear, and I wouldn't have gone through with it if it wasn't
given because of another, unrelated illness. Who would want to
know that their life would be over in a few short years? Becoming
afflicted is like being dead. Huntington's is not kind and does
not kill you quickly. It turns you into a human vegetable first.

My father has had Huntington's disease for 15 years. The
last 3 have been a nightmare for him. In one weekend he fell
twice and had 18 stitches in his head. He is covered with black
and blue marks that he does not feel because the majority of his
pain cells are dead. His last fall, which he was hospitalized
for, caused six broken ribs and a torn ligament in his foot. We
then decided he should see a neurologist in our area, who tried
him on a new medication. This medicine is making him a Mexican

jumping bean. He gets in and out of his chair every 2 minutes.
Which is better for him, stay in bed all day and be safe or to be
up and down like a yoyo and be in danger of falling all the time?
He does not speak to us at all except a "yes" or "no" occasionally.
He may not talk, but one day I said to my mother, "If Daddy were
well, he wouldn't have missed one of the boys' baseball games,"
and he had tears in his eyes. I feel the combination of drugs
and a strong sense of guilt keeps him from communicating with us.
Well, you would get tears in your eyes if you knew this kind,
gentle man, who was the greatest father in the world, and could
see what Huntington's disease has done to him. It is doing the
same thing to his brother and sister as well. It won't be long
before he will need permanent hospital care, and this is the day
we all dread. Most nursing homes will not admit Huntington's
patients. His mother was in Greystone Hospital for years, and
hopefully he will never be admitted there or any other state
hospital.

Huntington's victims are human beings and need governmental
help just as heart, cancer, and kidney patients do. If Huntington's victims don't affect you, think of those children at risk
who cop out with drugs, alcohol, and suicide. I feel the Government should allocate money for research to Dr. Chase and other
dedicated physicians, provide Huntington's victims with nursing
home care, provide Huntington's families with mental health facilities to help them cope with being at risk and cope with caring
for Huntington's patients, and provide adoption information to
those at risk who choose not to have their own children. Thank
you.

GUTHRIE: From your own description, why do you assume that
your father is going to be a human vegetable? From your examples
of his response (the tears in his eyes when he wanted to watch a
game), the fact that he is home with you, why do you assume he
is going to be a vegetable?

BUBBA: Physically he is progressing worse.

GUTHRIE: Oh, physically. "Vegetable" usually implies a
mental deterioration. From your description he seems to be still
a whole person in terms of his capacity mentally.

BUBBA: In his mind. He doesn't communicate at all, so you don't know what he is capable of thinking.

GUTHRIE: That is important. Have you tried better communication and demanded better communication? Perhaps you would find out more about him.

BUBBA: Definitely. He is well cared for---

GUTHRIE: No. I mean in terms of using his mental capacity.

BUBBA: We try, believe me. We have three children who come in and give him something to look forward to. My sister and I do the same thing, and my mother talks with him.

GUTHRIE: You're pointing out something very important: that we should not presume that this patient is going to be a human vegetable in the mental capacities side.

BUBBA: Only physically, I meant.

GUTHRIE: Good.

McKHANN: I should mention that sometimes we're going to have to be a little bit out of order, for certain people have told us they can be here at specific times because they have other commitments such as teaching, clinics, and things like that.

TESTIMONY OF
KURT HIRSCHHORN, M.D.
ACTING CHAIRMAN OF PEDIATRICS
MT. SINAI HOSPITAL

HIRSCHHORN: I am Dr. Kurt Hirschhorn, Acting Chairman of Pediatrics here at Mt. Sinai and Chief of the Division of Medical Genetics. I don't have to tell this panel or the audience of the type of tragedy that Huntington's disease provides for families. You've heard of an example just recently. I would, however, like to make a very strong point: that we're not going to relieve this tragedy simply by continuing to only hunt for ameliorating medications for the moment. We will not be able to resolve these questions until we find out what the basic genetic defect of the disease is.

I would like to begin by perhaps outlining one possible
strategy that might be pursuable if the Government can be persuaded to fund what might amount in the long run to a fishing
expedition, but one which might be worthwhile in terms of finding
the defect. The reason for approaching it this way, I think, will
become clear in a moment. If we think about what the eventual
possible solution is (at least in the next few decades, until
genetic engineering can perhaps become a reality, which can be
very far away), it is the possibility of making the diagnosis
from a cell culture, particularly cell cultures derived (1) from
potential patients by taking a skin biopsy and growing the cells
from the skin, because data from such cell cultures will also be
applicable to cell cultures that are derived from the amniotic
fluid which can be obtained during pregnancy so as to make a
decision whether the fetus that is in the uterus will be affected
or not. I will get back to what this implies in just a moment.

How can one possibly approach a defect whose basis we have
really few clues about from a cell culture point of view? One must
look for abnormalities in cells, but it is very unlikely that in
themselves we will be able to detect the actual biochemical defect
very readily for the reason that the disease primarily affects one
organ and therefore must depend upon differentiation of those cells
along neurological lines, and very specific neurological lines.
Therefore, I think that one of the ways of approaching this is to
attempt to make the cells that carry the Huntington's disease gene
express that gene in culture. One possible way of going about this,
as I see it, derives from the relatively recent successes in
growing a variety of parent tissues in tissue culture which
retain over many, many generations neurological functions. There
are a number of such culture strains available; among the most
valuable perhaps are those that are originally derived from malig-
nant neurological tissues known as blastomas, et cetera, which
retain such neurological properties for a very, very long period of
time.

There are other techniques now available that have been in use
for the past several years which allow one to fuse two different
types of cells together so that the resulting cell is a hybrid
between the genetic components of the two cells. If one now were
to take one of these normal or literally transformed nerve cell
cultures and fuse these cells with cells from Huntington's disease

patients, it may be--and I'll get back to why I say "may be"--
that the neurological functions in the hybrids would be retained
and that the addition of the Huntington's disease gene would alter
these functions in tissue culture as detected either morphologically
or biochemically in some manner so as to detect the presence of
the Huntington's disease gene in the skin cells or the amniotic
fluid cells, in the long run, that are fused with the nerve cells.

I say "may be" because our experience until now in fusing
undifferentiated cells with differentiated cells has had varied
results. In some cases the differentiated function has remained
and others have been extinguished. I foresee possible ways of
getting around this extinction by using cells for the fusion
purpose that have perhaps lost some of their chromosomes that may
be responsible for **extinction** of the positive differentiated
function. I think that such techniques are possible and can be
done in the future.

If we assume now that such experiments, which will clearly
take a great deal of effort and expense and manpower to complete
successfully, can be completed successfully (first of all, by study
of such hybrids and culture away from the patient, where changes
that are secondary to the disease may confound the picture), we can
begin to approach what the primary defect of the disease is and
perhaps learn something very fundamental that helps in the treatment of the disease.

For the time being, perhaps more important, we have the possibility of doing the prenatal diagnosis for the disease. A lot
of people have been talking about the carrier detection test for
Huntington's disease; in other words, an attempt to diagnose
individuals before they have the symptoms. Understandably, there
has been great resistance to this from the patients and their
families: People don't really want to know if they carry the gene,
if you get right down to it.

On the other hand, if one is able to offer these families
prenatal diagnosis under the circumstances where they are known to
carry the gene, I believe that both problems may be resolved simultaneously: that a family may want to know if their children
will be affected or not at a time when they still have an option
of terminating a particular pregnancy, and they will only want to
know this really if they themselves carry the gene. Therefore,

both of these techniques can be resolved with the same basic
experimental approach of trying to detect the gene in these few
experiments.

    This is simply one of the many possible approaches to go
after: (1) the basic defect; and (2) specific diagnosis and prenatal diagnosis. But what I would like to end up with is to make
you completely aware that that is not the end of the road in
terms of solving problems. We have now had a great deal of experience of well over 1,000 prenatal diagnoses for a variety of
genetic diseases. In our answers, and in most of the cases we
study, the results will come out normal because a great number of
these are studied for advanced paternal age, the existence of
Down's syndrome in the unborn fetus. Even in the advanced paternal
age some of the pregnancies will still be normal, although the
risk is 5 percent, which is higher than the general population.
In those 5 percent or so of families where we have found an abnormal fetus and the families have exercised the option of terminating that particular pregnancy--in retrospect, we should perhaps
have suspected this but, in fact, it came as a great shock to us--
these families were in terrible trouble.

    Following the induced abortion, there have been a host of
severe psychological problems in these families, leading anywhere
from a relatively brief period of depression to severe prolonged
depression, psychoses, marital difficulties, enormous guilt feelings, a variety of problems that we really did not expect. Here
we had thought, well, the family had the option of not having a
severely defective child and now has an opportunity of having a
normal child by trying another pregnancy, and that this would be
very welcome to them.   In fact, it was welcome to them on initial
talking; but now in a followup study, which has been going on for
well over a year now in our laboratory, the difficulties are
almost universal. I would say that of the 40-some cases that we
now have followup on, over 30 have experienced these difficulties.

    Therefore, one of the other pleas that I would have in terms
of support for research is really social science research: an
attempt to properly evaluate what genetic counseling is all about,
with the end result that genetic counseling is particularly, in
terms of prenatal diagnosis--but I think this is only part and
parcel of evaluating performance of genetic counseling and its

effect upon the family. I think that this is going to require
the combined approach between the geneticists and social scientists
in the design of proper studies so that we may at least understand
what we are doing and perhaps can improve our counseling procedures
so that the family does not experience these adverse situations
following the discovery of an abnormal child.

McKHANN: Kurt, I'd like to ask you a question which you may
not be able to answer but I think would be of interest to many
people oriented towards Huntington's disease. Here's a genetically determined process with a very long latent period which varies
from patient to patient, even within the family. Do you think
that's genetically determined, and if so, think that instead of
getting at the basic mechanism, genetic research at postponing
the disease is a possible direction to go?

HIRSCHHORN: Let me try to respond clearly. No one has any
firm answers to what you're asking. There are, however, a number
of other examples in genetic diseases where we know that the identical mutation will result in onset of disease at quite different
times (the classic example is sickle cell disease) so that the
interaction of genes and the internal and external environment is
clearly what is behind at least that particular difference in onset. We must remember that genes do not act in a vacuum.

All genes basically require for their expression external
environmental situations. Some genes, for example, will only
express themselves in the presence of male sex hormones. Even
though women carry the gene, they do not express it under ordinary
circumstances. I personally believe that the variation and onset--
at least that variation which is seen within families--is due to
internal and external environmental conditions. I completely
agree with you that one should search for the cause of this variation of onset. I don't believe that you'll find it on the genetic
basis. I think you will find it in perhaps a normal, perhaps a
nutritional or whatever basis (in other words, an internal and
external environmental basis), and perhaps one can control it in
terms of the delay of the onset of the disease.

McKHANN: In terms of what you are implying with your
question, is there genetic heterogeneity in Huntington's disease?
In other words, are all patients with Huntington's disease affected
by exactly the same mutation?

HIRSCHHORN: We have now all long learned the lesson that
the answer to that: you will find many different mutations that
will give you the same disease. This is true for almost every
inborn error that has now been studied, and I am quite certain
that we will in the long run, when we understand the defect, find
the same in Huntington's disease. But there are two kinds of
genetic heterogeneities. That's important to remember. One of
them is due to different mutations of the same gene, the kind of
thing, for example, that is responsible for the many different
kinds of abnormal hemoglobins we see around the world. They are
all mutations of the same gene, but they are different mutations
of the same gene. What happens there is usually you get more or
less severe disease. The other type of thing (as we have learned,
for example, in the mucolipidosis, a group of storage diseases
that can be associated with mental retardation), we know that a
group of different genes, each of them with a particular mutation,
can produce a storage disease with mental retardation. It can
mimic the other one quite readily. The approach to this dissection
of heterogeneity has now been learned for diseases where we know
the biochemical defect. Once again, I don't believe we're going to
solve that problem until we know what, in fact, the biochemistry
is of the production of the symptoms of Huntington's disease.

GUTHRIE: Do you think, Kurt, that there is sufficient
interest and funding by the Federal Government for the kind of
continuing social science research that you imply is needed for
this kind of help to families?

HIRSCHHORN: We've had a number of discussions at the NIH
about this on two committees that I've sat with. In searching
through the current funding, at least by the NIH, there is zero;
there is really nothing. Everybody gives very good lip service
to the necessity for this, but our own experience is that review
panels, perhaps because of their particular biases--I have no
particular criticism of them for this, but if the molecular biology
review panels see something that they interpret either as social
science or--and this is extremely important--that they choose to
interpret as clinical service, even though it is research, they
will knock it out of the grant or throw the whole grant out with
it and the person will not get funded. We have had this type of
experience ourselves.

I've always failed to understand, for example, why a research
grant that tries to resolve the problem with the use of experimental animals is allowed to have funding for the animals and the
animal caretaker and the food for the animals, et cetera, whereas
a clinical research grant that tries to get to the bottom of a
disease and therefore requires a necessity to see patients and
families and do something for these patients and families in return for cooperation, why this is different. But this is my own
personal bias. I think one has to establish a totally new kind
of granting mechanism for this, or else persuade NIH that social
science does have a role to play in resolutions of diseases that
have severe psychological and emotional problems.

N. WEXLER: Dr. Hirschhorn, the patients that get into
psychological troubles that you see through the genetics clinic,
do you have an adequate referral system for them there? The
second question, which is naive from a psychologist, if we could
find an H.D. patient with a neuroblastoma and we took that tissue
and grew it out in culture, could we perform the same kinds of
experiments because we would have the transformed tissue in which
the gene is presumably expressing itself?

HIRSCHHORN: Let me answer them one at a time. Insofar as
the first question is concerned, yes, we do have a very good
psychiatry department here, and we have used it for referrals and
for immediate help with patients. I don't think this is adequate.
We have a very good social worker with us, but I think what we
need is a psychiatrist or a clinical psychologist to work with
us directly on a full-time basis because these problems are
unpredictable. To go after them after the fact, I think, is not
totally satisfactory.

Insofar as the second question is concerned, I don't think
that you necessarily mean a patient with a neuroblastoma. I
think that the kind of work you are referring to can perhaps even
be done on ordinary brain tissue cultures from normally transformed Huntington's disease brain. However, we must remember
that what I was talking about really went one step further. I
think some people are trying to do this, attempting to detect the
defect in cultured brain cells, and this should be encouraged.
The point of using normal brain cells with a Huntington's disease
fibroblast is to alter a normal behavior into an abnormal one in

the presence of the gene in order to protect that gene in the
person from whom the cell is obtained.

TESTIMONY OF
MONSIGNOR JAMES CASSIDY, PH.D.
DIRECTOR OF HEALTH AND HOSPITALS
ARCHDIOCESE OF NEW YORK

CASSIDY: I am Monsignor Cassidy. I am Director of Health
and Hospitals throughout the Diocese of New York. My interest in
Huntington's disease comes from the first personal contact that I
have had with it, I guess, which I remember vividly--very vividly.
My first contact was over 10 years ago as a senior clinical
psychologist at St. Vincent's Hospital in New York, and coming up
with this particular diagnosis in a person who was a very talented
musician. I guess from a psychological point of view, our great
interest in it was the gross deterioration that was going on in a
very brilliant person.

We feel that the great difficulty is that we strive to deal
with the needs of people, and we feel that in this particular
disease the problems are different from many of the others. We
feel that we strive to do something for people with cancer, heart
disease, or other kinds of problems, and we usually can be rather
successful in the sense that we have a unique hospital that we
are very proud of in the work that we do with terminal cancer at
Calvary Hospital here in New York. The usual length of stay for
the people that are there is probably about 60 days; but yet it's
a very happy place, and it's something where we feel we can do
things for people who are very ill. We have several other skilled
nursing homes that deal exclusively with terminal patients.

The great difficulty with this disease is that there are so
many other implications: the family and the people who take care
of them. It's a different type of person you almost need to work
with this type of disease. I find that the doctors and psychologists and everybody else like to deal with successes. To work
with this type of patient requires a great deal of patience. Besides the great research we feel that the Government should really
be involved in because the disease is such a tragedy, we feel that
an awful lot has to be done in dealing with this particular type

of patient and to satisfy not only his needs but the needs of the
families that are involved in it.

I think we feel a greater need for something to be done with
this particular type of disease, even though, thanks be to God, it
doesn't have the same numbers that are involved in it as we find
in other diseases. The great difficulty we find is that there is
sort of a hopelessness that comes with people. As a pastor care
person is often very much involved in this, we feel that this
requires that people have a great sense of faith and a great sense
of their understanding of something that's bigger than they are.

Because this disease has certain particular implications,
rather than many of the others that we deal with and feel that we
are rather successful with, we feel rather hopeless in this. It
requires a different type of approach and a different type of
person to deal with the realities besides the research that's involved in it. We have been trying to do something in this area,
but it is very difficult to do in that I think that the great need
is the Government's help, particularly in funding research and
funding projects to be able to take care of these people and
their needs.

GUTHRIE: Do you have at this time any patients that you
know of in any of your hospitals?

CASSIDY: I could give you a name right now, but I can't give
it to you. We have 14 hospitals.

GUTHRIE: You have 14 hospitals. I was just going to ask
you, within that 14-hospital range, has anyone ever done a study
on the number of people or the number of days they stay? You
say yours do not stay long term, right?

CASSIDY: No. We had that problem before the chronic disease
hospital. Of the 14 hospitals, one is the general acute hospital,
so that people usually don't stay long. Now we find that there is
a need in society and we've tried to do something about it.

GUTHRIE: Yes. What do you do when somebody is in your
hospital and you don't want them any longer because you're not
equipped to handle them? What do you do with those people?

CASSIDY: Then we usually try to refer them out very often to
state institutions or somewhere else if we're not able to do anything for them. We may have one or two in a couple of our nursing
homes that the Sisters run. I have to give you the exact name,
Rosary Hill, which is a very skilled nursing home where the Sisters
work with cancer patients.

GUTHRIE: They would take a patient there?

CASSIDY: Yes.

GUTHRIE: I think, though, that you're pointing out something:
that even you have a problem as to where you want to place this
patient, other than a state hospital, whether they belong there or
not.

CASSIDY: Yes. I think it's just, too, that the family is so
much involved in it. I think the great difficulty when you deal
with this type of patient is that they're really intelligent and
know what's going to happen. I think that people can face the
certainty of death in a short period of time. You know, if you
went to Calvary Hospital this afternoon--it's a very happy place,
believe it or not--people know that their length of stay is less
than 60 days. But when you deal with this type of patient, it's
different, because when their intelligence starts deteriorating,
they are aware of it because of the great number of problems.

GUTHRIE: The people that you know of within your facility
as people who care, I would imagine that you would like to say
how they suffer.

CASSIDY: Yes. I think this is our greatest difficulty.
We feel that we would really like to do something for these people,
feel a need to, and we are just not able to do what we really
feel we'd like to; especially, some of the Sisters have taken some
of these patients when they really haven't had the background to
be able to deal with them as well as they could, because they felt
the need. But we feel that something should be done more specifically to be able to help them. I don't think they really belong
in the nursing home just being taken care of along with cancer
patients.

GUTHRIE: We have great empathy for people like you who are concerned and care and feel, again, inadequate to the problem. We appreciate your help.

McKHANN: I'd like to ask you a more general question that is modeled somewhat on the problems we see in Maryland in terms of the parochial school system, which is finding it is less and less able to cope with its own population, let alone any expanding population. Do you see essentially church-oriented hospitals expanding, contracting, or staying the same as an alternative to full Government role here?

CASSIDY: That's a very specific question we're very much involved in. I think that the Church here in the Archdiocese of New York feels simply that we should stay in the health care field. Even though I think most original hospitals were founded by religious orders taking care of people, now the Government is involved. We feel there is a need for the Church to be involved because a great number of ethical and moral issues are going to be resolved in the health field, and we feel that it's very important that we have some impact into it.

I think that even if I go to England, where it's almost a complete government system, it is interesting that the only hospitals the Catholic Church has in England are long-term care hospitals for taking care of this type of patient. We feel that it requires an almost religious dedication to deal with that type of patient. I think we can do a better job with that particular type of patient than maybe we can in an acute general hospital, when you're dealing with just maybe bodies and they're not really persons. I think that's where I feel the impact of the Church is going to be, dealing with some of these situations like this that require long-term care and a real sense of dedication given to these people. The struggle is going to be, "Is the voluntary hospital going to survive?" If the voluntary hospital can survive, we're going to survive. But that's the basic question, if you can answer that one for me [laughter]. We have made a very definite decision in this Archdiocese to make an effort to continue our hospitals. Here in New York is the best medical care given by voluntary hospitals.

TESTIMONY OF
STEVEN M. JAEGER
AND
PEGGY JAEGER
NEW YORK, NEW YORK

S. JAEGER: My name is Steven Jaeger, 15 Charles Street,
New York, New York, 10014.

P. JAEGER: I am Peggy Jaeger; the same address.

GUTHRIE: Are you husband and wife?

JAEGERS: Yes, we are.

GUTHRIE: I thought maybe you were sister and brother.

P. JAEGER: I had no introduction to Huntington's disease
until I met Steven (that was when I was 14 years old and we were
in high school together), and there were a lot of rumors in the
community as to what was wrong with his mother. People were kind
of whispering under the tables when they saw that we were hanging
out together. Friends and a lot of people told me that his mother
was an alcoholic; she was in an institution, and all these other
things. I kind of didn't listen to the rumors, but Steve and I
kept on being friends, and my parents sort of got concerned as to
what the situation was. Steve and I never really talked about
it, other than he told me she had Huntington's disease, and I
didn't really understand what Huntington's disease was. Finally,
I knew that she was not living at home, and I knew that on certain
weekends she would come home to visit, but I was never allowed to
leave the house. I never met her. I knew that she was dying,
that it was getting worse, but this had been going on for a while.
Other than that, I really didn't know anything about Huntington's
disease. Being curious as I was, I had asked Steve these questions,
but he didn't really know very much himself and he never really
felt that he wanted to discuss it.

As we continued getting closer and closer, there were a lot
of pressures, et cetera. I did find out that it was hereditary
and that each child had a 50-50 chance. At that point my parents
got very upset about the whole thing, saying, "There are other

people around. Why do you have to stick...?" They were very
torn because they really, really adored Steve. But yet they saw
that his father was suffering a lot, even though they really didn't
know the whole situation. From bits of information they heard
through the community, what they saw, they knew that his father
was suffering a lot and they felt like, "Well, this will all blow
over."

    Then finally people began to realize that this just wasn't
hanging out together, that we were getting involved. When I went
away to college--I had thought about it a lot in my own mind prior
to that, but I kind of just ignored it, thinking it would go away.
Then when I went away to college I kind of really did a lot of soul-
searching and said, "I think I better really think about it, think
about how it's going to affect me and affect my life." But I didn't
know where to turn. I didn't know who was going to tell me. I
knew that there was a medical library at the university, and I
could have gone to the medical library and picked up books, but I
didn't want to know all of the technical things and the very
embarrassing details. What I needed, I needed somebody to talk
to; not my parents, because they were too emotionally involved;
not my sister and not a friend; not somebody who knew me. I
needed somebody who I could really just talk to that would just
understand the situation and could relate to it.

    I had mentioned it to my physician (I had gone for a checkup
and this was right after Steve's mother had died) and I had said,
"By the way, Steve's mother died of Huntington's disease. Do you
know anything about it? I'd really like to know." So he said,
"Just forget about him. I don't even want to hear about it.
There are too many other people around. You don't have to settle
for this. You don't know what you're getting youself into." And
I just looked at him. Then he turned around and he said, "Well,
if you want a geneticist, I'll give you his name." And it was
like--I didn't want a geneticist; I didn't want a psychiatrist.
I didn't know what I wanted.

    I was in special education at the University of Maryland,
and Huntington's disease was mentioned in one of my texts, so I
figured maybe the head of the department I ran across would know
since she was very involved in all of the diseases. She was really
terrific but she didn't know very much either, so she sent me to
the head of the health department. I went to the head of the health

department and she didn't know anything either, and she gave me
the name of some guy in Boston who was supposedly very good in it
and said to write to him. I didn't want to write to him, so I
went through a lot of soul-searching and a lot of feelings as to
"Do I want to give up having children? Do I want to subject myself
to what his father went through?" And yet you can be optimistic
and you can be very--"Well, it's not going to happen." But you
also have to be realistic. There would be nights when we would be
sleeping together and it's like--everybody jerks in the middle of
the night. It's just a common thing. But like with him, "Oh, my
God. This is it."

So I said, "Can I live with that? Can I sleep with him at
night and not think of that and not worry every single day when
I get up?" It was just a continual internal battle, and I just
didn't know where to go. I had nobody to turn to. Okay, now I
know exactly what it's all about, and even today my parents know
what it's all about. But my parents still talk to me about having
children, Steve's grandparents still talk to me about having
children, and they won't leave us alone. They can't accept the
fact that maybe we don't want to have children because of this.
It's like when somebody has cancer and you're dying, people can
deal with it. It's there. You just have to deal with it immediately. But when it's like something a little obscure, people
just can't deal with it. My parents don't want to deal with it.
They don't want to know about it. There's no doubt in my mind that
if I need them, they'll be there; but to them and to a lot of
people it's just not something to deal with. I'm lucky because
I'm a strong person and I coped on my own. I've really found what
I'm looking for, and I think I've really adjusted and been able
to make my own decisions.

But I still don't know to this day what I'm going to feel
like in 3 years when all my friends are having children. My
sister has children and everybody's running around--and as much
as I say yes--and Steve and I have discussed it--I am willing
to give up not having children. It's easy to say. But right now
I'm not in a position to want to have a child, so it's very easy.
I can't afford it financially or emotionally. I'm not ready. But
I don't know in 3 or 4 years if I've just talked myself into believing these things or if I'm really going to believe in it. I
mean, I don't know what effect it's going to have on our marriage,

because I love children and he knows that. It's a very, very
hard thing to make these kinds of decisions. You do, you need a
lot of help. I guess what the answer is--I guess what maybe I
needed was somebody in the same situation, somebody else who had
married into a family and made their decisions.

S. JAEGER: My experience began with H.D. when my father first
told me that that was what was wrong with my mother. Before that
I was aware that something was wrong but no one knew or would say
what it was. I found out the name; I found out a simplistic
version of what it is. At the time I was about 12 or 13; I'm sure
I wouldn't have understood much more, and probably at this point
I wouldn't understand much more. But the problem that I always
felt was that no one really knew any of the answers, and even if
anyone knew all the answers, they weren't going to tell you; and
if they were going to tell you, the attitude was a very--the same
sort of attitude, "Let's just ignore it and it'll go away," or
"Let it run its course and then forget about it."

My mother spent many years in institutions, hospitals, and
nursing homes, and really nothing ever happened. She just got
progressively worse and worse and worse. There was very little
that the doctors could do for her, and there was very little that
was done for our family. I had a younger brother and sister, and
my father ended up having to raise all of us. I guess in some ways
I helped him raise the other two, but I was also growing up at the
same time. It was very hard on the whole family.

As an individual at risk it is very hard to even think about
your life in any meaningful way when you know that you have a 50-
50 chance of having H.D. when you're 35 or 40. Without any guidance,
without anyone to talk to, without anyone who knows your options,
what can be done, what can't be done, without people who are aware
of what the medical research is, the genetic counseling, the guidance, the psychological problems, without having these people
available it's very hard for individuals to cope with this.

My situation was probably a lot better than a lot of other
people because I was in a situation where we knew people who were
involved with the organizations like CCHD and with NHDA and we were
able to get in touch with people who had some answers or at least
who could talk to you and at least had the same experiences. This

makes it a lot better for somebody in my position who knows these people, but there have to be a lot of people who are not aware that their relatives are suffering from H.D. First of all, as one of the doctors stated, the diagnosis is so haphazard still that there are most likely people in hospitals suffering from some sort of chronic disease that is H.D., but they (the doctors) just haven't decided that that's what it is.

There are other people whose relatives have H.D., and other people who have H.D., but they're not able to be put in contact with these organizations and with other doctors who know geneticists, specialists, and neurologists who know what is going on. I personally feel that that is the major need as far as the families are concerned, and I don't think that organizations like CCHD and NHDA can really reach enough people on their own to alleviate that problem. There has to be some sort of more organized method of accumulating information, of funding research, and of setting up programs for family counseling and for genetic counseling. Without these things, I would think the families are never going to be able to go through this ordeal any easier.

GUTHRIE: Steve, I'd like to ask a question. Because of the way you have lived and what you know today--and you can change your mind 5 years from now or 2 years from now, whatever it is--do you have any thoughts yourself about your being told earlier in life, or is it better to wait until later? What is your feeling today?

S. JAEGER: I'm working under the assumption that I was told pretty much what was known at the time. Maybe I'm wrong. Maybe there was more known and more available to be told me when I was 12 or 13 years old. But I think at that age it was the proper thing to be told. It causes a lot of problems, but I think being able to face them sometimes at that age--maybe 12 or 13 is a little too young, maybe, but within that age span. Before you start to mature, before you become 18 or 19, but before you're going out on your own, I think you should have that information because it involves the whole family and you should at least have some idea of what is occurring while you're still in the family environment.

GUTHRIE: You're saying, then, that if you were young enough, you feel that maybe the person could cope better because he had more time to think it through?

S. JAEGER: I don't know if that would enable you to cope better. I think it gives you the opportunity to think it through.

GUTHRIE: To give you more time. That's what I'm thinking, and I wondered how you felt about that.

S. JAEGER: I think so, especially in the situation where it's known from age 10 that the family knows about it. If you keep it from the child for 7 or 8 years, you're depriving the child of the opportunity to grow up with it. There are a lot of psychological processes going on. If the child is shut out of it, then when the child is 18 and you all of a sudden spring it on the child, it's full-blown. I would imagine it is very major then.

GUTHRIE: Yes. There are people, you see, who speak the other way. That's why I've asked your opinion, how you feel. You shouldn't be told until you are about to be married, or something?

P. JAEGER: Steve, could I, from the other end? I totally disagree because I think it's very unfair to subject somebody to that. Why shouldn't these people be entitled to make their decisions before they actually get emotionally involved with some-body else? I think that would be so traumatic, to have to cope with everything at once.

GUTHRIE: You're saying the opposite of what Steve is saying?

P. JAEGER: No. I feel they should be told when they're younger, when they live in the house and have the support of the family and can grow with the family, et cetera, and can make their decisions before they come home and say, "I'm in love and getting married," and then, "Well, it's time we sit down and discuss it." I just think that would be too much. It sort of happened when Steve and I had stopped seeing each other for a while. The reason was because Steve had felt he didn't know if he wanted to get married, because he felt he didn't know if he could handle it in the sense of, "Do I want to put somebody through what my father

went through, the financial burdens and everything else? Is it
fair for me to ask somebody not to have children?" He said he
didn't know if he ever wanted to get married, and I said, "Well,
I don't want to push you in any way because that would be worse,"
so we stopped seeing each other, and it was the first time. So
he turned around and his father said, "What happened to Peggy?"
Steve said, "We're not seeing each other." He said, "Why?" and
Steve said, "Because I don't know if I ever want to get married."
Steve, wasn't that the first time you actually said that?

S. JAEGER: Yes. That was probably the first time since the
initial talk and the initial things that occurred in the family
when it was determined that H.D. was involved.

GUTHRIE: Thank you very much.

TESTIMONY OF
JANE SMITH
CONNECTICUT

SMITH: Good morning. My name is Jane Smith. I am 27,
married, the mother of one child, and I am a high school mathe-
matics teacher. My mother died of Huntington's disease 4 years
ago, and I would like to speak to the emotional trauma that a
family goes through. I have a letter in front of me that was
written to me from my aunt (my mother's sister) while I was a
freshman at college. When my mother was diagnosed as having
Huntington's, there was a split made in our family, and relations
with her family and my family were just severed. This was the
first time that I had heard from her in years. It was sent
special delivery, registered mail. It says:

"The first thing I have to ask is, have you ever heard of
the Golden Rule: 'Do unto others as you would have done unto
you'? I certainly hope you are never faced with such rottenness."
(I was 18 years old when I received this letter. It put me in a
state of shock.) "Do you have any idea how miserable and lonely
your mother is? God knows, she would never have put one of you
out, including your sister" (who is mentally retarded), "and she
was told to by medical authorities. Your weekly letters are
really of no help to her, and I imagine it eases your consciences,
but as she says, 'Why do they bother, or do they think they have

to write me?'" (Mom may have said this, but I think she said it to make her sister feel better rather than make herself feel better.)

"Big deal, where she is. For $50 a week she's getting an inadequate diet, one attendant for 47 people, a bed between two people who hate her because she can still move about and constantly tell her to get out, shut the door, put out the light, not to have company in the room, et cetera," (which is true, but it was impossible in our situation to keep Mom at home). "Amazing to me to think that she worked for 24 years for this" (and by "worked" she means working as a housewife). "What a lousy world, or is it the people in it? Do you realize now that her actions were furthered by her father keeping her incapacitated with liquor to meet his own needs?" (This is completely untrue. Mom never drank. It was just her reaction to Huntington's that always made people think she was incapacitated, and obviously my aunt didn't know the facts.)

"If she were to pass away tomorrow, would you all attend and sit there and cry because she was your mother, or what? And too, who is left to take care of these details? Believe me, my way of life is to help those in need while they are here on earth, so as long as I can I shall make sure she has the material necessities," (which turned out to be untrue as the years passed): "But, believe me, someone better become the next-of-kin." (I'm not sure what she meant by that.) "You certainly don't expect her divorced husband to attend to these things. Well, maybe he will so he can get his hands on what money is left." (In this, she was referring to a $60,000 trust fund which was left to my father when his mother passed away. My father had to divorce my mother so as to—I'm not sure of the exact reason; he explained it to me—so that he could have her put in a home and have the trust fund set up to take care of her. It was also because our home was in complete turmoil, and he knew that for my younger brother something had to be done to have a more stable home.)

"Boy, I hope you kids are being paid enough for this turning-the-cheek-the-other-way attitude." (By "being paid enough," I haven't any idea what she means.) "Is it enough so you can forget to visit your mother or be too busy with your own worlds to have her visit you, to give her the human contact she desperately

needs from her own children? Is it enough so you can always go
to sleep without seeing her desperate face? Is it enough, really,
so it can make you forget you have a mother? Thank God I don't
have to walk in your shoes."

When I received this letter, I just couldn't believe it.
Here I was, away at school, away from my family, and to think that
a relative would accuse me of having deserted my mother, which was
not the case at all. I was a distance from her and I could not
visit her daily, but I did visit her as often as I could.

I also have some letters which she wrote to a lawyer (there
were nine). These letters were written 5 years before her death,
when she was initially removed from our home. She was first in a
private home with nursing care; after that she was in a rest home
for a couple of years, and her last few years were in a nursing
home. To the lawyer, she says:

"When my husband came to pay my board, I asked for money,
but 10 new cars we have confiscated. He hasn't sold his as yet.
He drives by. He and his family are living in Hanover. I have
all cars. He has seen only to pay board. If can done but sit
back and read. He still a garrison in Dover, and he and children
live in Dover. He's seven or eight new cars, a camper truck. I
have enough on him. He has sold his house. I enough on him to
jail. He still does give me money. He got divorce in" (I think
it says "Bermuda"--I can't read it--which is not true), "but I
live in Massachusetts. He must get around." (I can't read the
rest of that.)

As you can see from this, she was experiencing tremendous
hallucinations. These are completely false statements. There is
no basis to this. I do not know where she got this information.
I remember when she was first removed from our home, going to
visit her. She would sit on the porch and just any car that went
by, "There he goes now! There he goes now!" Her hallucinations
were very difficult for me to deal with at that time. I was still
a teenager. I have another letter here somewhere. Would this be
of any use to you, this letter?

McKHANN: I think that we probably don't have to hear the last letter. I just would like to ask one question. As you think back over this, what kinds of people would have been the most help to you in handling this?

SMITH: I think at that time this aunt could have been very helpful to me: someone just to sit down and talk with. I didn't understand what my mother was going through. I think just someone aside from my immediate family to sit and talk with, anyone.

PRATT: Did the family have any contact with a professional counselor?

SMITH: My father does not believe in doctors or any kind of professional help in that capacity, so he was not involved in anything and he did not make any attempt to get us involved. We were completely removed from help of that sort, and I was too young at that point to seek it.

PRATT: Do you think it would be good now?

SMITH: Yes, I do believe so. I think that at that point, not for my younger brothers and sisters; they were just too young. But I think for an older person, yes.

PRATT: What age were your brothers that you thought they were too young?

SMITH: They were 10, 11, and 12.

TESTIMONY OF
NANCY PLERHOPLES
WILMINGTON, DELAWARE

PLERHOPLES: My name is Nancy Plerhoples. I am 30 years old, married, with no children. I am a trained social worker, but I am testifying as a layperson. My paternal grandmother died of Huntington's disease in 1965 after years of debilitation and after a lengthy hospitalization. Huntington's disease was known to run in our family, and my grandmother's chorea movements were first diagnosed when she was 64.

My father is 61 now and is subject to mood swings and nervous tics. He has difficulty holding a pencil to write. My father says that since there is no cure for H.D., he sees no reason to consult a neurologist to get a formal diagnosis. His family doctor says that he "probably" has H.D., but my father desperately wants to believe that he does not have it. I am afraid for him and for myself.

People who have not seen H.D. firsthand have a hard time understanding why we are so afraid. Living with a victim of H.D., watching the unsightly physical deterioration, coping with mood swings and intermittent bizarre behavior, and finally, not being able to effectively communicate with the victim have touched my entire family.

Knowing that my aunt and father have a 50-percent chance of contracting the disease brings another wave of fear. When the disease does strike, a new cycle of suffering and fear begins for the victim and his children. Knowing that there is no cure for H.D. and being aware of how limited the medical treatment is, it is no surprise that suicide attempts among H.D. victims are not uncommon.

My family experience has led me to believe that there are several categories of objectives pertinent to helping H.D. victims and their families. The first set of objectives requires fully utilizing existing knowledge. These include: (1) education of health professionals; and (2) education of H.D. victims and their families.

A second group of objectives has to do with expanding current resources. These objectives are: (1) availability of professional counseling for H.D. victims and their families; and (2) availability of medical care.

The third set of objectives is tied to research efforts and includes: (1) finding control drugs to treat symptoms; (2) early detection of H.D.; (3) basic research; and (4) finding a cure for H.D.

I think that the education of health professionals is of primary importance, because they are the key to a well-informed

family. Many decisions have to be made about the kinds of care
and family planning. It is crucial that the affected families get
correct information and have access to medical people who can
answer questions as they arise. It is also important that these
medical resource people be sensitive to family fears and handle
questions with sensitivity.

Because we are aware that H.D. runs in our family (we can
trace it back three generations), we have not been subject to the
lengthy and emotionally painful process of incorrect diagnosis,
which is all too common among H.D. victims. However, one well-
meaning physician assured my aunt that since she had not contracted
H.D. by the time she was 40, she had nothing to worry about.
Apparently this doctor was not aware that H.D. appears in the
early sixties in our family. Even well-informed families find
coping with H.D. difficult. Often, doctors do not take the time
to help patients and their families sort out feelings and offer
the family support on an ongoing basis. While I intellectually
understand that my father's outbursts of rage are to be expected
with H.D., I find myself wanting some guidance in knowing how to
react to him and outside help in dealing with my feelings towards
him.

Family planning is also an important area for me now. My
gynecologist is encouraging me to have a tubal ligation; but my
husband and I are reluctant to make a final decision, and we
would talk to a counselor if one were available.

Quality medical care from diagnosis to long-term custodial
care must be available to all families at a reasonable cost. My
personal concern now has to do with financing long-term care. Our
family cannot afford to pay for several years of care for my
father in a private nursing home, and we are not eligible for the
State's medical assistance program. The Public Health Department
in Delaware runs an excellent hospital for the chronically ill,
but one must be indigent to be cared for there. As it stands now,
one must be very poor or wealthy to get quality health care.

Through research we need to understand the nature of H.D.
We need drugs to ease the symptoms, to alleviate both patient and
family discomfort. Even controlling the gross chorea movements

would be a blessing. We need a means for early detection; this combined with family planning would help limit the disease.

These immediate needs must not preclude support of basic research. The more we know about all neurological disorders and genetic diseases, the closer we may come to finding a cure for H.D. Also, we should remind ourselves that suffering is not limited to the H.D. family. We share many problems with families afflicted with other neurological disorders. Hopefully, by supporting basic research, we can look to a time when all neurological disorders and genetic diseases can be cured or eliminated.

GUTHRIE: Because we're running short, I think we're going to hold back our questions, aren't we?

McKHANN: I think we'd better. That was a very nice presentation, though.

TESTIMONY OF
NORMAN A. LEOPOLD, D.O.
ASSISTANT PROFESSOR OF NEUROLOGY
HAHNEMAN MEDICAL COLLEGE HOSPITAL

LEOPOLD: My name is Dr. Norman A. Leopold. I am the Assistant Professor of Neurology at Hahneman Medical College Hospital, and the Codirector of the CCHD in Philadelphia. I originally designed the presentation for those much less knowledgeable about Huntington's disease than you that are before me now, but I think it represents my feelings about Huntington's disease not only as a neurologist, but as someone who cares for patients with Huntington's disease and sees their problems every day, and as someone who is interested in clinical research.

I see Huntington's disease, if you wish, as not a disease, N-O-T. It is not accurately diagnosed by the medical community; it does not have adequate therapy; physicians are not yet able to diagnose this illness preclinically; it has not received adequate research support; it is not yet accepted well by the patient or his family; and it is not known or understood by the public.

What is it about Huntington's disease that makes it associated with so many negative factors? If you observe patients with

Huntington's disease you will see they move to excess; they squirm
and make us feel uncomfortable, agitated, and anxious; they may
fling their arms, contort their bodies, and distort their faces;
their mentality, their judgments, and their emotions may be impaired; their speech may be slurred, and when it is comprehensible
the language is often abusive; they often have been raised by a
parent in whom they have seen the same or more extensive symptoms.
Awaiting their future with gloom, they often hide from the outside
world, fearing first the glances of their coworkers, and eventually
the eyes of their children.

Even the unafflicted family members live uneasily, as each
know they have a 50-50 chance of developing the same illness. The
patients are burdened by immense guilt and depression that may
lead to suicide, or their behavior and appearance may so disrupt
the family that legal dissolution of the marriage or permanent
institutionalization is the only resolution. Even then the tragedy
is not over, as institutions for the chronically ill reject the
H.D. patient often because they may cause serious disruption of
the routine of other patients and burden the staff with unwanted
work as the Huntington's patient develops increasing functional
dependency.

The appearance of choreiform movements often heralds the
isolation of the H.D. patient. No adequate therapy is yet available to abolish these movements; many patients can be improved, but
still the signs are present. This problem is often personally
resolved by self-imposed social isolation; yet the remainder of
the family desire, and require, socialization. Anger, hostility,
and frustration are experienced by the family as the patient
slowly, year by year, deteriorates. A significant financial loss
often causes a further strain on the family, especially when the
patient is the primary source of financial support. Often the
wife is then required to seek work; even if she obtains adequate
monetary compensation, she must leave her children at home to a
person who may be physically, emotionally, and intellectually
incompetent.

Huntington's disease is obviously a complex illness that often
destroys the patients and their families as well. It is a familial illness, transmitted from one generation to the next. But
once a diagnosis is made, we often refer not to Huntington's disease patients, but to Huntington's disease families.

This has been an area of greatest neglect by the medical community.
The needs for the family include family and genetic counseling,
psychiatric care, various home services, occupational training
and placement, and other services.

Family and genetic counseling are extremely important to
inform the entire family about the disease and its long-term
implications. These have not been readily available to the H.D.
family. The information provided must be done with care and
often with psychiatric support, as the knowledge of being an at-
risk individual can be emotionally devastating, leading at times
to severe depression and even suicide. Further family counseling
may be necessary intermittently over the next 5 to 10 years as
the patient deteriorates.

Psychiatry can play an enormous role in the management of the
H.D. family as the therapy provided to the family may be as important as the medications administered to the patient. The changes
in personality often occur in H.D., ranging from severe depression
with suicidal tendencies to anger with physical violence. Psychiatric support is essential for the family if they are to understand
and cope. Today, most psychiatrists are not yet willing to become
involved in the care of the H.D. patient or their family. Further,
the cost for additional professional care is often prohibitive.

Home services of various types are not yet available to the
H.D. family. The family with young children and the affected
father are the most in need of these services. The loss of income
can rarely be recovered when the mother, often previously untrained, is forced to seek employment. Public welfare is often
the only viable alternative. Home services might provide enough
support so that a full-time job can be pursued with the comforting
knowledge that the family is not being neglected. Further, I
propose to you that such families might be provided with this
financial support for the education and/or retraining similar to
those educational benefits that may be provided under the GI bill.
The war that takes place in the home of an H.D. family can be as
brutal as any and may last not for months, but for generations.

Medical research into the mechanisms of H.D. has been in
progress for over 70 years now, but the data, I think, is mostly
an accumulation of "not" information. However, the new techniques
that are now available can extend our knowledge. The areas of

ignorance are numerous, and many more scientists are now involved
in research, both clinical and basic, that is directed at Huntington's disease. The advances in neurochemistry that we are aware
of in the past 3 to 4 years have provided the basis for understanding some of the abnormal movements and mentation in Huntington's disease; yet these drugs can only partially suppress the
obvious symptoms. Some brain chemicals are reduced in Huntington's
disease, but attempts at replacements have not yet been successful.
The answers to Huntington's disease are obviously not going to be
found easily.

As a clinical neurologist, I have been engaged in neuro-
endocrine research in Huntington's disease for every year since I
was a first-year resident, approximately 6 years now. The abnormalities in Huntington's disease that were first reported by me
and my coworker Dr. Kanalski were not at all expected, and we are
not quite sure how they relate to Huntington's disease. That
research, however, has continued and expanded so that unaffected
at-risk family members are now being tested, with the goal of
trying to establish a presymptomatic patient. This research has
been supported entirely through private contributions through the
CCHD. Tests determining which of the at-risk patients are actually
presymptomatic patients are one of the three major research areas
of the scientific community here today. If a definitive test can
be found that will allow presymptomatic diagnosis, then the completion of the two remaining tasks (that is, the development of a
symptomatic cure, as well as eventual prevention) will of course
follow. My own research also has begun to expand into areas of
other choreatic movements, hoping to find the same abnormalities
in this particular group of patients.

When I began, I stated that Huntington's disease was <u>not</u> a
disease. The logo of the Committee to Combat Huntington's Disease
is a person twisted in knots and is representative of the affected
individual. It is hoped that through the work of the people here
and the programs that we might be able to establish we can eliminate not only the "nots" but also the "knots" of Huntington's
disease.

GUTHRIE: Could I just ask, what do you do after you have
made a diagnosis? What do you do with a patient who comes to you

and you know that you have said, "Yes, you have Huntington's disease"? Do you have a procedure?

LEOPOLD: When a person first comes, we never tell him immediately without having gone through at least some basic tests that they have for Huntington's disease. I think if we did that, most of the people we would see we would probably never see again, we would never be able to talk to again at any further time. They would probably just pick themselves up and walk out. They often come to us and they want to know if they do have it. We do suggest that there is a possibility that they do and we have signs which are indicative of Huntington's disease, but we would often prefer to just run tests to make sure that there are no other signs that might be available. At the time when we do feel that the patient has Huntington's disease, we do tell them and we also tell the family that the diagnosis, based upon the history and physical examination, is strongly established.

I find that the family or the wife, if that is the case--only the two of them--is apparently resigned with the choreatic movements, and I have found that the times we give the patients medication to reduce the movements to please them, we have negatively influenced the psychiatric pattern of the patient. In those cases we do not give the medication--or maybe a lower level of control. I think that depends upon the family situation. We try to have family counseling, but we can only do it as physicians because there is nothing available to us without the family having to pay large sums of money for it.

GUTHRIE: You're missing that team approach, I gather? There is no team?

LEOPOLD: There is no team. We've approached the psychiatrists with this kind of problem and people say, "Oh, yes. We think that is interesting, and we will be willing to help." But when the time comes to get them to come in, there is no one there: the seat is empty.

GUTHRIE: But you would recommend that you would like to have it?

LEOPOLD: Oh, of course. Sure.

GUTHRIE: A good psychiatrist, a good geneticist, a good sociologist.

LEOPOLD: Sure. You can't do it by yourself.

GUTHRIE: This is the suffering of the doctor.

LEOPOLD: Yes. But it's much less, obviously, than the suffering of the patient.

GUTHRIE: Yes. Thank you.

TESTIMONY OF
FLORENCE SIEGEL
REGO PARK, NEW YORK

SIEGEL: Good morning. I am Florence Siegel. I am an elementary school teacher in the New York public schools, and my husband is a victim of Huntington's disease. I have been asked to kind of be more specific as to the kinds of things that this Commission could recommend to help patients with Huntington's disease and their families.

One of the most important things I have found in all of our problems and troubles in searching for help was that information about Huntington's disease was very limited. If one or two doctors were aware of it, the information was never passed on in terms of an institution or a health or mental clinic (the medical profession in general was extremely limited); also, how to go about handling the patient with the disease. We, in turn, have seen a neurologist who had but one other patient with this disease previous to the time my husband had come to him, so he, too, was a stranger as to how to handle the case, other than neurologically and mentally. Professionally, he had no other way but to give out medication and to be sympathetic, but there were no programs, no therapy, whether physical therapy, mental hygiene, health, et cetera. We ourselves have to go out personally, individually, and look for this to solve our own problems, in terms of our problems in the mental health field, in terms of getting help for the family.

We do have two children and we didn't know where to go. We had no resource, except the telephone book, and that's exactly

what we did. We just called up one mental health clinic after
another when a crisis situation occurred and went our own way
Saturday or Sunday, and we couldn't find anybody who was able to
help us. We did find one person, a social worker, who was willing
to come in on Saturday afternoon because of the call that I made
and because I said that the situation was immediate. Even the
local hospitals had no facilities to help us at that particular
moment. We could have gone and they would have given my husband
a pill, but that's not what we needed at the moment: he needed
someone to talk with.

Finally, when we did locate a psychiatrist who was able to
work with my husband and the family, the psychiatrist herself
knew nothing about the disease. She was completely unfamiliar
with the disease and really had to go back through her medical
books and associates to find out, because she was a complete novice
in how to work with this person. Also, in terms of families with
children at risk, how do you talk to them? How do you handle
them? Who do you go to? Who is there to help? These were all
the questions that we needed answers for, answers which we had to
seek out ourselves through much trouble, suffering, tears,
et cetera.   In terms of how the Government can help, they can help
by funding professional people to be trained to help those of us
who are suffering with these kinds of neurological ailments, to
help the families who are desperately in need.

Also, in terms of the general medical staff (nurses, doctors),
these, too, need orientation in the field of what to do. They're
all working in the dark. It's all been, from my experience, trial
and error. Even now, my husband, who is at the VA hospital on
23rd and First Avenue, they are helping in the best way they know
how; but again, it's trial and error. Nobody knows how, what will
work, what won't work. Even if they have found something that
might help him, I don't know if the information is being passed
on. There's information, I believe, down at NIH; if it could be
forwarded to Veterans' hospitals who are assisting and who have
patients with Huntington's disease, these suggestions might in
turn help them. The information, the kind of research, whether
it's practical or medical, is not being filtered through the
communication system at all in terms of the medical profession,
at least from my point of view.

McKHANN: You had one point in your document, in the very last part, on page 5, where you talked about some of the financial aspects. Could you comment on that?

SIEGEL: Oh, yes. Of course, there's always the problem of finances and money. As with all people who have diseases which are incurable, the problem eventually comes to the point where the person has to be placed in some kind of permanent facility. Families like ours, we're extremely limited. It was an impossibility. In the position that I have I do have a certain amount of medical coverage which, in terms of a nursing facility, would probably last--I forget the limit of the contract. My husband, in turn, has Social Security. This is a 90-day bit in the nursing home. After that, from the various phone calls I had made when I felt that he needed to be hospitalized, I found out that after the 90 days I would either have to take him home or I would have to place him a state institution.

If I wanted a private facility, I would have to dissolve, liquidate, every bit of finances that we had, every bit of income up to, I believe, $2,500, and I would be allowed under $300 a month to live on. Therefore, I would have to quit my job and could no longer earn my salary because it would be over and above the required amount. I could not afford to place my husband in the private facility, or even the State facility, or even the city, because I couldn't afford $1,200 a month. At the time, I had a daughter at home that was still going to school, and I had all the other personal needs of any human being who is alive and well and trying to live as best they can. So the financial situation had become extremely impossible.

Somebody had mentioned the Veterans' hospital, and of course my husband does happen to be a disabled veteran. There, again, we found a problem: You couldn't get in unless someone helps to get you in. I thought this was kind of outrageous, too. After all, we're not at war. The facilities are there and should be available to people like my husband, to families like ours; they are not overcrowded and the help is available.

GUTHRIE: Can I ask a question, Florence? Because you mentioned the experimental work in medication at the NIH, what do think would be your personal reaction and what do you think would be your husband's reaction if an experimental drug were given to your husband that made him very much worse?

SIEGEL: As I understood it, when applying to NIH, it was a gamble.

GUTHRIE: No. I'm asking, what would be your reaction? Because we hear about the problems of suing doctors, and whatnot, how do you think you would feel and how do you think your husband would feel if an experimental drug were used that made him very much worse, not better?

SIEGEL: I guess I personally would wind up chalking it up to experience and figuring we took our chances. It would be extremely difficult to answer and pinpoint it now, but the way the situation is at the moment, I don't know whether it really matters one way or the other because our chances are so limited.

GUTHRIE: But you would not, then, want to go around and sue the doctor? I mean, this is the kind of problem that doctors are facing.

SIEGEL: Not under the circumstances, knowing full well that it was an experimental program, no. I mean, this is a gamble we took and we would take.

GUTHRIE: Would be willing to take gladly, right?

SIEGEL: Exactly.

GUTHRIE: That's important for people to know, I think.

SIEGEL: Yes.

N. WEXLER: Mrs. Siegel, were you ever advised, as some families are, to divorce your husband to make him indigent?

SIEGEL: No, I wasn't advised. I knew that was available. Let's say that is the last road that any of us would wish to take. I guess that if I had to, I probably would, because I could not see going on welfare and giving up a position that I liked when I was independent. I would--I think I would.

N. WEXLER: In some states it's not available, because you
would be sued for his alimony support.

SIEGEL: You're probably right. I don't know what the laws
are in New York State, but I think if that is the road I had to
take, I would.

GUTHRIE: I have another important question about the VA.
Did you ever apply to the VA?

SIEGEL: Yes.

GUTHRIE: You did. Did anyone say yea or nay, that they
would accept him on the basis that this was a service-connected
or nonservice-connected disability?

SIEGEL: No. At the time we went there, it happened to be
3 days before he was finally admitted with the help of a doctor.
When we got there--I remember it was Thanksgiving weekend--we sat
there, and he went from one doctor to the other, and they were all
very nice about it. We finally got down to the psychiatrist because that was what they decided he needed. The psychiatrist,
whose knowledge was very limited, did not understand the disease
and recommended a medication that was wonderful for Parkinson's.
I explained to him that this was contrary to what was indicated.
He said, "Well, that's all right. Let him take a little of it."
Well, there we were. We were there from 9:00 in the morning until
4:30 in the afternoon--and my husband was not eating; he was in a
terribly debilitated state at that time; he was willing to sit
there--and nothing happened. They gave us an appointment for a
week later. They saw him; they realized his condition and said,
"Go back and try this," and that's where we were. There was
nothing that we could do.

GUTHRIE: They never actually asked the question of whether
it was service-connected or nonservice-connected?

SIEGEL: No. They had his service record. I had brought it.
As I said, he is a disabled veteran. They know what was service-
connected, and the question never came up.

McKHANN: Thank you very much.

TESTIMONY OF
LEWIS JAFFE
ELKINS PARK, PENNSYLVANIA

JAFFE: Good morning. My name is Lewis Jaffe. I am from a
Huntington's family and have been active in CCHD since its inception. I really came to make a pitch that's been made much better
by others. In the last few weeks especially it's come to my
attention that wives of Huntington's patients are in very, very
bad shape in almost every situation that can be realized. Most
women have had the shock of having to take care of a patient that
they were completely unprepared to handle. They lose their income,
they have no facilities to handle the patients, and their lives
have become almost immediately deteriorated.

There was one woman who was supposed to be here today who
wanted to tell her story. She called me Monday morning and said,
"Lew, I can't make it. My husband fell down the steps. This is
the third time in 2 weeks. I can't leave him." This woman's
trying to hold a job. She has no one at home but an elderly
mother who can't help her, and she just cannot leave. There are
other women with whom I come in contact through CCHD who call and
say, "Can you help? Can we find someone? Can I find a way to
make a living so I can work and bring in a few dollars while my
husband's home?"

I believe that there should definitely be occupational
training for wives. I believe that there should be some sort of
day care centers for patients because they are desperately needed.
My observation is that the male spouse is able to handle the
situation somewhat better than the female for some reason or other.
He seems to be out of the house more; he's not tied down as much.
The female spouse has terrible problems. We really have to look
at some of these things, because I firmly believe that there are
facilities available. With very little training, at no great
expense to the Government or to the community, we could make life
a lot more palatable for the family if we could just get this
little help.

GUTHRIE: You're recommending something rather interesting,
Lew. You're talking about an outpatient center just like the aged

centers, in a sense, where people with the disease may be able to go for recreational therapy, to play chess. Isn't that what you're saying?

JAFFE: That's exactly what I'm saying.

GUTHRIE: A place where people could go, and then the mother or the wife, or whatever it is, could go out to work. That's an interesting recommendation. I like that.

McKHANN: We're just asking what your thoughts are about any modification of the Social Security mechanism as a source of income under these circumstances.

JAFFE: I haven't really thought about that very clearly. It seems to me that there should be some way that Social Security could help with the training program for the unaffected spouse so that she may either be compensated for going to school or something like that, because most of them have been out of the labor market for a long, long time and are just not able to handle the job.

McKHANN: Let me ask you a more general question that hasn't come up yet. I haven't heard much discussion of the role of non-affected family members; for example, siblings of an affected parent.

JAFFE: This is something that is very dear to my heart. I'm not a very religious man, but it seems to me that God blessed that child not to have Huntington's. I find that, in general, the unaffected sibling has a tendency to run. Unfortunately, even the at-risk children have a tendency to find an excuse for leaving the house and leaving the unaffected spouse with more responsibility than there really should be. If life could be made a little easier in the family, I think there would be greater family feeling than there is. But everybody unaffected has a tendency to run away, to ignore as much as they possibly can, unfortunately.

GUTHRIE: But as an unaffected sibling yourself, what do you feel? Other than the fact that you do work so hard for CCHD, and do stand by your family, and do all the things that you do, how did you feel when you found out that they had it and you didn't?

JAFFE: I really don't know. I can't honestly answer that question. I knew it for a long time before it was clinically confirmed. In my particular case, my sister obviously had Huntington's, at least to our family, but she would not go to get a clinical diagnosis. It was only by saying that all three of us would go that we got her to go, because she was very, very adamant about not having it, as so many other Huntington's patients are. My brother was different. We never had that kind of problem with him. He was a typical case, almost, because he was very, very quiet and easy to get along with. But my sister, we had plenty of problems with her.

You've heard all these other personal problems and I don't have to go into them, but one of the things that was said and I think should be reemphasized is that there is no psychiatrist that I know of around that is in any way capable of handling a Huntington's patient. Fortunately, CCHD helped our family in a time of need. We stuck together. We got backing from the people who were at the meeting; they helped us. But the doctor that we took my sister to was completely unfamiliar--we took her to one of the largest mental hospitals in the city of Philadelphia and the psychiatrist in charge said, "I remember seeing a Huntington's patient my freshman year in college," or some sort of thing like that.

GUTHRIE: Did you discuss this disease in your family?

JAFFE: We had very little discussion of Huntington's. My grandmother, mother, uncle, sister, and brother all have Huntington's, but only under the most tense situations do we ever discuss it. It's never discussed with the patient.

GUTHRIE: Even now?

JAFFE: Even now; never discussed. Maybe that's our protective mechanism, but it's not working 100 percent because I have two nephews who had many, many problems that are psychiatrically connected with Huntington's.

McKHANN: Thank you very much.

TESTIMONY OF
MARGARET JONES
WEST HEMPSTEAD, NEW YORK

JONES: Good morning. It is very difficult for me to talk
about my experience with Huntington's disease. The emotional
stress is more than significant, especially when you repress the
horror that the knowledge of this disease brings to you.

Several years ago it was considered a possibility that a
relative of mine had Huntington's disease. The family's reaction
was normal. While one relative called or wrote to everyone,
trying to obtain further family information to receive a more
competent diagnosis, other relatives debunked everything she had
to say, attributing the behavior to eccentricity.

For many years my father had been in and out of therapy and
hospitalized twice for extreme depression. He also had outpatient
shock treatment and several debilitating episodes, one of which
ended with him in jail. He has been on antidepressive medication,
none of which I felt was ever adequate.   The diagnosis had become
organic brain disease; more specifically, atherosclerosis. Then
about 2 years ago my parents started seeing doctors concerning
nervous movements that were becoming more and more apparent. I
had grown accustomed to seeing the movements and had attributed
them to his mental problems and nerves. We went to different
doctors for months. I don't know how many we saw or how many medications were tried, but nothing worked.

My father was hospitalized at Mt. Sinai, and through a combination of luck and fortitude, I managed to find the most fantastic group of doctors. They set about to do what no one else had
done before: make a proper diagnosis so that my father could
finally be treated. The end result, obviously, was a diagnosis
of Huntington's disease, and the inconceivable had become a
reality. Two years before, while everyone was talking about our
eccentric relatives, unbeknownst to me, another physician had
made the identical diagnosis concerning my father's sister.

I behaved with true splendor, gathering and reading all available information and asking doctors every conceivable question. It took about 2 months for me to become so severely depressed that I ceased functioning almost completely. I simply couldn't live knowing all I knew about the disease, knowing tomorrow I might be next, thinking the depression that had gripped me was telling me I had it already, thinking my daughter might get it (how do you tell your child?), thinking that since I was single and had hopes of someday remarrying, who would want me? One day I tried to kill myself. I was lucky: A psychiatrist talked with me, explaining that my thoughts, not the disease, were depressing me; there was just as good a chance that I might not have it.

My brother told me that he had lived with the knowledge for 2 years and every day he looks in the mirror and tells himself, "Today I am 36, and look at me. I still don't have it." He still believes that if you don't show signs of the disease by 40, you don't have it; but I know better. At present he can't accept it, and he stays away from anyone who knows what we might be carrying. Presently, over 30 potential carriers exist in our family.

Mother knows nothing about it; she thinks my father is mentally ill and has nervous tics. We have been advised by a social worker and psychiatrist that she is incapable of handling the knowledge at this time. But some part of her knows, for she keeps asking relatives and doctors if there is any chance that my father might have Huntington's.

Last week my father refused to take his medicine and then tried to kill my mother and himself. Today he is again in the hospital. He's 65, and my mother is 62, and all they have are their house and Social Security; all their savings have gone for the last hospitalizations. I had to tell my mother to keep him in the public hospital in the hopes that she won't lose the house, even though the care and the quality of physicians are much better in private hospitals. They're talking about institutionalizing my father now, and I have difficulty handling that and have no idea where the money will come from. Medicare doesn't pay for everything, and my folks have just missed out on Medicaid. I haven't seen my father since he's been hospitalized this time; it's too painful. Every time I see him he asks me to help him kill

himself; somehow I think he's right. I hope, if it becomes
necessary, someone will be that kind to me.

The doctors have said that my father's progression with the
disease is about 5 years. I hope that they're wrong, since that
would mean that we have so much longer to wait. It's terrible
living with the guilt of wishing your father dead. It would end
his pain; it would take away a visual representation that would
end some of my pain, and then we could have an autopsy that would
ascertain the diagnosis, for there is a thread of hope.

Why isn't there a place we could go to for diagnosis? Why
isn't there a test to determine if someone is a carrier before
they have children? Why can't we get reasonably decent financial
assistance? Why don't we have the medications that can help make
life bearable to the dying? We have seen the effect. Why have
they not delegated enough funds to find the cause?

I wrote a poem the last time I saw my father and he asked me
to kill him. I'd like to read it to you:

> "There is no life,
>   (I wrote your name across a mountain
> Only pain ending in everlasting death,
>   (And left to find the quiet sea
> Only the death that ends the pain.
>   (Where the birds and I can share its sound
> There cannot be a dream where there is no hope.
>   (And treat each other with cautious pleasure.)
>
> "There is no sufficient reason to live.
>   (Why do rainbows fade so fast?
> There is no life,
>   (I just admired its colors and wanted to share
>   its splendor.)
> Only the death that ends the everlasting pain."

GUTHRIE: I'll just ask one question. You came here today and
you read your paper. Are you willing to go on living?

JONES: Absolutely.

GUTHRIE: You have hope?

JONES: I've reconciled it. You know, it's something that transpired quite some time ago, and I've managed to reconcile it all. I think the biggest problem was the fact that I had literally no one to turn to. I lived alone with my daughter. My brother couldn't accept this disease, and I could not speak to him. My mother was not permitted to be made aware of it, so there was literally no one to talk to. I was the one who was handling everything dealing with my father, since there was no one else, and I think that it was just too much for one person to attempt to handle. Unfortunately, there was absolutely nowhere to turn. I didn't know about you then.

GUTHRIE: Can I also assume that your smile and your presence here are because you believe things are going to happen?

JONES: I'm positive that things are going to happen. I don't think that there's hope for my father, but I feel there is tremendous help for other people, and we really don't know how many there are.

GUTHRIE: That's right. If they all could know and go through some of the experiences that you've gone through, if they could turn to help and hope, we could get some answers, couldn't we? Thank you very much for helping.

TESTIMONY OF
FLORENCE BERGER
MAPLEWOOD, NEW JERSEY

BERGER: My name is Florence Berger. My husband has Huntington's disease. His father was diagnosed when our youngest child was 2; therefore, I anticipated and waited and waited for the symptoms to occur. I felt that I saw them in him long, long before anyone else was aware of it.

We went from one neurologist to another because he was having problems dealing psychologically with the fact that his father was put into an institution. The psychologist suggested going to a neurologist to find out whether his problems were physical or psychological so she would know in which direction to go. Every neurologist that we went to told my husband that there was nothing

wrong with him, even though he came with the information that his
father and his father's sister had been definitely diagnosed for
Huntington's disease. I saw things in my husband and the
neurologists said it was my imagination: I was anticipating it;
I was looking for it. It was there, very, very faint, but it was
there. I resented the fact that information was withheld as far
as having children, not for me but for other members of my family.
For me, our children were here, but other members had not yet had
their children and were encouraged by doctors that the risk was
not there.

The rest of my story has basically been told. The one thing
I would very much like to emphasize is that we are now at a point
where my husband is at home and has been at home for 2 years. He
was down at NIH for a time and went back down a few weeks ago to
be involved in a program. I received a phone call from them and
was told that he had to return home because he could not function
without his medication in order to be able to participate in the
programs. They had to be drug-free, and he could not function
without the drugs. This took away hope from him, from us, from
the children. (We have three children, 26, 22, and 18.) There
is no place for him to go at this point. He is certainly not
ready to be put into an institution. We do not want to put him
in an institution.

It is most important at this time, when he can still function,
to keep him physically and mentally alert and active. There are
no places. We do not want to put him in an institution. We want
him at home. We want him to be with us and we want to be with
him. But how can you see this happen to a person and see them lay
in bed from morning until night and not be aware of what's going
on? They keep telling you that they're going crazy for the lack of
something to do, and there's no place to take him and no facilities
for him to go to. If there were only places where he could go for
the day and come home to us at night and be with us. When they're
put in institutions, nothing is done for them. They need the
stimulation of activities. They need the stimulation of people
who understand what is wrong with them. They need the understanding,
and they need the love, the consideration, and the feelings their
families have for them, and for this not to be taken away far too
soon just because they can't stay at home and there's nothing to
do for them at home.

When I had to go to work, I specifically went to seek employment with a physician because I felt that this would put me in a position to have access to much information. Most fortunately, I work for a physician who is a wonderful human being and has been wonderful to me, though he knows nothing about the disease and has not seen any patients with it in his training. He has told me that I know far more than he does, but he is just helping me in other aspects.

If only there were places for people to go and still return to their home. I feel that this is very, very important because I feel that the person that has the disease should not be removed from their family. I feel that it is a very, very important thing, because when you're put into an institution you're just part of a facility. Until this is absolutely necessary, just for the lack of having a proper place for them to go, to put them in this type of facility is very, very cruel and very heartless. And yet what other alternatives do we have? There is nothing.

GUTHRIE: Do you have anyone that comes in during the day while you work?

BERGER: No. My husband's not to the point where he cannot be left alone. He can function.

GUTHRIE: He needs something to do.

BERGER: He needs something to do with his time. He is not to the point where he needs someone to do things for him. He has difficulty shaving; he has difficulty doing certain things. I was out the other day, and my daughter had to go out for a little while. She came back and I said, "Did you make Daddy lunch?" She said, "He said he'd make his own lunch," and she told me what he made. He's very capable of doing things. He is.

GUTHRIE: I think you're emphasizing something very important, that the H.D. patient has maybe years of activity, personal contact, mental capacity beyond what most physicians believe; therefore, we must encourage again the right to live as fully and as well as possible as long as possible.

BERGER: Yes. Also, I feel that as far as the family is concerned, many patients are put into institutions because there is no other alternative, and they are robbed and the patients are robbed of many years of some kind of relationship.

GUTHRIE: Good family living.

BERGER: Yes. There is no reason for a father or a mother to be taken out of the home at the point, for example, that my husband is at. His children love him and he loves them; they want him to be part of their lives, and they want him to participate in everything that they do. They do not shun him and they do not close him out, nor did we do this to his father. It was out of our hands. I wanted to keep his father in our home, but was advised--because at that point I had small children and could not. But we used to take him from the facility every weekend, Saturdays and Sundays, and bring him home to have dinner so that he could have the contact of family.

GUTHRIE: I have one question that goes back to the first thing you said that I find very interesting. Florence, since you are the only one who recognized early symptoms in your husband, have you any idea what you saw or felt or knew that nobody else could recognize?

BERGER: Having a very close relationship with his father--not that much time had elapsed--I saw the same things in him.

GUTHRIE: Like what? How was that? Help us out.

BERGER: Different emotions, speech. They always told me my father-in-law was nervous. I would say personality, interaction, but it was very, very limited at that point. Maybe I was reading into it when it really wasn't there.

GUTHRIE: Maybe you were. That's what we're looking for: What are these early signs? Maybe you were reading something that was there.

BERGER: I saw as much as I wanted to deny; and though we never discussed it, I feel that he felt it also. Something was said before about the unaffected sibling. His brother has never come to see him. I will call him. (I have a very close relationship with his brother's wife.) Part of the reason is his fear of even

dealing with it. He can't deal with it. He asks his wife
questions about himself constantly, if she sees things. He does
not even want to come to our home to see these things in my husband because he is fearful.

GUTHRIE: For himself.

BERGER: For himself at this point, being 5 years younger
than my husband. My husband will be 50 next month.

McKHANN: Thank you very much. I think we will be breaking
now for lunch. I'd just like to make a couple of comments before
we do. The purpose of these hearings is to get ideas and directions that we can take back to our parent committee to work on
or look into. I would just like to mention a few of the things
I've heard that have come out of these discussions this morning,
some of which I don't think we have discussed among ourselves
at all.

I think we knew about the lack of knowledge in the medical
profession and the lack of training, but we certainly have had
that reinforced. I think we knew about how difficult it is to
get information, and we certainly have had that reinforced
considerably.

I feel Dr. April's ideas about the need for model centers,
which are not acute hospitals and are not skilled nursing homes
either, gave us some very clear-cut ideas about how they should
function. I'm just skipping through this to bring out some of
the high points.

I believe we are aware of the high cost of this illness, as
is true of many chronic illnesses. I think the question we have
to address is what mechanisms are there to alleviate that.

Dr. Hirschhorn's genetic ideas: I will just tell you how
we are functioning. We have subcommittees of our panel which are
looking at specific areas, and Dr. Hirschhorn is a member of one
of the two we have in the genetics area. We'll be pursuing these
lines of investigation in greater depth through these subpanels,
if you will.

Father Cassidy brought up a very interesting role for private hospitals, particularly if the Government is going to put its emphasis into acute medical care, and also how an oriented religious group can provide something that perhaps other people just plain can't.

I think another point that has come out is this whole point of day care centers. I believe one of the things that we can do is to look carefully at what the people in the mental retardation area have done and transpose some of their ideas into an older population. Even though the populations are different, the needs are very, very similar.

I think that those are at least some of the points that we have heard, and I am sure that we will hear others; there will be other points that will come up from the other public hearings. I would like to point out that we are getting this little by little, and we'll put it back together.

TESTIMONY OF
PATRICK DUNLEAVY
AMITYVILLE, NEW YORK

DUNLEAVY: My name is Patrick Dunleavy. I would like to
read a letter that was submitted to the Commission by my wife.
She's here, but she would prefer that I read it for her. The
words might be a little out of context as they were written by
my wife.

"I am happy to have an opportunity to present written
testimony to the Federal Commission for the Control of Huntington's Disease.

"Before being diagnosed as a carrier, my personal knowledge
of Huntington's disease was exactly nothing for me and my family
of three brothers and four sisters. My father was the carrier
of the disease, and to the day he died in 1959, at age 75, he
never knew he had it. When he was about 60 years of age, my
mother and all of us saw some nervous movements which we never
really bothered about: It was just Pop's nervous way. He always
had his feet going as well as his head and shoulders, but his
mind was perfect.

"One day coming from work, he fell down the subway stairs.
Luckily he didn't hurt himself. When he arrived home, we called
the doctor, who told us he had hardening of the arteries at the
base of the brain. In another few years his condition worsened,
his mind got very foggy, and he was sent to Pilgrim State Hospital.
He spent a total of 6 years there, was examined many times by
various doctors during that time. He died quietly in his sleep
in 1959, and never in all those 6 long years was H.D. ever mentioned
by the hospital staff.

"When we went to Dr. John Whittier at Creedmoor Hospital for
family examinations, he collected our family tree. He also obtained information from Pilgrim State Hospital about my father's
confinement there, and not one word about H.D. No one had any
knowledge of the disease. Can you believe this at such a large
hospital? They had an honest excuse: They never 'heard' of the

disease. How dreadful that was, but it was a fact. They didn't know. Poor Pop. If he only knew the legacy he left us, his eight children.

"Up to 1968 we never knew we were H.D. carriers and we, as a family, grew, married, and had our own families. However, one sister, Betty, the most beautiful-looking girl in the family, stayed single. She had a very good job in the personnel department of the New York Times. She was a very smart dresser and just had it all together. She had to voluntarily leave the job because she was not able to handle it when things got busy. She obtained other less demanding jobs, but they didn't work out either.

"She went to Dr. Francis Gagliardi in Jamaica, a psychiatrist, who diagnosed her condition as nerves. In the meantime, Betty was slowly deteriorating in front of our eyes, and the sad part is that she was aware of what was happening to her. Her last job was at a local library, and she was asked to leave because she was thought to be an alcoholic. Oh, how embarrassing and cruel, because she never even drank. It was humiliating and crushing, and that was the last job Betty had.

"She kept going to Dr. Gagliardi, as she developed fits of crying all the time. It was a miserable sight for the whole family. Since there was no help available to her, she felt like some kind of freak, and I don't blame her. The doctor suggested going to Kew Gardens Hospital for a series of tests over a 2-week period, which included shock treatments. They found nothing mentally wrong. Then he mentioned H.D. to my mother for the first time, and she said, 'What's that?' He delved into my father's background and said it was H.D. He told her it was genetic, and she froze, sick and unbelieving. She had watched one of her children change from a beautiful girl right before her eyes, and the thought of the ugly disease hitting the family was devastating.

"My mother decided to share it with everyone in the family but me: First, I am the youngest; and second, I have six children. My sister Betty was given medicines and sleeping pills to help quiet her, and she was able to cope so much better. It was the years wasted in not knowing what she had that really wrecked her. She knew now it was not her fault and could accept it. She is still at home with my mother and two sisters who care for her and love her.

"As my own children grew we would visit Grandma's house, and they were always shocked by Betty's physical condition. In all honesty, I told them it was just nerves. I thought her actions were very much like Pop's at times, but I never put them together. Then about 3 years ago they told me that Betty had H.D., and I said, 'What's that?' I decided to keep it from the children for a year, thinking they might better be able to accept it then. I just decided it was a bad dream and that it would all go away. My husband wanted me to tell them so badly because we were always a sharing family. Finally one night I shared it with them at the kitchen table. We all cried together, were scared together, and were angry together that such a thing could happen.

"In checking into what help was available, I discovered that Creedmoor State Hospital had a testing program. We all participated in the test over a period of 3 weeks. Results: I have it; my oldest brother, age 62, has it; and the other five are still at risk. The whole experience was devastating for each of us and our families.

"I am 48 years old, wife, and mother of six children. In June 1975, I was diagnosed as having H.D. It was a very bitter moment, not for me, really, but for my children. Here I am, happily married and my children almost grown (Anne, age 24; Dorothy, age 22; Theresa, age 20; Mary, age 18; Christine, age 17; and Patrick, age 15), all very healthy and happy; just a warm, beautiful family. We always had fun together. Our kitchen table was our place to share our laughs, our tears, and our talks, but mostly the laughs. The night before I decided to take the tests at Creedmoor, I had everyone sit at the kitchen table and I pre-pared them for the worst. Then a week later I had to tell them with tears in my eyes that I had H.D. I explained that it was genetic and hereditary and that they had a 50-50 chance of also having the disease. I also had to tell them there is no cure for the disease, and I felt so helpless. I cried for them and they cried for me and my husband cried as well.

"I decided that as long as there was no hope for me, there must be something I can do for my children. I went very often to Dr. John Whittier at Creedmoor Hospital, a very beautiful person, and participated in a number of tests, mainly digital dexterity, blood tests and some skin grafts. I felt quietly thankful because it was the only thing I could do and it filled me with hope. Then it stopped: Creedmoor testing program was abolished. We were told it was due to lack of funds. With this went my hope.

"I have always had a deep faith in God, and am able to accept my cross, but I am very angry for my children, angry that there are so few people in this beautiful country of ours who care about me or my children and other H.D. victims. Please help us now, because soon I, too, will be staggering and falling and people will think I am an alcoholic because no one knows. So I want to shout it from the rooftops: 'Please find some help for my children. They must be healthy.'

"I am willing to testify at the local hearings in New York on September 22 if you feel it will help."

GUTHRIE: Can I just comment (because I think it's important for the record) that Dr. Whittier's program, although it has been so-called terminated, is being moved, and that the big problem now is not only to help in the move, but to see to it that his program may continue with the staff that he had and will need in the new facility. This is something that we have learned about, we're very concerned about, and it is our hope that we will be able to see to it that those of you who have used his facility will have that opportunity again, just as soon as he gets settled, which will be at the end of this month, hopefully.

DUNLEAVY: Do you know where it will be?

GUTHRIE: Yes. It will be at Leary Long Island Research Institute at Stonybrook. The problem is that it is so far away. The other thing is that I have spoken to him very recently, and the problem is getting the staff he will require in order to carry on the work that he has done. He does require a certain number of personnel, which at this moment is not available because his is one of several divisions at Stonybrook. All of us in this community will have to make an effort to see that he has the opportunity to continue. Because of that, I'd like to then ask the next question, if I may. I assume, from what I've heard from your testimony, that he has been helpful, that he has given you hope, and that his center is of importance to people like you.

DUNLEAVY: Absolutely so. Yes.

GUTHRIE: And you would like to see that others have that opportunity as well?

DUNLEAVY: I definitely would, because we feel that knowing it is not the greatest news in the world to get. At least you have a place where you can get a definite answer, yes or no. The fact that he is participating in certain tests, I think this is also encouraging in gathering data that may find some successful answers to the problem.

GUTHRIE: Does it mean more to you personally to know that there is a place that is specifically called a "center" for this kind of disease? Does it help you, rather than just going to a hospital?

DUNLEAVY: I'm the father of these six children who are all at risk, and I would like to know that they can go to some place when the symptoms start showing and be helped and maybe help others who might get the thing in the future.

GUTHRIE: So that the word, a specific "center" for this disease, is important to you?

DUNLEAVY: Very much so.

GUTHRIE: Not just any old place where somebody might know something about the disease.

DUNLEAVY: Right. And also the fact that I'd like to know that there is a lot of money being spent towards developing a cure, which I hope is the end result of the study and the findings of this Commission.

GUTHRIE: Yes. Will you thank your wife for all of us?

DUNLEAVY: Yes, I certainly will. Thank you.

TESTIMONY OF
ABRAHAM N. LIEBERMAN, M.D.
ASSOCIATE PROFESSOR OF NEUROLOGY
NEW YORK UNIVERSITY SCHOOL OF MEDICINE

LIEBERMAN: I'm Dr. Abraham Lieberman. I'm a 1963 graduate of
the New York University School of Medicine. I completed a neurology
residency at the New York University School of Medicine. I served
for 2 years in the armed forces in Japan, and upon completion of
my tour of duty I spent another year doing pharmacology. Since
1970 I have been on the staff of the New York University School of
Medicine, where I am now an associate professor of neurology. My
major fields of interest are diseases of the basal ganglia, the
most prominent of which are Parkinson's disease and Huntington's
disease. I have written several papers and have some 40 publications on Parkinson's disease and this area.

My interest in Huntington's disease goes back to 1970, when
I had just completed my training in pharmacology. At this time (as
now) I was working with a Dr. Leonard Goldstein, who is a professor
of neurochemistry at N.Y.U. He, with Dr. Julius Axelrod of the
National Institutes of Health, had independently developed a blood
test serum which at that time we thought might enable us to predict
who had the disease and who did not. At that time my knowledge
of Huntington's disease was that of any neurologist in a residency
program: You're apt to see several people with the disease
briefly, don't really meet their family members, and you see them
for a brief period of time and come to the conclusion that it is a
terrible and awful disease and are very happy when they're sort of
shunted off to the back wards of the hospital and they don't have
to bother you any more, because there's nothing you can do for them,
there's nothing you can say to their family members, and you're
just very happy when you don't see them any more.

At that time I had no particular expertise in the field, and
we thought that it would be relatively easy to find some people
with the disease and come to a determination as to whether this
blood test was useful or not. The first problem that came about
was to find people with Huntington's disease. Almost every large
medical center will have one or two patients with the disease, but
to find large numbers of people in various stages of the disease
is very difficult. We began by calling various people we knew in
state hospitals; there were three people in one hospital, four

people in another hospital, and five people somewhere else. At that time we ran around to various hospitals and we'd find a few people with the disease and draw blood specimens on them.

The Committee to Combat Huntington's Disease (which we really didn't know about but found out about through one of the patient's families) was a very great help to us because they were able to put us in touch with families that had the disease who were then able to tell us where we could go to find other people with the disease. They were also a great help because we wanted to see people who had a large spectrum of the disease, people in the early stages as well as the late stages. People in the early stages of the disease are usually at home and usually don't leave the home. Unless you know someone who can approach them for you, it's very hard to meet these people because they are reluctant to talk about the disease and they don't want just any doctor coming by and talking to them out of idle curiosity, so we found this to be very helpful.

We also encountered a number of problems that we never would have realized if we were not actually involved in taking care of people with the disease. We thought we had a test at the time that would enable us to predict who had the disease and who did not at a very early stage. One of the things we found out was that there were a number of people with the disease who wanted to know if they had the disease, but there were a number of people who didn't want to know if they were at risk, if they had the disease. I think a lot of people don't want to know that they have or that they're going to develop an incurable disease.

The problems of this are problems that you cannot appreciate unless you are intimately involved with this disease. When it became apparent to us that this blood test really was not specific for predicting the disease, it was very hard to shake yourself loose from the disease, because one of the things you realized was that a great deal was known about the disease descriptively-- there were beautiful descriptions about the disease--it was fairly easy to diagnose if you had an appropriate family history, but there was really nothing of substance that could be done for this disease.

One of the major problems is that this is a disease of the brain itself, and it's very hard to get an idea of the biochemistry

of the disease because you just can't take a fiew pieces of brain
tissue from living people. It's not a disease where there are
obvious abnormalities in the blood or in the liver, where at various stages of the disease you can take sample pieces of tissue and
get an idea of what's going on. You just can't take a piece of
brain from a living person, and you can't do it serially, so this
is an enormously difficult disease to study.

Pathologically, you could tell where there was more involvement with a certain area of the brain than with certain other areas
of the brain, but basic biochemistry of these areas was very difficult to evaluate. One of the problems was that in order to make a
biochemical determination of the brain tissue, it has to come in a
fresh state. Most of the patients with the disease are very eager
to be helpful, and this was never a problem. It was never a
question that a person who had the disease was reluctant to
participate. It was always a question that a person who had the
disease died (he usually died in a state hospital), and by the
time interested people at major medical centers were notified of
it, there had already been changes in the brain which really made
precise biochemical analysis just not accurate. This is really a
major problem. It has been one of the things that I think is
really hindering us from understanding what is going on inside
the brain.

As I say, once we'd gotten involved, we really then couldn't
get away from people who had the disease. We thought that we would
like to see some drug that we had available that could be useful in
treating people with this disease, and then we ran into a whole
other set of problems. To use drugs you have to be able to follow
people on a daily or a weekly basis. You can't just take a sample
of tissue or blood specimen or urine specimen and then just go off
to your laboratory and run a test. You have to give the medication to a patient and you have to examine them at frequent intervals, and it's a much more complicated problem. The problem was
that the patients who had the disease were usually in state hospitals or chronic care facilities, and the people that had the drugs
and the ideas and the interest were usually at major medical centers
and were far removed from the people with the decision. It is not
practical to go every day or every week to a state hospital to
see how a trial is going, and to do it on an outpatient basis
created its own set of problems.

There were patients who were willing to come to the New York University School of Medicine, but many of them had difficulty moving, difficulty getting around, and it became a major problem for the family to bring them to a medical center on a daily or weekly basis. Aside from the fact that there were no charges for services rendered--there were no charges for the tests--it involved transporting patients; it involved making arrangements to have someone stay with children. It was a major task for family members.

The people who had the least involvement, who had the disease but were mobile, these were people you didn't necessarily want to treat. The population that you wanted to treat was in state hospitals, where it was not feasible to treat them because you were not going to supervise them on a daily basis. The people who were outpatients and needed treatment could not readily come to the medical center, and the people who could come were those who needed the treatment the least. This has been something that has really prevented us from developing a fairly good means of utilizing the drugs that we have to the best purpose.

For 2 years I was on the staff of the Manhattan Veterans' Administration Hospital, which is directly connected with the N.Y.U. Medical Center and is on the same campus (it's on 23rd Street, and the Medical Center extends from 23rd Street to 32nd Street). The most useful experience for us and the patients came about when we were able to take some patients out of the chronic care facility and admit them to the VA hospital and treat them. This was possible only for those patients who had already been veterans. I must say this, that the one thing that was of great comfort to many people was the Veterans' Administration Hospital. Many family members who are unaffected and know that a father or a son or an uncle has the disease become desperate as to what they're ultimately going to do because the patient, particularly towards the later stages of the disease, becomes just about impossible to manage in a home situation: The movements become very violent; they are constantly falling; they are constantly having difficulty with feeding and swallowing, and they are difficult for trained personnel to take care of, much less family members. Inevitably, what happens is people start looking for chronic care facilities, and they generally are not available to them; or if

they are, at really exorbitant costs: $500 a week to take care of
a patient is really beyond the means of 99 percent of the American
population.

   The VA hospitals are one of the best interests to us,
particularly because they provide long-term care. It was a great
comfort to the patients and the families to know that ultimately,
when worse came to worst, there was a place where the patient
could go, where the patient would be treated humanely under
reasonable conditions.

   Since 1972 I have not really been directly involved in
Huntington's disease. My interests have led elsewhere. But I
think that over a 4-year period of time I developed certain ideas
and perspectives on the disease and what I think would be most
helpful. I think there were two basic things:

   1. Support of basic research to do one of two things: to
develop a test which will be 100 percent reliable in predicting
who is at risk for developing this disease. There is some evidence
that we may be very close to such a test. A test like this would
have to be such that the person who has the test performed on
them does not necessarily have to know the results. To some
people this would be a staggering, crushing thing to know, that
within 10 years they would develop Huntington's disease and die
of this. It would have to be of such a nature that the affected
person would not have to know the results. And, too, it would have
to be something that could be done through amniocentesis so that
through the infant, the embryo, one could predict for a woman who
was at risk if her child was or was not going to develop the
disease.

   This might be an answer to the disease, since it is a
genetically determined disease. It could be determined who could
develop the disease, and taking appropriate measures after that
might lead to a virtual absence of the disease. But this would
not be something that would come about for two or three generations.
We would still have the major problem of the people who have the
disease now, of children who are going to develop the disease, and
a large population of people who are going to be at risk with the
disease, certainly, for the next 50, 60, or 70 years. Even if
tomorrow we develop a 100-percent safe way of predicting who was
going to have the disease and take measures to prevent those

fetuses at risk from developing the disease, we would still be left with a large group of people who are going to develop the disease, and we still have a large responsibility to this group of people.

GUTHRIE: Excuse me. May I interrupt for a minute and remind you that you've left out a group of people who do not know that this disease is in their family, so we can't just wipe it out by having amniocentesis.

LIEBERMAN: No question. In this area there is some very exciting research with neurotransmitter agents, but this is really an elementary level and is certainly several years away from leading to positive, practical steps that can be taken to help victims of the disease. It's getting there, but it has to be encouraged. It's not something that is going to lead to a cure of the disease tomorrow. Working in this area is a tedious proposition, and it's a very difficult area to work in, so one is the area of basic research.

What practical steps might be taken that would be useful to medical people who are involved with the disease, to help them bring the studies in the laboratory closer to practical application? I think one thing would be regional centers for the disease. I say "regional" because it's a large country, and it's just not practical to have one center in Washington, D.C. or New York and have people who have the disease in the State of Washington fly out once a month to visit their relatives, so I think one would have to be regional centers. This does not mean you have to put up new facilities. There are several large Veterans' hospitals and existing facilities that could serve this function, but I think one would be regional centers for the disease. These centers should be in close proximity to major medical centers where there are scientists with basic laboratories who are doing research in the field. The centers would provide blood specimens, urine specimens, and brain specimens for people who work--when I say, "provide brain specimens," anyone who has the disease knows that this is not something that anyone says lightly, and they fully understand these implications, so this would bring the laboratory close to the people with the disease.

Regional centers, too, would provide a place where people who have questions about the disease, where people who think they

are at risk with the disease, where they have family members at
risk with the disease can come and receive the best knowledge of
the disease, so they don't have to hunt around and go running to
different doctors who finally send them to somebody who knows
somebody who knows somebody who has seen three or four cases of
the disease, and they can come to a place where there are people
well trained in the disease. This would also encourage other
physicians to know more about the disease. Frankly, I think if
they heard the testimony of many of these people (why don't their
physicians know how to diagnose or recognize the disease and know
very little about the disease except what they've been taught in
medical school several years ago), it would encourage physicians
to actively work in the disease; it would encourage medical
students and residents to see people firsthand with the disease,
to talk to their family members, and to really stimulate them to
go into the field.

My interest in the disease came about because I happened to
see some people and I was interested in blood tests. If the blood
tests hadn't come along and one person with the disease did not
happen to be in the hospital and happen to have abnormally high
blood tests, I never would have gotten interested in the disease.
There are just too many other things going on in medicine for you
to focus in on this disease.

I think providing centers like this would train neurologists,
medical students, and physicians to know more about the disease,
make them spot the disease and hopefully spot a few people with
bright minds to go into the field and make a major contribution
to the disease. I think that centers like this where people who
have the disease can ultimately go will take a great burden off
many families, because many of the families will keep family
members as long as they possibly can until it is just impossible
to take care of them because the movements are too severe, be-
because they can't swallow, because they just can't handle the
temper tantrums and the outbursts. I think also the family knows,
"Gee, if worse comes to worst, I can at least go to this place
and I'll be helped, where they'll take care of my father or my
mother or my brother," et cetera. This would take an enormous
burden off many family members.

I think that once you have a population of people with Huntington's disease in various stages at a few medical centers, this will encourage other people who have drugs or techniques to go to these places and say, "Look, we've got this drug and we think it works. Let's try it over here." You'll never find a more willing group of patients because you'll tell them, "I've got something that may work. There's one chance in a thousand. Got terrible side effects, but it may work." Everybody participates. There's no question. "Anything, because if it's not for me, maybe it's for my kids." I've never found a group of people who, when they could, would be more willing to participate. I think that's about the essence of what I wanted to say.

McKHANN: Let me ask you to stick around for just a moment, would you? Dr. Yahr has a 2 o'clock appointment, and I have a couple of questions I want to ask you.

TESTIMONY OF
MELVIN YAHR, M.D.
MT. SINAI HOSPITAL

YAHR: I am Melvin Yahr. I am from Mt. Sinai Hospital and I am Chairman of the Department of Neurology and Director of the Center for Parkinson's and Allied Diseases, which includes Huntington's.

I have not prepared a formal statement, and I am delighted to have had the opportunity of hearing Dr. Lieberman, since he has pretty well spelled out the problems relative to caring for patients in this community, some of the research directions that we would like to develop, as well as the center concept for the diagnosis and treatment. I would be delighted to answer any questions you may have.

McKHANN: I was wondering, Mel, if you would comment from your own perspective, since there has been a fair amount of publicity about it, on the current state of the idea of data and other transmitters being either specifically or secondarily involved in this process, and whether you see this as a promising line of therapeutic virtue?

LIEBERMAN: I think that there is enough confirmatory evidence that this is a reality as to a defect in the nervous system. I

suspect that we have not fully resolved whether it's primary or
secondary, though it looks like it's primary. But it does give
us a handle on the way to look in a definitive way at a very
important neurotransmitter system that has a functional aspect
in relation to the fact that it is regionally distributed in the
nervous system. That has a lot of importance, I think. If one
looks at the Parkinson's story and its eventual therapy, it had
something like the same kind of beginning, so it may be a
beginning that has a great deal of importance.

GUTHRIE: I'd like to ask Dr. Yahr, in your concept of a
center I assume that you would like to be seeing more than just
an H.D. patient because of the value of the relationships of
these various neurological disorders to each other?

YAHR: Yes. I think, Marjorie, that's a very good idea, and
I'd like to expand a little bit about it. I think the problems
of Huntington's disease, as we know it today, are intimately related to what we know about the nervous system in general, and the
only way we're going to advance our understanding of Huntington's
is to advance our understanding of the brain. I think any center
that restricts itself and becomes just disease-oriented does
itself and the public a disservice because, first, you can't
attract scientists that limit their perspectives and their hori-
zons in their investigation; and secondly, you can't even attract
good clinical scientists to do the same. They want to be able to
have a more comprehensive involvement with neurological disease,
even though they may emphasize a single disease.

For a long time, when we organized our Parkinson's program,
we used that kind of a concept in attracting scientists. We
weren't attracting scientists to work in Parkinson's disease. We
were attracting scientists to work in mechanisms, in causation,
in pathogenesis, the etiology of diseases of the nervous system
as they related to basic motor dysfunction, to sensory dysfunctions,
to the cognitive functions of the brain, all of its functions, with
the emphasis that some were part and parcel of the disease
process. I like the center concept that brings in close contact
people who are doing investigative work in the nervous system. It
becomes disease-oriented as you gain more information. I like the
center concept that brings the basic scientist and the clinician
closer together so that the clinician can spell out for the basic

scientist some of the clinical problems, and the clinician can translate the new information that the basic scientist develops in a clinical utility. I think that kind of center--what you call it makes no difference--what it actually does and what its work is should not be restricted or limited and only oriented to one disease.

GUTHRIE: I think it's a problem that we face, and that's why I asked the question of many of the H.D. families who feel that they want an H.D. center.

YAHR: I can well understand why they want it. I think if one begins to talk to some families, people that have H.D., and begins to tell them how you need genetic input, how you need biochemical input, how you need the input of psychologists, how you need the input of people who understand how motor mechanisms work, what these abnormal movements are, it requires a great deal of expertise and talent from a variety of fields. What you may learn in one field may have great influence in Huntington's disease even though it may not seem that way when you first start out studying it. I think that we need a larger conceptualization of what a center is. You could call it a "Huntington's Disease Center," but its work has to be a basic mechanism in the nervous system.

McKHANN: Mel, let me ask you a question that is one of logistics. This is a commission on Huntington's disease and related conditions. There's been a previous commission on epilepsy that's in progress; there's been a previous commission on multiple sclerosis. My guess is there's going to be a few more before we're through. All of these commissions are going to come up, I think, in part with variations of this center concept. What are your thoughts about this in terms of how they should be implemented? My concern is that they're going to get parcelled out as disease entities and not turn out the way you're describing.

YAHR: I think you may be right, Guy. I think I would say this, first, about the commissions in general. I think the commissions have done a great service, at least the one on multiple sclerosis (and the volume is about that thick; I've read through it, I must admit, not in enormous detail). I would share your apprehension if what eventually happens as a result of the Commission is that we segmented neurology into experts in these little fields. First of all, we don't have the manpower to even begin

to do that, and we couldn't even if we wanted to. Secondly, you
would have a number of individuals who would only be like the
blind man feeling one side of the elephant and never knowing what
the elephant is like until they get the whole perspective: They're
not going to know what the whole brain is like, and if you don't,
you're not going to make much progress. I would share your apprehension. If what occurred was that we ended up with centers
directed for various specific diseases and only for that, I don't
think we would do the public very much of a service in finding a
cause and cure for the disease.

I think that the center concept can be utilized as an
umbrella for various things. There may be very little difference,
for example, in the kinds of folks working in my laboratory in
Mt. Sinai here, in the work we're doing relative to Parkinson's
disease, or dystonia, or even some aspects of multiple sclerosis
in terms of the nervous system, and what you might want to do for
Huntington's chorea. It would be better to have an all-inclusive
group working in this area, at least from the investigative standpoint, than specializing it out to Huntington's disease. I would
hope that what the commissions could do in regard to the specific
disease process is to increase the clinical resources within the
community for caring for patients. Dr. Lieberman mentioned this,
and I would agree 100 percent with him.

We don't have at our fingertips and available for the patient
genetic counseling, appropriate psychological testing, the long-
term care facility, the availability of specimens from the patient
that he himself might want to give. We've had Huntington's
patients tell us, "Look, I believe in the idea that when I die I
want to give my nerves, my spinal cord, and my brain, just like
people will do for an eye bank or a kidney bank," and then we
don't have a facility in this community to house such an individual
so that we can retrieve these kinds of biological specimens in the
shape and form that we could best use them. Even though these
people are committed (they believe in it and we want to honor
their wishes after they die), we can't get these specimens to do
the best kind of research with. Within our community no facilities
exist of the kind of supportive things for patient care and for
supporting the research effort with human material.

N. WEXLER: Regarding human material, I know you've had some
experience with tissue banks. I wonder if you could just comment

on your opinion of the necessity for such banks and any problems
or recommendations that you would have to this Commission regarding the tissue bank?

YAHR: Yes. I think you and I talked about this, and I want
to take this occasion to publicly thank you for having secured
some specimens and having them sent from California for me. They
were specimens that I had been trying to get for about a year and
a half. As a result of our meetings and your intervention they
arrived in a week and are now on hand. I want to thank you.

N. WEXLER: Thank you for that. I really wanted to get the
necessity for the bank on record.

YAHR: Some years ago (I guess about 15 or so, perhaps longer),
when the Parkinson's program started, one of the needs that we had
was for Parkinson's brains, to study their biochemistry. The
head of the Parkinson's Disease Foundation, Mr. William Black,
came to me one day and said, "Why don't you have a brain bank?"
Someone standing there said, "Well, a bank is something you can
make deposits in and then take something out. Now this would be
a bank where you only put the brains in, but you won't be able
to get any brains back, and they'll be for the scientists." We
did start the brain bank at that time and we made it a resource
not only for our own use, but for the use of any other scientist
who had a reasonable investigative program for working in the
field. We collected the material at various states, both the
fresh state and fixed state.

I'm not certain that I can give you any directions in how
you regionalize this, but communities could have banking facilities, if you will. Banking facilities usually consist of deep-
freeze equipment as well as the resource to obtain the specimen in
its proper state. The way we did this was to contract, in a sense,
with various people, pathologists who knew brains, and also have
our own team available that would go any hours of the night or
day, because you have to get these specimens within 2 or 3 hours
of death to make them worthwhile. We have the deep-freezing
equipment and all the kinds of safeguards you need with deep-
freeze equipment should the power supplies fail or electrical
shortages occur, et cetera. I maintained it at Columbia for about
10 years, and since I've been at Mt. Sinai we've reproduced the

facility and supported it out of our own resources so that we
have available now for study material that we feel is very
critical for advancing our information about these diseases. But
we do have trouble. I reiterate what Dr. Lieberman said. We have
trouble in this community getting Huntington's brains in people
that expire, except if you happen to have your facility next to
a Veterans' hospital or somewhere near the nursing home facility
where you can make these arrangements. Am I answering your
question?

N. WEXLER: It seems like that would be a huge expenditure
for each institution to support. If the Government were to back
that kind of endeavor---

YAHR: I don't think you need this at each institution. I
think there ought to be a centralized facility that could bank
this material, and you could just as easily bank it for Huntington's disease, multiple sclerosis, vascular disease, and any other
disease of the brain. You could have one centralized facility.
I think the importance of establishing that kind of facility is to
get a commitment from the people who do it to make it available
to the appropriate investigators when they have a reasonable program that they want to pursue. I think these are the kinds of
implements you need, but I don't think you have to duplicate this
in 10 different places. I don't think everybody needs their own
repository of this material. I think one centralized facility
within a delineated geographic area is about what you have to do.
Don't forget, you don't only have to retrieve the specimens,
these specimens are worthless if you don't retrieve appropriate
clinical information so you actually know what the disease was,
in what phase of the disease the patients were, what drugs they
took, and a whole host of other carriers of clinical data.

N. WEXLER: If the patient dies in some back ward or some
nursing home, you don't have access to that material, do you?

YAHR: You may not, though we have on occasion developed
relationships with such facilities and have had access to their
records and developed our relationships to the point that we
would know the drugs that were given, when they were given, within
reasonable limits: fairly good information.

N. WEXLER: Thank you.

McKHANN: Thank you very much. I wanted to get your comments on a point that comes up in terms of the question of testing the potential of the patient at risk. We've talked about the idea of amniocentesis and the aspect of information to the patient. There's one issue that hasn't come up. I'd be interested in your comments about it; that is, it is conceivable in approaches to therapy that it would be important to be able to detect the disease early. I wonder if you see that use for such a test. That might not only be a test that could detect a patient's potential to get the disease but also conceivably, if it were not based solely on the genetic defect, relate to a degree of activity of the disease.

LIEBERMAN: Of course, it would be valuable to detect, before certain changes take place in the nervous system, a person with the disease at a very early stage. I think one problem with Huntington's disease is that if you examine the brain of a person with Parkinson's disease, from which we're reasoning by analogy, that brain looks relatively normal, except for some changes in one small area of the brain, the substantia nigra. The brain of the patient with Huntington's disease shows marked structural changes: It is smaller in weight, the ventricles are enlarged, there is a decrease in cerebral substance in the frontal and parietal regions, and there is a marked shrinkage of the caudate nucleus and other structures in the basal ganglia. In many ways, by the time you're seeing a symptomatic patient with Huntington's disease, you're seeing a patient in whom major structural alterations have taken place in the nervous system.

I think at our present state of knowledge no one thinks that with a drug we're going to replace a volume of brain tissue. Parkinson's disease has lent itself to treatment because there is a tremendous amount of disability and it is correlated with very little in the way of structural change. I think if you're going to develop effective drugs for the disease, you would have to develop these drugs at a point where the disease really did not become evident, because probably by the time it became evident so many structural changes had taken place that there is very little you can do, except maybe slow down the progression; of course, this would be of great value. The problem is developing such a test. In any event, it's one of the reasons you asked about GABA. Again, there are many aspects of Huntington's disease that are sort of

the mirror image of Parkinson's disease, but that analogy should
really not be carried too far because they are distinct diseases
with distinct differences. It may be that these differences are
more important than their similarities.

    McKHANN: Thank you very much. We're going to move along
now. I would like to mention something to the people who are going
to be appearing before us the rest of the afternoon. From our
point of view, the major point of these public hearings is to get
an idea of the range of problems; but more important, the potential solutions. I bring that out because we've heard a number of
the problems that exist, and I think we have to get solutions, or
someone's idea of solutions to the problems, in proper context.
We don't need to keep hearing the same problems all over again
because I think we've heard a pretty good spectrum. I think if
people can keep that in mind, we can focus down on part of the
testimony that will be most helpful to us.

TESTIMONY OF
STEPHEN KEMPSTER, M.D.
NEW YORK, NEW YORK

    KEMPSTER: I am a psychiatrist with a private practice. I
originally submitted a report on Huntington's which was kind of
rambling. I spoke to Dr. Reuben, or he spoke to me, and he
emphasized what you just emphasized: that we all have our very
painful soap operas of our contact with this disease.

    In any event, I got involved with this 25 years ago. A
young man was leaving his family and had at the age of 23 many
of the usual problems that young men have: the separation. He
was a little bit timid in respect to women; he also wanted to
make contact with them. It seemed like a fairly ordinary psychiatric problem. Then as I listened to him, I discovered that his
mother had had Huntington's disease and apparently had developed
it about the time of his adolescence.

    Over time he resolved to a good extent those psychiatric
problems that I've addressed myself to. Then he finally met a
woman and wanted to get married. He brought her in and I emphasized the importance of their having some kind of neurological
evaluation on him--he must have been 26 at the time--and somewhere
along the line it didn't happen. He saw a cousin who was an

internist who, in turn, reassured him but did not pass him on to someone with expertise in neurology. I didn't discover that until some time later. Maybe this is part of what we're talking about when we discuss Huntington's: there are all kinds of flukey things that go on. Why this cousin didn't refer him to an expert neurologist is almost characteristic, I think, of the disease. It stirs up all kinds of strange things, professionals in the noninvolved families, in the involved families; all sorts of things that shouldn't happen, happen. Anyway, over a period of time he developed overt Huntington's.

Meanwhile, I became aware that he had a sister who had married without revealing her at-risk state, nor had her father or anyone else. His earliest symptoms were more of the dystonic Parkinson's line, that sort of thing. Her earlier symptoms tended to be more in terms of the kind of growing reclusiveness, paranoia, ineffectiveness, et cetera. In respect to this family-- I won't spend too much time on it, but I think it's probably not unrelated to a lot of what has been talked about. Eventually, the two siblings developed the disease and they had to be hospitalized. Their spouses divorced, got married, and tried to put together a family where there were five children at risk.

At that point I became very humbled by the situation. I guess those who are familiar with Huntington's are aware that it's really a very singularly catastrophic kind of disease. All diseases, like cancer, et cetera, are catastrophic, but here's one where you sit on it for 30 years, or whatever. Very often children are not apprised, so there is a lot of mystification in the family; they don't know what's going on. On the other hand, let me say, at what point should they be demystified? I don't think that we really have studied that enough to know what the hell to do. Sixteen? Fifteen? Fourteen?

One of the issues, I think, is the ability to diagnose very early the person who is not only at risk but is predictably going to develop Huntington's. Then we create another problem: How do we use the information? I think that these families are in dire need of enormous counseling (genetic, psychiatric), but it should be something that is really worked at. It's probably that kind of thing that will take at least two, three generations to work out. (I put down two; Dr. Lieberman said three generations. I'll go along with him.) I spoke to Dr. Whittier over the weekend and I said, "Well, one of my thoughts was to call it a catastrophic illness." He said, "Every illness is a catastrophic illness." I've been thinking about what would be a good word, and I haven't really quite come to a conclusion about it. There are many very terrible things that happen to people. In hereditary diseases people grow up normally, get married, have children, and then maybe in their twenties or thirties they begin to deteriorate and it's all downhill. In looking over the literature on what we're doing in the way of treatment, at best the measures that they have are palliative but really do not change the thrust of the progression.

As a psychiatrist I have been involved in family therapy, and I am very much aware of the extent to which the family is impaired. There's a terrible spillout: not only the immediate kin but extended kin get involved in this. Nobody knows what to do. Everybody feels helpless. Everybody is helpless. There are all kinds of things that are impinging on the families of these people (those who are affected, those who are not biologically affected) that are generating, I think, their own kind of calamities. This particular family that I've been dealing with is in what might be called a state of reprieve because the oldest child is 25.

McKHANN: We're going to have to move along. I was just wondering, from the point of view of a psychiatrist, if you have a specific suggestion?

KEMPSTER: I do. You've cut me short, which is all right. Being a midwesterner, I don't talk quite as fast as I should. I don't think I think that much more slowly. But my thought is that these people, these families ought to be offered really substantial and sophisticated psychiatric and genetic counseling, because at the present time it is my guess (and that of other people) that many of these people are not even located. They don't come out of the closet. I think that just in straight economic terms, let alone the humanity involved, there are probably, let's say, 10 undiagnosed Huntington's people who are considered schizophrenics, or whatever, and the social cost is enormous. If the families at this point are in that terrible position, that if they reveal what they are about and nothing comes back, they simply endanger themselves. If they don't reveal it, then they walk around and become suspicious and paranoid, and what have you. Meanwhile the scientists don't know that much.

My guess is that the beginning point is to make this kind of offer. We could establish some kind of special definition of this disease. It would be possible for you to get certain kinds of special help and more people would then be prepared to expose themselves. But there is a danger, because the simple exposure is, "All right, you are told of the disease, and you might have the disease that might lead to your death at the age of 39, and you deteriorate and you have to be hospitalized." How do you help people cope with that? I think we have to offer something, and it would have to be something substantial to enable them to cope with it; otherwise they get caught up in a kind of denial and secretiveness which is psychopathological in its effect. I'm not knocking basic research. I think that's very important to the extent it could be implemented if a here-and-now service were provided. In other words, instead of waiting around for people with a particular interest in doing this kind of neurological or pathological research, if you had five times as many people who were also getting something that was immediately useful, it would become more probable that the basic genetic issues, neuropathological issues, would be better attended to. In other words, in terms of phasing it, I would say you start it, and I think once you get it moving the other things will much more readily happen.

McKHANN: I think we're going to have to move along. Thank you very much.

TESTIMONY OF
LYNNETTE ROSSER
GENETIC COUNSELING CENTER
CHILDREN'S HOSPITAL

ROSSER: I am Lynnette Rosser, here today from Children's Hospital in Pittsburgh as a clinical social worker in the Genetic Counseling Center who has been an interested CCHD member for several years. I appreciate the opportunity to provide testimony from this vantage point and do so respecting the contributions of family members heard this morning, and feel almost as though there's a need to apologize as there's no way to match the eloquence and towering truth of their words.

Since Huntington's disease appears for most people in middle life, I have sometimes encountered a puzzled look in the question, "But Huntington's disease isn't a children's disease, is it?" I

would like to focus my remarks briefly on this notion of Huntington's disease as it relates to children, in the broadest sense of
the word. From the child's point of view, H.D. may first affect
him by way of presence in the home of a grandparent with H.D. The
greater assault to a child's world comes later if a parent develops
H.D. One family may develop and find the resources to deal with
the physical and emotional changes and share, as Mr. Dunleavy
described, the pain and the tears and the anger with the children.
Another family may find that its members withdraw into silence and
pain and a loss of support instead. In still other families there
may be severe disruption as families splinter apart, and children
in these families are often encountered in foster homes and in
adoptive homes and are of concern to us in genetic counseling
centers.

     The ability of a family to not only survive but also to
provide good nurturing for each other and for their children
depends upon responsive, coordinated services available to them
in crisis and over the long term, such as home care, outpatient
services, transportation, emergency hospitalization, quality
nursing homes, and financial support, such as national health
insurance. Models for this do exist, as we discussed at lunchtime, for other people. When we talk about centers, I think of
things in a children's hospital, such as a cleft palate center.
This is not a separate building or a separate center, but there is
a time set aside for cleft palate patients in which resources are
mobilized on that day, in that place, for that kind of patient,
so that, for example, the parents of a 6-week-old baby with cleft
palate returning from a followup genetic counseling appointment
have already been to the cleft palate clinic, have met the physicians, the surgeons, the speech therapist, the dentist, have gone
to a meeting of the Cleft Palate Parents Association and been in-
vited to be an officer. Now that, to me, is early intervention
and effective mobilization. I think it's the kind of thing that
we're interested in arranging for Huntington's families: that a
multitude of forces can be mobilized around families when they
most need it and can be there for them later on.

     Since Huntington's is a genetic disease, children at risk of
having the disease-causing gene will inevitably come to the painful task of integrated intellectual knowledge, reality problems,
and great reactions into their life plans. I believe that if

services are set up when families are identified, at times of
crisis they can return to a resource that they know, that is
trusted, and can be there. We've had the experience with one
family in which the father has Huntington's disease. The mother
has two sons who are going into college, and she suspects that
one of her sons is developing the disease. We have tried to work
with them about how to handle this in terms of medical and psychological management. How it's worked out now is that she returns
with her sons regularly on an annual basis. She calls earlier
than her appointment, speaks with a psychiatrist she knows about
how things are going, calls him once in a while if a crisis comes
up, visits the pediatrics neurologist for a checkup, and has kind
of a family conference with me and with the other people that are
involved. I think this kind of a model for prevention can be
useful. I know the Commission is empowered to explore prevention,
and I think this is one way: services have to be there for people
who are not yet patients.

I sometimes remember the words of children who have spoken
as they are trying to deal with it. One little girl, who was 11
years old, was very quiet. She was with her parents, and then
she felt brave enough to ask the question: "Do nosebleeds mean
I am going to get the disease?" something that was quietly on her
mind. Another child, who was 14, sat very quietly and said, "I
pray to God I don't get it." I think it's important that we don't
overlook the children in what they're dealing with.

Most literally, H.D. is a children's disease, of course, because there are some children with the active juvenile form of
Huntington's disease. There is no need to underline the importance
of sensitive care of a team of specialists with situations like
this. We've talked about neurologic diseases and heard some very
moving testimony about this. I was pleased to learn that at
Children's Hospital they are now arranging to have a social worker
assigned full time to the neurology clinic. I'm hoping that we
can arrange a closer kind of relationship with families.

Lastly, it is a children's disease because it involves unborn
children; it involves young couples at risk, struggling with decisions about family planning on the basis of limited knowledge of their
futures. It is true, as many have said, that there are those who
do not wish to know their carrier status, but there are also young

people who very much would like to know and who have sought to
find out as much as possible about what their futures would be.
I'm thinking of two young men who explored this very thoroughly
and then decided that it was not possible to know enough about it
and decided to have vasectomies. I think if we have more knowledge in the future, these kinds of decisions would be able to be
different for them.

In conclusion, I believe that the families that are directly
involved with the disease are best able to define their needs,
and that professionals and volunteers in dozens of fields ought
to be available to help make certain treatment, education, and
research are realities. Again, I'm just giving my concern about
children and remembering the words of an H.D. mother who, when
asked after a conference, "What was the most difficult part of
this for you?" said, "The children. The children."

GUTHRIE: Because of your feelings and experience, what would
you answer to a family who says, "I don't want to tell my children
anything. After all, we don't really know yet, so why should I
tell them anything, let alone come to a center to be fortified for
something they may not ever have?"   What would you say to that?

ROSSER: I don't know. I think you have to go very carefully
with the expressed needs and wishes of the family. You want to
stay with it to make sure that they're really considering everything that's involved. From hearing the things different people
said, I would be very reluctant to push this sort of thing, but
I think I would want to explore with people like this, "How much
am I trying to protect myself, in terms of pain, and how much am
I trying to protect the children?" As I remember you saying once,
when families are not communicating about these disorders, you
don't know what the other people know. You don't know what their
pain is, they don't know what your pain is, and you're depriving
yourself of possible support, in a way.

GUTHRIE: If you're familiar with a center (you've been going
there all along), I can see how much easier it would be if this
problem occurs. But there are families who say, "But it may not
occur, so why should I bother doing all of this in advance?"

ROSSER: Okay, this was another idea of mine. I picked it up the other day at home. My husband works with older people, and he had gone to a conference where he had all these folders on multipurpose senior citizens centers, and there they were providing so many of the services that H.D. parents could use. They were talking about day care, hospitals, transportation, a multitude of things that many H.D. families would be eager to receive. This is why I appreciate CCHD so much: their need to have things avail-able for people who are not willing to identify themselves as patients. I think you have to be able to reach people and talk with them and be in touch with them all the time without insisting that they accept the role of patient. This is why I do think the idea of a multipurpose center is a useful one.

McKHANN: Thank you very much. Let me make one point. We have at least some 14 people to go on my list, so we really are going to have to stay within some kind of 5-minute time limit. Again, I'd really like to emphasize the input of suggestions and solutions to problems from different vantage points. I think we've heard a wide spectrum of problems, and many of you have been here. If you have new problems to bring us, fine; but I think we have heard a lot of the problems that exist.

TESTIMONY OF
MARCY FEIGENBAUM
SUPERVISOR, INITIAL RESPONSE UNIT
WESTCHESTER COUNTY DEPARTMENT OF SOCIAL SERVICES

FEIGENBAUM: My name is Marcy Feigenbaum. I supervise a service unit which deals with specific problems of the aged, blind, and disabled; and in doing so, for the past 7 months I have been supervising a case worker who has worked actively with two gentle-men who have Huntington's disease. They are 59 and 63, respectively. Their situation might be somewhat different from others we've heard today, only to the extent that they are the people in the woodwork who aren't coming out, not because they made a conscious choice but because their style of life is such that they are the forgotten people. These are people who are receiving SSI, which is Supplementary Security Income. I don't know if everybody here is familiar with that, but it is a Federal program which supple-ments Social Security. These people are living on a very, very meager income with absolutely no community support whatsoever.

We literally found them in a third-floor walkup in a very, very dilapidated building in an old section of Yonkers. They had received no medical care whatsoever in many, many years. The only reason that the H.D. was discovered was because the brother who was 59, who for many, many years was thought to be schizophrenic, had cut his leg badly last March and was taken by ambulance to a local hospital. The doctor attending him recognized his name because there is a third brother who lives upstate who had been treated by this doctor at Montefiore Hospital about a year and a half ago. He recognized the name, took a look at this gentleman, called the other brother in, tested both of them, and discovered they both had H.D.

These two brothers have never married. The brother who is upstate is married, has two children, and I believe his daughter also has children. From what I gather, this brother who lives upstate is the most chronically ill of the three, but he was always the most functioning. These two brothers were living in an apartment with practically no furniture; they were not eating properly; there was nobody involved with them. The younger brother, who was thought to be schizophrenic, supposedly has not washed or bathed in about 6 or 8 months because he has little men within him who tell him not to touch water.

The elder brother, prior to his debilitation which he has experienced recently, used to be able to support the younger brother and do for him whatever he could. He has since become much more disabled. We have been able to get a visiting nurse in (first on a 2-day-a-week basis, and now it's once a week). We've also secured a homemaker (a male homemaker, I might add), who comes in 4 hours a day, 7 days a week. We have also gotten a Q.E. (which is a qualified examiner) to the home to do a diagnostic workup of the other brother. As can be expected, the results were he declared that he had mild psychosis and the rest of his report just reiterated what we told him, so it really was of no help whatsoever. His only basis for saying H.D. was because of what we had said to him, so clinically he just put down, "mild psychosis."

We've also secured a doctor who has gone to the house to at least look at the younger brother because we were afraid that since he was not touching water the skin condition would

deteriorate greatly. We have gotten many supports into the home.
We are in the process of trying to get them relocated. When we
first started working with them, the younger brother would not
consider moving to any other apartment. At this point the older
brother's condition is so bad that he can't navigate the few
flights of stairs, so we are trying to get them relocated. The
problem is that obviously they are not the most desirable tenants
when you present people like this to a landlord. We've had many
fires in Yonkers recently and there is a tremendous housing
shortage, so it is a tremendous problem. Once we find something,
it must be on the ground floor, and, of course, we'll have to work
with the younger brother towards accepting this idea.

Ultimately, our long-range plan would be for some type of
nursing home placement, when and if it is indicated. At this point,
neither brother is accepting the idea. I might also add that the
middle brother who lives upstate, evidently his wife has had
contact with my worker's client. She said that her husband is
becoming so unmanageable that they want very much to place him in
some type of institutional facility, and she has not been able to
find an appropriate setting for him. As far as these two clients,
even if we get them to the point where they are accepting of some
sort of institutionalization, we will find the same problems that
we have with chronically ill M.S. patients or Parkinson's disease
patients, and that is, obtain a facility that will accept them.

I don't think I'm going to go on with some of the details,
because, as you say, you are trying to cut it short. As far as
suggestions, my first suggestion, which is something I feel is
necessary in terms of any illness or getting any type of center
or program for anything, is education, education not only for the
family and for the individual, but for the professional. In our
dealing with this particular family, we found that very few social
workers, very few doctors, none of the psychiatrists with whom we
worked, had ever had any dealings with H.D. It was solely this one
doctor--and only by fluke--that recognized the symptoms. I think
you have to start on a professional level; then you have to work
with the family (not only the individual, of course, who is ill,
but primarily with the rest of the family) in terms of accepting
what is there, in terms of counseling, and in terms of just helping
them accept something which is going to be inevitable.

GUTHRIE: I'll just very quickly comment that because of your
role in this kind of work you emphasize the word "education." I
think all of us agree. I think one of the things I'm asking you,
as a social worker, have you made any effort to do any education
within the framework of your own colleagues?

FEIGENBAUM: It's interesting you should ask that. I have
done a lot of public relations work for my department around areas
of the aged, blind, and disabled. This is the only particular case
of H.D. I have come in contact with. Since it has manifested itself to me, I have talked about it, yes. I have not done any
public speaking about H.D. I have about other problems of the
aged and chronically disabled.

GUTHRIE: But you see the need for your own colleagues to do
something about it?

FEIGENBAUM: I definitely do, and I will whenever I see the
opportunity. I have discussed it; I have obtained literature from
my cousin on H.D. and have distributed it all over, so that much
I have done.

GUTHRIE: I want to make a comment. I would venture to say
to you that some of the other professionals that you speak of who
have been looking at patients didn't know they were looking at one.

FEIGENBAUM: Right; exactly.

McKHANN: Thank you.

TESTIMONY OF
ARTHUR D. BLOOM, M.D.
PROFESSOR OF PEDIATRICS
AND HUMAN GENETICS AND DEVELOPMENT
COLUMBIA UNIVERSITY

BLOOM: I am Arthur D. Bloom, of Columbia. I thought that
what I would try to do is communicate to you some sense of some of
the medical genetic needs in the New York area particularly, in
addition to just speaking generally about medical genetics.

I'm acting now as Citywide Chairman of the Task Force on
Genetics, which is sort of an offshoot of the National Foundation

of the March of Dimes. This is an organization of all of the
clinical geneticists within the Greater New York area who are
directors of genetics units. I'm not going to focus on Huntington's
disease, but rather the general problems of delivery of genetics
services in New York, of which delivery of services to patients
with Huntington's disease is obviously a part. To do that, I want
to give you some data. We recently completed a questionnaire
which was filled out by the directors of 22 genetics units in the
Greater New York area, plus an additional six satellite units.
The data covers the period January of '76 and the questionnaire
was designed by Dr. Stein, from the School of Public Health, and
myself.

The first piece of information that I think is relevant is
the issue of outpatient care for genetics, and the question here
that was asked was: "What is the ethnic distribution of patients
in your service as seen in the outpatient clinic?" The distribution was as follows: 72 percent white, 17 percent black, 11 percent Hispanic, 8 percent other (which is a new species).

With an estimate of about 7,300 patients seen per year in
outpatient genetic settings in the Greater New York area, the distribution for inpatient genetic services was somewhat different,
with 52 percent of the patients on the inpatient side of genetic
units being white, 26 percent being black, and 22 percent being
Hispanic. What happens is the blacks and Hispanics basically
have access maximally when they are hospitalized. Essentially,
what this means to genetics services is when they have babies--
and primarily, babies, of course, were affected with genetic
disorders. In a sense, the other side of the coin is that, of
course, there is a selected advantage for the white population in
the Greater New York area, as throughout the rest of the country,
in accessibility to genetics services. This is something that is
of great concern to this Citywide Task Force; namely, the apparent
failure of our groups to reach the urban indigent population.

If one looks at the data that we've generated now on payment
for clinic visits, roughly 51 percent of the patients seen in
these genetics units pay for the service with insurance, insurance
and their own funds, or their own funds alone. An additional 24
percent make no payment whatever and are totally underwritten by
the unit, the hospital, whatever. An additional 21 percent paid

for their genetic services by public funds so that roughly one-
fourth of all patients do not pay and roughly one-fourth pay for
these services out of public funds. What I may suggest is
financing of these services.

Medicaid reimbursement, as well as Blue Cross and Blue Shield,
is well below the actual costs of services. That includes services
such as clinical and laboratory diagnostic services, laboratory
services alone, and the genetics side of it. We look very heavily
to the National Foundation of the March of Dimes for covering the
costs of maintaining genetics units and the delivery of genetics
counseling in the Greater New York area, as throughout the rest of
the country. While their input is really critical for the functioning of many of these units, it obviously is inadequate, so that
I see a major need existing, both in New York and across the
country, for really significant State and Federal funds for the
general area of the delivery of genetics services.

I think that the Huntington's disease patients present
particular problems in the late onset of the disease, the difficulty in diagnosis in the early stages, reproductive problems.
We all face this over and over again in our genetics counseling
units. I see the Huntington's problem, really, as a part of the
overall problem of how we're going to implement and improve the
delivery of genetics services across the country.

Just one other point: Since we are heavily concerned with
births in general in the genetics business, the number of births
in New York City in 1975 was in excess of 100,000; of those, 52
percent were white and 48 percent were nonwhite and Puerto Rican.
This population that's being born is clearly not having ready
access to these genetics services, unless they happen to be born
in a hospital where these services are available.

McKHANN: Would you comment, Dr. Bloom, on the accessibility
of genetics services to families where the expected problem is
going to occur in children versus families where the expected
problem is going to be with an adult?

BLOOM: Yes. I think that we have particular difficulty in
reaching adults. Most of the clinical geneticists across the
country are pediatricians; and while that's all well and good, it

does mean that a large proportion of the cases that we see will, of course, be in the pediatric age group. We do see lots of adult patients, but there is essentially no other central unit within the hospital that focuses on the genetics of neurologic disorders in the adult. There is, obviously, the Neurologic Institute which has primary concern for the care and treatment of adults who have neurologic disease, but the interaction is not all that good in most of these units; or you may have a neurology clinic which takes care of the primary neurologic problems of patients, but many of them do not work hand in hand with geneticists as a rule, so that's a big problem.

GUTHRIE: May I assume from what you're saying that you would be interested in including H.D. patients, young or old, for genetic counseling in all of these centers that you're now concerned with?

BLOOM: Yes, and the reason, I think, is that hopefully we become a bit better as we gain experience in doing the genetic counseling so that one of the things that's of great concern to us is, "How effective are we?" I think we are very good; sometimes not so good.

GUTHRIE: Could you give us an estimate of how long it would take, in terms of how many sessions in counseling this would require, when you assume the burden of the H.D. family?

BLOOM: Right. The number of hours is very considerable and obviously would require a detailed pedigree to be taken and, depending on the size of the family, it usually takes an hour to 2. Depending again on the number of individuals involved, the number that have to be counseled is inevitably complex, depending on their understanding of the genetic principles and the efficiency with which we transmit them, so that there are many hours spent in the counseling of a single patient or family with Huntington's disease. It's a real problem because these dominantly inherited disorders are not at all well understood, either by us or by the patients. The variable expressivity of these changes makes them very complex and hard for people to understand.

GUTHRIE: Then would you say that you have enough staff at this time to do this kind of job?

BLOOM: No, not at all. I think we are limited severely by
the modest kind of funding that most of us get from the National
Foundation, and we can't really begin to deliver the kind of care--
and I think that the figures I gave you indicate that that's a
citywide problem.

McKHANN: There's been discussion about the potential development of national genetic registries. Do you think that's feasible
in this country or only in a less mobile population, like Sweden
or something? That's point 1. The other criticism I've heard
leveled at this is the question of invasion of privacy. Could
you comment on those two points, because we may have to address
that issue?

BLOOM: Yes. I think the invasion of privacy is obviously a
very difficult one in these times. I think that there is a
feeling among geneticists that the registries are extremely useful. They have been tried. There are registries for patients
with chromosomal disorders, for example, here in New York State.
That's an effective means. I think that fundamentally the approach
ought to be very detailed information and computerization, in a
sense, of people involved, people who make up the pedigrees themselves at the institutions that are involved in genetic care
delivery. There is no problem in putting together computer
programs which will enable one to list individuals on every pedigree one takes. Those individuals can then be culled at will if
one wants to ask a specific question of them. This worked very
effectively---

GUTHRIE: Wait, wait. Stop there. What do you mean, "culled
at will"? Can you go out and address a family with a genetic
disease without realizing that you might be betraying the confidentiality of that family?

BLOOM: Okay. We have to draw some lines. Those lines are
not yet drawn. Okay? What I'm saying is that if there are individuals who show up 5 or 10 or 20 years later, they can be identified as being part of that pedigree, and therefore their genetics
can be easily traced. This system, I think, worked well in Michigan, where they have a fairly good program and large numbers of
Huntington's disease patients are followed in much this way.
Whether one could actually put it in a national registry or not, I

have my strong doubts in this day and age. I'm not sure there
would be all that much advantage to it, and I think that the potential invasion of privacy might give people a lot more problems
than it's worth.

    N. WEXLER: I would like to briefly follow up on Marjorie's
question. Do you have the kind of interdisciplinary staff that
you need? If Medicare or Medicaid does reimburse, for approximately how many counseling hours will they reimburse?

    BLOOM: The reimbursement is basically for the physician's
consultative services. That's fundamentally the way it goes. In
New York, Medicaid reimbursement for genetic counseling, which can
take many hours, obviously, is $24, which doesn't begin to cover
the complex of individuals involved in the delivery of these
genetic services. It is multidisciplinary by definition. It has
to involve not only the physician, geneticist, usually a genetic
counselor, a genetic associate, a master's level person, often
involves social workers, often involves psychiatric support.
There is a whole team of people that is required to deliver these
services. Very few units have all of these people available so
that we're working pretty much at our limit at the present time,
and it's very hard to see how much further we can go. Yet the
need exists so that increase for it is obviously desperate.

    GUTHRIE: It would be interesting if you could document for
us at some point what it should cost, what it might cost, by
using the team approach to following through maybe one family.

    BLOOM: Right. I think it would be an astronomical figure,
and I'd like to play with that.

    N. WEXLER: You're on.

    GUTHRIE: I'm also concerned about your approach to the
confidentiality. We have great problems---

    N. WEXLER: We also have great time problems.

    GUTHRIE: All right. I just think it's important to comment
that we're very pleased that you're doing what you're doing, but
we also have the problem of letting families that wish to remain
anonymous have that privilege.

BLOOM: Of course.

McKHANN: Let me just ask Nancy if she could be sure that
that particular question gets directed to that genetics subgroup,
this problem of invasion of privacy.

N. WEXLER: Yes. They will be dealing with that.

TESTIMONY OF
GRETCHEN J. DARLINGTON, PH.D.
CORNELL UNIVERSITY MEDICAL COLLEGE

DARLINGTON: I'm Gretchen Darlington. I'm at Cornell
University Medical College. The recommendations I would like to
propose to this Commission stem from my experience as a researcher
in somatic cell genetics and as a participant in the 1974 workshop
which was sponsored by the Foundation for Research in Hereditary
Disease.

The first suggestion I have is that Federal funding of an
interdisciplinary committee modeled after the workshop program,
one which is composed of researchers and physicians, would be, I
think, most productive. The purpose of such a committee would be
to identify questions associated with genetic disease and propose
scientific approaches to resolve the questions raised. Genetic
diseases such as Huntington's disease pose special problems; for
many of them the biochemical defect is simply unknown. This
often means that treatment and care are based on trial-and-error
methodology. Prenatal diagnosis is really impossible without some
genetic determinant which can be identified. The research aspect,
in turn, must be broadly based and exploratory in nature; more,
really, a search for clues to the genetic basis of the disorder than
an application of technology to eliminate the effects of the
disease.

As a participant in the 1974 workshop, I found that the
combination of backgrounds and expertise truly stimulated the
identification of new avenues of research in a number of fields.
The only difficulty in these meetings was the frustration in
knowing that the proposed projects could only be investigated if
research funds could be found, and that brings me to my second
recommendation: This is for research support. Moneys for pilot

projects and to sponsor fellows or investigators on sabbatical
leave for 1 or 2 years would be particularly helpful in this
area. The kind of research that must be done, I think, to identify the basic deficiency is different from the majority of research
projects that are undertaken. Certainly, preliminary investigations of this sort don't compete well in the present Federal
funding programs that now exist.

Furthermore, many investigators cannot really afford to
invest much money or energy in projects that are more speculative
in nature and may not represent the major thrust of their laboratory's research program. Seed money, I feel, serves to stimulate
new approaches to problems, and support for young investigators
serves two purposes: It directs research to a particular problem,
of course, but it also focuses the attention of a young person on
the problems of genetic disease at a formative stage in their
scientific development and extracts a kind of commitment from
them, I think, in their further work. It seems logical to me that
the establishment of a program modeled after the workshop and the
funding of pilot research projects would very naturally go hand in
hand.

Finally, I would like to underscore the comments that have
already been made concerning regional care facilities. I think
it's worth noting that where one finds active treatment centers,
you are much more likely to find active research programs associated with them. When patients are scattered in care facilities,
it's very hard to focus any kind of research program directed to
a particular disease. This concept has been presented, and I
think it will be expanded by Mrs. Klass, who will follow me.
Strictly from my very limited point of view as a researcher, a
regional center would identify and localize a patient population
for researchers interested in studying the disease. I think, in
turn--and I think it's important to say--that it would provide a
way for those families who are interested in contributing to
research to do so. Very often I think they feel frustrated by an
inability to come in contact with people who are studying the
disease.

McKHANN: Thank you. Let me ask you one question. It's the
same question I asked Dr. Yahr. Let's start from the point of
view of Huntington's disease. If you're conceiving a regional

center, I think it wouldn't be too feasible to have a center only
for Huntington's disease. How do you orient it?

DARLINGTON: No. I agree with you.

McKHANN: You make it a center for genetically determined
disease, a center for neurological disease, a center for diseases
that occur in certain age groups? How do you get around that
problem?

DARLINGTON: I'm not sure we have to be so rigid as to define
them in one category or another. I guess my own personal inclination is to incorporate Huntington's disease with neurological disorders. I suspect that the major research thrust will be in that
area, and that might be a more logical localization for these
patients than in genetic centers.

McKHANN: You're going to get drummed out of the genetics
union [laughter].

DARLINGTON: Yes. But the second reason I feel that way is
that strictly in terms of services for the patient and care for
the patient, if one tries to compete with genetics centers, you
have such diverse needs that I don't think a genetics center could
meet those needs; and for a similarity of services, a neurologic
center would seem most appropriate.

N. WEXLER: In line with that, I know that there are approximately 500 to 700 genetic neurological conditions. There is a
sense among some investigators of subdisciplines of neurogenetics,
and there was even one suggestion that a journal be formed in
neurogenetics. Do you think that that would be a substantial
population?

DARLINGTON: That seems quite feasible. I think regionally,
depending on the frequency of that disease within a certain geographic area, one may need to specify a genetics-neurological
center.

GUTHRIE: That's the figure, 500?

N. WEXLER: According to the Tower, it's 500 to 700.

McKHANN: Thank you very much.

TESTIMONY OF
PHYLLIS KLASS
ASSOCIATE DIRECTOR
GENETIC COUNSELING PROGRAM
NEW YORK HOSPITAL-CORNELL MEDICAL CENTER

KLASS: My name is Phyllis Klass, and I'm the Associate
Director of the Genetic Counseling Program at the New York
Hospital-Cornell Medical Center.

I would like to expand a bit on Dr. Darlington's suggestion,
and previous speakers', on regional centers for the care of patients
with Huntington's disease and their families. This approach seems
to me to offer an ideal way in which all the services needed by
the Huntington's family can be made available to them. Prototypes
of such clinics or centers already exist for other genetic
diseases like muscular dystrophy and hemophilia. My experience
as a member of the staff of these clinics has impressed me with
the benefits to be gained by such a unified approach. In this
setting, physicians, nurses, psychologists, social workers, and
genetic counselors work together as a team to provide continuing
support of services.

I'd like to turn now to my particular field, genetic counseling. The tragic consequences of Huntington's disease to a patient's
entire family have been eloquently described. The fact that Huntington's is a genetic disease is one major reason for the stress
it puts on family members. Not only must they cope with all the
feelings engendered by having a loved one with a degenerative
disease, especially one with behavioral manifestations, but they
must also deal with the possible genetic implications for themselves and for each child in the family. Psychological difficulties
within and between individuals are a normal consequence.

However, there should not be superimposed upon the normal
stresses those that result from a faulty understanding of the
genetic mechanisms involved. Frequently, a so-called "family
disease" reduces the self-esteem of its members by implying a
family taint or curse. Now this superstitious view can be overcome by a clear understanding of the mechanism by which harmful

genes which we all carry can cause disease. Genetic counseling
seeks to lessen the stigma of genetic disease by substituting
factual information for the mystical explanations concocted by
many families. Lessening the stigma can have a second advantage.
It may allow a greater openness in discussing the existence of the
disease with members of the extended family. This would avoid the
secrecy which is frequently imposed by Huntington's families and
would permit unsuspecting relatives to be informed of their own
possible risk.

There is yet another problem area to which genetic counseling
addresses itself. Individuals who are at risk for developing
Huntington's disease must wrestle with the decision of whether
or not to have children or, indeed, whether or not to enter into
marriage, for fear of becoming a burden on a spouse. A genetic
counselor does not attempt to answer these questions, but he does
provide a setting in which the individual can formulate a plan that
is best for him. The counselor does this by offering himself as a
source: a source of facts as opposed to superstition; a source of
understanding because he knows the disease; and a source of continued support because of his specialized training in counseling.

GUTHRIE: Of course, it's good to relieve the stigma of the
family, but how do we relieve the stigma as it pertains to the
society around, which is what really causes the stigma?

KLASS: I think to some extent people, by their action and
the way they feel about themselves, cause the response in others.
I think if we can hold up our head high and feel comfortable
within ourselves when faced with this problem, we make other
people comfortable with it, too.

N. WEXLER: I think your counseling procedure at Cornell, in
my experience, is quite unusual. For example, you have extended
counseling sessions to carry people over several years' duration,
if necessary. Could you briefly tell us what the range of services
are that you perform?

KLASS: I think what you're saying, Nancy, when you're talking
about my work with hemophilia and muscular dystrophy, which is outside of a genetics clinic setting--and that's what I think is an
appropriate model for Huntington's disease or neurogenetic diseases,

which might be a good title, because I think it's in that multi-discipline center with neurologists and psychiatrists or psychologists, and all of that, seeing the family on a continuing basis over years as we do with muscular dystrophy. This is where it's important to be. The genetics clinic and its personnel can contribute to that by being another specialized service and being part of that team. But I really think that the center of that team belongs in a separate unit. Did I answer your question? In those settings I can see families many, many times. The funding is different, too.

N. WEXLER: Who supports that?

KLASS: Muscular Dystrophy, for instance, supports genetic counseling.

GUTHRIE: Do you see an advantage, perhaps, of having families not with the same disease work together through a center? You mentioned muscular dystrophy. Do you see an advantage or disadvantage of H.D. families meeting at the same time in group sessions with other families with similar disorders but not the same one?

KLASS: It's difficult to manage that sort of encounter sometimes. We once tried to start a family group for parents of children born with different sorts of birth defects. We had a similar group for parents of mongoloid children. That works out beautifully as a continuing group. When we tried to put together parents of children with different physical defects, it did not work easily, because each parent was trying to say, "Well, my defect is worse than yours, and this causes different problems for my child and for me," and there was too much conflict to be of help to them. I personally think that if we at least held them together with neurogenetic diseases, that may have some validity. But I do feel that families help each other a great deal.

GUTHRIE: Very much.

KLASS: Very much so. In a center like this, they need one another, to go up with one another. While that can have its heartaches, certainly, it has an awfully lot of support built in.

N. WEXLER: Is this group long-term counseling, the parents'
group?

KLASS: Our Down's Syndrome Group? Yes, it is.

GUTHRIE: We asked before, and I would like your opinion also
on how you feel about bringing people in families where they really
don't want to tell the children, they would really like to delay
it, into counseling?

KLASS: You see, this is where I think it's difficult if
your only contact is with a genetic clinic, because in a typical
genetics clinic you may see the people who are seeking the advice
perhaps once or twice, and your relationship with them is somewhat
limited. If you're seeing them in a continuing care facility,
you're building up a relationship, you're growing with them. As
their needs change, and as your relationship then becomes greater,
you may change their mind or you may respect their wish to keep it
the way they wish it.

GUTHRIE: One important question I want to ask, do you ever
recommend sterilization or procedures of that kind that some
family might not like to hear, or are you basically information?

KLASS: I have never recommended sterilization to any patient
that I can possibly think of. Only when a patient asks me, "This
is my decision. What are my options for dealing with it?" then
under those circumstances one might say, "Contraceptive devices,
sterilization"; in other words, help them implement their own
decision. I wouldn't dream of making that decision for anybody.

McKHANN: Thank you very much.

TESTIMONY OF
MARC AST, M.D.
BERNARD W. SCHLESINGER FOUNDATION
INSTITUTE FOR HEREDITARY RESEARCH

AST: Good afternoon. I'm going to be showing some slides for
the purposes of this presentation. I will try to coordinate the
speaking and visual part as professionally as possible.

I'd like to report some recommendations from research that
have been developed from a Huntington's disease research group
composed of Stuart R. Snider, Erica Metzig, Steven Rosenberg,
Danny Tobin, and myself, affiliated with the Columbia Presbyterian
Medical Center and the Bernard W. Schlesinger Foundation Institute
for Hereditary Research. In this presentation I will be presenting
some material which is very familiar to all of you, but it is
important in terms of presenting some new strategy which we have
developed in further detection and research.

Huntington's disease, a chronic disorder characterized by
increasing choreiform movements and progressive dementia, is
inherited in autosomal dominant fashion with complete penetrance.
All carriers of the gene develop the disease, and the disorder never
skips a generation, as we know it. The age of onset ranges between
25 to 50 years, with most cases appearing between the ages of 35
and 40. At birth every child of a person afflicted with Huntington's disease has a 50-percent risk of developing the disease; of
the "at-risk" population, one-half are expected to become afflicted.
If we look at the at-risk population, the offspring of H.D.-
afflicted individuals, with increasing age more and more of the
population develops the disease. However, as age increases, the
risk for the remaining unaffected members decreases. I would just
like to indicate briefly a point that hasn't been emphasized
clearly enough. For example, at age 30 an at-risk individual has
approximately a 46-percent chance of developing the disorder. At
age 60, the probability that an at-risk individual will be
afflicted is only 9 percent. The onset of the disease usually
occurs after reproductive life begins.

McKHANN: May I ask you a question about that? That's true
across the entire population, but does it vary from family to
family?

AST: There are, of course, the individual variations of
late- and early-onset families.

McKHANN: I guess the question I'm asking is does that
variation breed true or not?

AST: In general, you can say yes. However, we have
encountered in our studies that certain events, traumatic events,

early in life can precipitate an early onset in delayed-onset families. The factor of stress and fatigue is a significant variable, and looking at variants in terms of age of onset. Have I answered your question?

McKHANN: Yes.

GUTHRIE: That does not affect the childhood form, only the adult form?

AST: Right. The onset of the disease usually occurs after reproductive life begins. Thus, one of the most important and pressing problems is the identification of the genetic carrier; this will make possible proper counseling of individuals in whose families the disease has occurred. Furthermore, identification of the genetic carrier is important if it becomes possible to intervene preventively by biochemical or other means.

A wide variety of studies have been undertaken to find some means of identifying the carrier of the H.D. gene before the onset of the disorder. Clinical studies, for example, have attempted to find test responses of an H.D.-afflicted group. However, all attempts at early detection (clinical, genetic, or biochemical) are fraught with pitfalls. A brief examination of one clinical study using electroencephalography illustrates this problem.

In 1948 electroencephalographic methods were used to predict the presence of the H.D. gene before symptoms occurred. At first, test results were encouraging. H.D. patients showed significant EEG abnormalities, or a positive response. Of the at-risk off-spring of these patients, approximately one-half showed EEG abnormalities (that is, a positive response). The remaining one-half showed a negative response, or no EEG abnormalities. Two facts here are crucial:

1. Some at-risk siblings showed an abnormal test response similar to the H.D.-afflicted group; and

2. The pattern of the positive and negative test responses (50 percent positive/50 percent negative) matched the expected distribution of the H.D. gene in the at-risk group.

Therefore, if the EEG test is valid, the 50 percent of the at-risk siblings showing a positive response would be the 50 percent who have received the H.D. gene; those with the negative test response would have escaped the H.D. gene, and as a result would not develop the disease.

An 18-year followup study (by Chandler) showed EEG to be unreliable in predicting H.D. Twenty-three of the offspring originally tested ultimately developed H.D. Of these H.D.-afflicted individuals, approximately one-half had shown a negative test response 18 years earlier, the remaining one-half a positive test response. As a predictive test, EEG proved to be no better than guessing.

There have been many other proposed tests, including finger oscillometry, electromyography, premorbid personality and genetic markers such as fingerprints, also the levodopa provocative test. The techniques either have failed to provide reliable and consistent results, or have not yet been evaluated.

What is the pitfall? The problem encountered by all early detection or predictive studies is that the evaluation of any test takes anywhere from 15 to 30 years. The testing of young at-risk offspring necessitates a long-term followup until a sufficient number develop the disease to confirm or disconfirm the test. Obviously, reduction in evaluation time would be beneficial in every way, at least in allowing the prompt elimination of ineffective tests so that research can be directed toward the development of an effective test.

We suggest a methodological change, a new research strategy developed primarily by Steven Rosenberg of our research group. This new research strategy might effect such a reduction in evaluation time and at least permit a preliminary evaluation of any proposed predictive test. Let us return again to the "Age/Risk" table.   Let us refer to the degree of risk as a function of age. From these statistics it is possible to define a new population of probable noncarriers of the H.D. gene, termed "escapees." Escapees are individuals who were formerly at risk but have remained free of symptoms and are age 50 or over. From the table we see that this group has an 80-percent to 100-percent chance of

escaping the illness. Adding the escapee group to the patient
and at-risk groups, we find the following distribution of the H.D.
gene:

1. Patients, by definition, are all carriers of the H.D.
    gene.

2. At-risk offspring are 50 percent carriers and 50
    percent noncarriers.

3. Eighty percent to 100 percent ideally of the escapees
    are noncarriers.

We see that the at-risk group will, in time, divide evenly into
the H.D.-afflicted and escapee groups.

A predictive test would optimally produce response patterns
which correspond to the pattern of inheritance of the H.D. gene,
and we can see it again in the slide, just assuming that the
markings are for positive and negative response:

1. All H.D. patients would show a positive response.

2. Fifty percent positive and 50 percent negative responses
    would be seen in the at-risk offspring less than 50
    years of age.

3. Approximately 80 percent to 100 percent negative
    responses in the escapees.

Accordingly, as far as the distribution of positive and
negative responses is concerned, H.D. patients would be representative of at-risk carriers of the abnormal gene as they will be when
they become symptomatic, with both patients and their heterozygote
carrier offspring showing the positive response. Probable noncarriers or escapees, on the other hand, would be representative
of the at-risk offspring who are noncarriers as they will be when
they pass 50 years of age (i.e., the critical age of onset of the
disease), with all of the latter and nearly all of the former
showing the negative response.

Consequently, the examination not only of affected patients
and their at-risk offspring, but of probable noncarriers or escapees

as well, would simulate long-term followup of offspring at risk.
This would permit rapid evaluation of predictive tests through
comparison of the proportion of negative over positive responses
in the probable noncarrier and the at-risk samples. I believe this
point is clear now. Just to repeat it once more, we can look at
the older individuals, those who statistically have--to the degree
that probable noncarriers exceed at-risk offspring in the proportion of negative responses over positive responses, to that degree
is the carrier detection test effective.

If the proportions of positve and negative responses in the
two groups are equal, then the test can be discarded as ineffective.
If we return to the earlier study cited, the EEG study, if they
had selected a group of escapees and had applied the test in 1948
according to our model, one-half of the escapees would have shown
abnormalities and one-half not. Instead of having to wait 18
years at a great expense, they could have told very quickly within
a matter of months whether their test was an effective test or not.

The model can be tested by a simple statistical method,
comparing the two dichotomous variables: positive versus negative
responders and probable noncarriers versus at-risk offspring.
Where sample sizes are sufficiently large, a more complicated and
more powerful analysis can be made. Data may then be quantitatively
ordered to expand the two categories of probable noncarriers (that
is, unaffected, age equal to or greater than 50) and the younger
at-risk offspring to several levels of age ordered quantitatively.
A hypothesis would then posit that from 10 to 19 years of age, the
unaffected at-risk would show a lower proportion of negative and a
higher proportion of positive responses than the offspring aged
20 to 29. In turn, those aged 20 to 29 would show less negative
and more positive responses than those aged 30 to 39, and so on,
decade by decade. The higher the age level, the higher the proportion of negative over positive responses should be in the unaffected
offspring of Huntington's chorea patients. Various statisticians
(for example, Fleiss) provide a statistical model applicable to
such an analysis.

Lastly, of course, to ensure the positive association between
negative responses and age of at-risk offspring is not an artifact
of increasing age, escapees would have to be compared with carefully
matched normal controls. The importance to genetic and social

counseling and to possible early therapeutic intervention of rapidly separating ineffective detection tests from the potentially effective is obvious. This hypothetical escapee methodology could be tested quite simply by application to another disease for which there is a presymptomatic detection technique of proven validity. The goodness of fit of the observed values for affected patients, at-risk offspring, and probable noncarriers or escapees, aged 50 or above, to the expected values established by the genetic pattern of the disease would decide the matter of the correctness of the hypothetical model.

To summarize then, in a sense we see that H.D. studies may have been said to be only one-half complete. These studies compare only at-risk and patient groups. We have, so to speak, added the other half by comparing the at-risk group to the newly defined escapee group. We recommend that all future research studies in H.D. (specifically, early detection studies) incorporate the escapee methodology. Furthermore, we have here a clear instance where all of genetics research benefits from the investigation of H.D. The model proposed here can be applied to any genetic disorder.

A final note is in relation to the recruiting of patients and families for testing we have done. We have recently developed a simple, noninvasive test of coordination which works according to the escapee methodology. In recruiting subjects we have found that though many relatives are willing and even anxious to participate, the majority are unwilling and at times even hostile. We believe that in addition to supporting research on H.D., all concerned organizations should devote an equal time toward encouraging participation in these studies by families who would be immediate beneficiaries. Organizations should actively aid in contacting family members and strongly urge them to participate in research studies. It is not enough simply to inform them of the existence of these studies.

TESTIMONY OF
SYLVIA P. RUBIN, M.S.
GENETIC COUNSELOR
COLUMBIA UNIVERSITY MEDICAL CENTER

RUBIN: I'm Sylvia Rubin, genetic counselor at Columbia University Medical Center, Department of Obstetrics and Gynecology.

I would like to present to the Commission my viewpoint based upon my experience and expertise as a genetic counselor for many years. I have had considerable experience in giving genetic counseling to patients affected with Huntington's disease and their families at risk for Huntington's disease.

As you are probably aware from the testimony of many persons, the particular horrendous nature of this disease is the fact that a person born with the gene for Huntington's disease does not know this until he or she is in perhaps the third or even fourth decade of life, generally after they have already had their children. The very earliest manifestations of this disease are usually not apparent until after the individual has had his or her family. These children then in turn each have the terribly high 50-percent risk of being affected with Huntington's disease and indeed will not know this fact until perhaps the third or fourth decade of their lives. There is no definitive test as of this date to determine if an individual has the gene and will therefore have Huntington's disease sometime within their lifespan.

The particular relentless, devastating nature of the physical and emotional manifestations of H.D. make this one of the most multifaceted and complex of all genetic diseases to counsel. Immediate and continuing genetic counseling for patients and all family members is an essential and integral part of medical service and management of these individuals. The full comprehension of the disease, including all the multiple medical, legal, social, and psychological problems it encompasses, is a long and continuous process. Funds must be available to help these families have such a necessary service. The benefits are not just for the families affected or at risk for this disease, but for all society. They are part of our society and cannot be excluded. If they can be helped through research to find the cause of this dreaded disease or detect who are at risk for being affected, then perhaps we can help prevent future generations from being so affected. More productive lives would be led by all, which in turn would benefit society as a whole.

In listening to the previous people talking--I hate to be too repetitious, so I think I'm just going to get right to a specific recommendation that I would like to make. First of all, funds must be made available to facilitate the prompt recognition and followup

for patients and families affected with H.D. This includes the
education of physicians to recognize H.D.

Second of all--I know this has been mentioned before, and I
really feel this is important--a central agency, perhaps in connection with CCHD, which families can be referred to that would provide continuous care with all the multidisciplines that have been
discussed here; namely, neurologists, psychiatrists, psychologists,
genetic counselors, and a legal counsel would be very important as
well. These persons would provide continuous followup care for the
individuals in question and provide the multifaceted support required for as many years as necessary. I think I'll just leave it
at that because anything else I say will be repetitious.

GUTHRIE: If someone sent someone to your center for
counseling, what do you charge them?

RUBIN: This would be our usual fee which would be for any
patient. Of course, if there is any problem, if there is a question
of not being able to afford anything like that, then the fee would
be waived.

GUTHRIE: Do you realize, in answering it that way, that 90
percent of the families with Huntington's disease are impoverished
because of the problem of Huntington's disease so that they would
be coming to you and asking for your services without fee payments?
What would you do then?

RUBIN: I would not refuse them.

GUTHRIE: Not even 90 percent?

RUBIN: I feel that strongly about it.

GUTHRIE: Would the center support it?

RUBIN: I believe so. Yes.

McKHANN: Let me ask you a question in a little different way.
Under the current pattern of reimbursement--and let's not use that
90-percent nonpaid figure, let's say 20 or 30 percent--is it possible
for someone involved in genetic counseling to be self-supporting,

or does some outside agency have to essentially put in part of the money for genetic counseling to keep such an outfit going?

RUBIN: Exactly. I didn't mean to imply that this wouldn't happen. Yes, absolutely. Funds would be necessary to support a genetic counselor such as myself in a situation like this where you say 90 percent or even quite a lower figure would be coming that could not pay for it themselves. Of course, as you already know, the medical cost is horrendous, and you can't possibly put a price on the emotional burden. That's impossible. Funds must come from somewhere to support this. Absolutely.

GUTHRIE: Are you in agreement or disagreement with the idea of having a neurogenetics center that would include, then, the H.D. families and all the others who would need these services?

RUBIN: Yes. I think what I have suggested could be incorporated into something like that. I would like to make a comment on something that was asked of someone previously. You specifically asked about incorporating other diseases in with this, and I would like to put my input in with that. I do not think that this is a good or feasible idea. I really don't, because in my own experience I have found--similarly, I believe that Mrs. Klass, or whoever it was, spoke about it--that this is not a good idea. Different genetic diseases cannot be grouped together as far as getting families together to discuss their many problems because the problems are different; they are not the same. Of course, one individual feels their problems are more horrendous than others, and rightly so. They are to them. They are 100 percent to them, no matter what anybody else affected with another disease may have. For this reason it does not work. It works when I myself, whatever the disease is, try to get families together who have the same disease, but not a different one. It just does not work.

GUTHRIE: They're supportive of each other, in a sense?

RUBIN: Exactly.

GUTHRIE: That's important, as part of the genetic counseling?

RUBIN: Certainly. But it can work in cross-purposes and against the purpose when you get different diseases together. We have been trying to do that. It just does not work.

N. WEXLER: Would it be possible if you had a care center where you had certain kinds of recreational and rehab facilities for different genetic diseases but had separate counseling groups, et cetera?

RUBIN: That's different, because what you're saying is that the needs that have been set up for that particular agency would be the same means for individuals affected with different types of things. That's different. That may work, yes, if you have a counseling service available there that is specific for that---

N. WEXLER: Separate but equal?

RUBIN: I guess, in a sense, that's right.

GUTHRIE: Yes. In the VA hospitals there are patients who have a number of neurological disorders all together in rehab and physical therapy and speech therapy. Yet I'm sure that, as you say, in the counseling it might have to be separate.

RUBIN: Oh, exactly. They have the same physical problems that necessitate similar treatment, yes; that's exactly it. But as far as grouping them together for counseling or being able to compare their problems with each other, that's a totally different story.

PRATT: Have you encountered much need for legal counseling?

RUBIN: Oh, yes.

PRATT: I believe you were the first one to mention it, and I should think there'd be a great need.

RUBIN: That's very important, and that's why I included it very specifically, because there are many legal problems that---

PRATT: I should think there'd be a terrific number.

RUBIN: Right. People lose their jobs, people lose insurance policies. I mean, you could spend an hour or much, more more just on that alone.

PRATT: I think that legal's important.

RUBIN: Extremely important.

N. WEXLER: Do you have any experience with children who are at risk and who are up for adoption and whether or not that would affect their adoptability? I know you didn't mention that specifically.

RUBIN: No. I personally haven't had that kind of experience involved with that. Sometimes this is a totally unknown factor: You may not know. I have had experience with couples whose families have children who have been given up for adoption, and then afterwards found out that that family had Huntington's disease and cannot trace that child. This involves new legal aspects that come into play right there, of being able to obtain adoption records and that kind of thing. The moral and legal applications there are enormous.

N. WEXLER: If the child itself were at risk, I was wondering whether or not that would preclude it from being adopted easily?

RUBIN: I can't answer that question from any legal aspect.

GUTHRIE: You spoke of the role of a voluntary agency doing some kind of counseling of its own perhaps, or being supportive of what you're doing. Could you go on and give me a little idea, for instance, what could a voluntary agency do?

RUBIN: I don't use the word "voluntary." Some agency that would be set up--by "voluntary," do you mean someone that is---

GUTHRIE: I meant a health agency, like CCHD, which you mentioned.

RUBIN: What I specifically was referring to was something that would be funded.

GUTHRIE: They might fund?

RUBIN: That would be working with someone, of course, like your agency, CCHD, but not necessarily funded by CCHD; and hopefully Government funded.

GUTHRIE: Say that louder.

RUBIN: GOVERNMENT FUNDED. Government funded.

TESTIMONY OF
FRED E. OCHS
SUPERVISOR, QUALITY OF LIFE PROGRAM
JEWISH COMMUNITY SERVICES OF LONG ISLAND

OCHS: My name is Fred Ochs, Supervisor of the Quality of Life
Program at Jewish Community Services of Long Island, a family
service agency affiliated with the Federation of Jewish Philan-
thropies. Within the past year our agency inaugurated a new
program designed to provide social, cultural, educational, and
recreational services to individuals between the ages 21 to 64
who are homebound as a result of chronic physical illness. At
present, we are serving approximately 55 clients with such varied
diagnoses as muscular dystrophy, amyotrophic lateral sclerosis,
multiple sclerosis, rheumatoid arthritis, emphysema, Buerger's
disease, bilateral amputees, stroke victims, and patients with
severe cardiac conditions. To date, we have not provided services
to a patient with Huntington's disease. However, many of the
factors involved in any chronic illness apply equally to persons
with Huntington's disease and their families.

Intense involvement with individuals and families by our
staff has created a sensitivity to the effect catastrophic illness
may have on patients and their families. As a consequence, we
have chosen to focus on the specific area of the homebound, because
we recognized this as a most neglected area. Individuals who are
homebound are frequently overlooked by the community and health
professionals, particularly when such persons are considered poor
candidates for rehabilitation. National organizations often focus
on research and cannot divert substantial funds for direct services
to patients. In a period of scarce resources for social services
in general, a program that is designed to enhance the quality of
life may be viewed as a luxury. One must ask, however, "Can such
a program really be considered a luxury?" While it is important
to hope that research will in the future develop techniques that
will deal with a variety of disabilities, we must at the same time
question what can be done to help a homebound person create a
meaningful life for the present.

Individuals develop much of their self-esteem as a result of
interaction with other human beings. They receive recognition

through the approval by others of some aspect of their personality. When chronic illness strikes, however, it is often at a period in life when recognition and self-esteem might be expected to be reached or be at a peak. Patients who develop a chronic disease at such times not only have had their bodies betray them at a most unexpected moment, but often find themselves in a social vacuum, where even friends and relatives tend to avoid them, severely diminishing opportunities to build and sustain a relatively healthy ego. The husband or wife of such a patient, even if interested, quite frequently is required to work because of financial strain and therefore may be out of the house for long periods of time. Children may be away at school, or married and out of the home. Such patients are an abandoned population. They suffer greatly from a lack of meaningful human contact, and it should not be too hard to imagine the impact severe illness compounded by reality-based depression might have on a family.

An overwhelming majority of clients in our program express a need for contact with others and to feel useful in order to combat crushing feelings of rejection and abandonment. They view our services as vital in their efforts to overcome such feelings. To this end, our agency has arranged for a social worker to interview every person who applies and to evaluate their interests and capabilities. A customized program of activities is then developed and brought into the home at a time most convenient for each client. We have set up a weekly socialization hour, made possible by a telephone conference call hookup with another group which meets, plays, and is taught chess, in addition to developing and perfecting other games suitable to the telephone. Many of our clients are involved with painting and sculpture under the supervision of an art therapist assigned to the program, or are being taught a foreign language by volunteer and paid instructors coming to the home at regular intervals. Volunteers also have served as friendly visitors and shoppers for the homebound. A volunteer edits a newsletter that goes out to clients and to which they contribute. A barber and beautician are available to the homebound, many of whom express concern about their appearance, and counseling is offered in selected instances. New activities are being investigated and planned for future inclusion in the Quality of Life Program.

We feel that the activities outlined above can make a difference in the individual's will to live. We are calling for

more such programs to be instituted and the quality of life to be
viewed as a major factor in dealing with any homebound individual.
Perhaps what we should be advocating is Government subvention of
programs aimed at improving the quality of life for those no longer
able to function independently in the community, yet not deteriorated to the point where institutionalization is required. As we
all know, such a period can, and often does, last many years.

Jewish Community Services of Long Island is hopeful that the
community at large, both lay and professional, in both the public
and private sector, will recognize the need for such services. We
hope, too, that others will not only emulate our program and make
it available to all in need, but that they would contribute their
own ideas and efforts to the enrichment of such a service throughout the country.

GUTHRIE: I just wanted to ask, who supports this program?

OCHS: This particular program has been funded by a private
foundation, which has its limits, as you are all aware.

GUTHRIE: I asked the question in terms of when you spoke of
"we could emulate this program," and I certainly do approve of
that. I was wondering where one might look for funding. That's
what I'm concerned with.

OCHS: I'm not particular where the funding comes from,
whether it's, as I mentioned, private or public sector. I think
it's a most important activity and should be supported by everyone.

PRATT: I think it's a very interesting program. You said 50?

OCHS: At the moment there are 55 and growing. We're only in
existence less than a year, this particular program.

PRATT: What have you spent in that time?

OCHS: I wish I had the figures for that.

PRATT: Do you have any breakdown at all?

OCHS: Not really. It's very difficult for me because I'm not
really involved in that aspect of the program. I imagine it would

be hard to compute at present because it's an ever-expanding program with new ideas being developed involving additional expenditures. We are trying to expand the program so that the cost per capita would be less.

GUTHRIE: Is it conceivable, based on the last discussions that we had, that this program might be part of a neurogenetics center; in other words, an outpatient program, a homebound program in conjunction with a center?

OCHS: It is certainly conceivable.

GUTHRIE: ...might lead the way so that we are going in steps for the different kinds of care that people need. Your people might eventually have to go into a hospital, but this would be a transition, and a very helpful one, I assure you, from what you're saying.

OCHS: Yes.

McKHANN: How many people do you have in personnel to service your 50?

OCHS: We have the art therapist, an additional social worker, and the rest have all been volunteers.

PRATT: How many volunteers?

OCHS: Plus paid specialists on occasions when we can't get a qualified volunteer.

McKHANN: Do the clients themselves contribute to this program?

OCHS: At the moment we have no fee for this program. We anticipate that when the funding runs out we will be instituting our usual policy of a sliding-fee scale. That undoubtedly will mean that the vast majority of clients will be paying no fee or a very small amount.

GUTHRIE: Very interesting program. I love the words, "quality of life."

TESTIMONY OF
SHARON STIRLER
NEW YORK, NEW YORK

STIRLER: My name is Sharon Stirler. I am from New York City,
and I am at risk at 32 years of age. I am affiliated with both the
Huntington's Disease Association and the Committee to Combat Huntington's Disease. I'll just give you a couple of minutes on my
background, and then I'd like to concentrate on the problems of
the people at risk.

My mother is the first diagnosed patient with Huntington's
disease in our family. Since then my cousin and I have worked to
trace it back five generations, which were given to Dr. Whittier
to work with. My mother has been in a nursing home now for about
7 years and is totally incapacitated. She does not speak, feed
herself, walk, sit up, or in any way communicate. It really has
been a long 7 years. I have one brother, and he really is not
prepared at all to talk about Huntington's disease or his feelings
about it at this time.

Until I came to New York from Iowa, I did not know there was
anyone even working toward educating families, research, or doing
anything about it. I felt totally alone. It wasn't until I was
18 and had already left the home that my mother was diagnosed.

I want to make one comment. You were asking before of one of
the people who testified about babies being adopted if they were
at risk. I have another concern. What if you are a person who
wants to adopt a child, but you yourself are at risk? I think one
of the big concerns of people at risk has to do with the legal
things. I have been, as many people at risk do, avoiding going
home and reading all my life insurance and health policies to see
if there are clauses discriminating against Huntington's disease
and people at risk. I think there are many legal problems for at-
risk people, but I certainly have avoided looking into some of them.

McKHANN: Excuse me. I'm going to interrupt you there for
just a minute to mention something to Dr. Wexler. This issue
hasn't come up before but that's something that this Commission
could specifically look at, I think: this question of things like
life insurance, compensation.

N. WEXLER: In fact, we did talk to an insurance agent about preparing a position paper for us on this, but I think your point can be reiterated also about the capacity of a person at risk to adopt. That's something we should look into.

STIRLER: Another problem of all of us at risk is how do we relate to the patient as long as they are in the home? I'm saying my case because once my mother was in the nursing home, it was really difficult to relate at all. How do we give them support and yet deal with our own feelings? I went into psychotherapy when I finally arrived in New York, and it came as a result of a series of TV programs that came on all in one year, one after the other, which spoke about Huntington's disease, and even though the information was often inaccurate, the word was mentioned. I did go into psychotherapy to try to place this in perspective. I can stay fairly calm most of the time, but every once in a while there comes an overwhelming depression. I get it in various ways. But I do feel that the psychotherapy that I had was of immense value to me. This is a person who is not specialized in dealing with genetic diseases of Huntington's disease specifically, but was immensely helpful.

In conjunction with this, I want to mention that I myself at one time tried to run a rap group for at-risk young people. (I am a school psychologist.) People came once or twice and they could not bring themselves to come back. They were very interested. They felt pleased that we had gotten together. First of all, I did not have the experience; I wasn't doing therapy. Second of all, my point is that I think all of us at risk go through periods of extreme denial. After my mother was diagnosed (I was a graduate student at the University of Iowa), I was able to get free genetic counseling there and an EEG. Of course, these were interesting to me, but I put them away for almost 8 years before I even let myself consider how this all affected me, and that came at a point when I was considering marriage. As a result of all my emotional conflict about these things, I turned down the marriage proposal.

I think that whole thing of whether you should have children, how you relate to the other people in your family who are at risk, who are not at risk, who are afflicted, how you relate to important others in your life in terms of whether you share your feelings with them or you try to keep them to yourself, the whole support system is very crucial. As I said, I was sticking to that at-risk

group rather than the afflicted group. Just knowing that research
is going on, that organizations are working, is somewhat supportive,
but I really think it needs to be an intensive kind of support.

A point I would like to make is that funds must be available
through the Government or insurance or however, other than private
resources, to provide this kind of supportive therapy constantly.
I am sure you are all aware of the costs of therapy sessions today
and the fact that many insurance policies won't cover any sort of
therapy at all, so I feel there has to be some other kind of funding
for these support services. As Mrs. Guthrie mentioned, the families
are often drained dry in just providing patient care. I just want
to comment that it was a great relief to my own family last year
when I was able to help my father get the funds through the new
Government Social Security---

GUTHRIE: SSI.

STIRLER: ...that my mother's nursing home care is now paid
for. It took a great financial burden off my father and family.
Let me just look at my notes a minute. I think that's really what
I wanted to say to the at-risk group: the legal problems, the
continuing emotional problems, and the need for funding for some
of these things.

N. WEXLER: A brief question. If you had known that there
were psychotherapists available who were also knowledgeable about
genetic and neurological disorders, would that have influenced
your decision about psychotherapists?

STIRLER: Most assuredly, because many of the people in my rap
group mentioned that although they were in treatment, in psychotherapy, their therapists were unable to help them in any way. In
fact, they withdrew from helping them deal with the whole matter
of Huntington's disease. I feel I was just lucky in my choice
that it did not work out that way. I think it would greatly influence my or anybody else's choice if they knew that they were
knowledgeable.

N. WEXLER: Had you looked for somebody like that in the
beginning?

STIRLER: No. I'm afraid it didn't occur to me at that point. I was just desperate.

N. WEXLER: It's possible they don't exist. Thanks.

TESTIMONY OF
IMOGENE SAINBURG, R.N.
DIRECTOR OF NURSES
HARTWYCK NURSING HOME

SAINBURG: I'm Imogene Sainburg. I am Director of Nurses at Hartwyck Nursing Home in Paramas. We are a 35-bed nursing home facility. I was asked to present the nursing home's point of view in the care of the Huntington's patient.

I would like to present a couple of things in my own background first to explain some of my feelings and my reactions. Many years ago I did work in experimental neurology and neurosurgery out in Ohio in a research unit at Ohio State University. We did have at that time a couple of Huntington's patients that we were working with. I also have done a great deal of counseling with disturbed adolescents, and therefore family counseling, which sort of explains my interest in the counseling aspect of this whole thing.

Hartwyck has had in its history two Huntington's patients. The first was there before my particular time, and the last is the one that brought me to Mrs. Guthrie and CCHD and brought me to grips again with Huntington's disease. I'm going to give you a little bit of the history of the woman, not as much as I have written here because obviously we don't need that much. This woman is a 54-year-old widow with five living children. She has a history of approximately 10 or 11 years of severe Huntington's symptoms. She was brought to the nursing home in January 1975, and prior to that had been cared for by her son and daughter-in-law. I think at the time she was brought in, she was brought not so much because of the severity of the symptoms but because of the contin- uing reminder of the disease to the family.

When she came to us her symptoms were not so severe that she could not be contained in an open environment. I've heard several times this afternoon, "nursing home care, nursing home care." I think one of the big problems is Huntington's disease is a disease

of the middle age. This woman was 54, and the average age of my
nursing home patients is 87. She was put in a room with three
other women, the average age of which was 85. My social and recreational program is geared to the 80- to 90-year-old. Many of my
patients are senile or have certain physical disabilities and
impairments which are commensurate with their age: their hearing
and their mobility are impaired; their sight is impaired. They
are not tremendously tolerant of people who are somewhat different
than they are. This comprises one of the largest problems we run
into in nursing home care of the Huntington's patient. Many times
this woman would be very upset because one of the older women
would say, "For heaven's sakes, sit still. Why are you slopping
your food like that? Didn't anyone ever teach you to eat?" Now
this is no help to that patient, nor is it a help to the other
patient.

Another problem we've run into is that these people are
physically active. She did like to walk. She loved to walk
around the block and around the block and around the block. However, the neighbors began getting very upset because her balance
was very unsteady. After a couple of calls from the local police,
stating that there was some person up there who belonged to us who
was disrupting the neighborhood, she did have to be confined to
the grounds, which upset her tremendously. She became extremely
depressed because her family did withdraw totally from her. A
nursing home, by the very fact of its existence in the area of care
that we are--that's a very poor statement--does not have a social
worker on duty. We do not have active counseling available. We
do not have psychotherapy available. Most Huntington's chorea
patients (or Huntington's disease patients), when they are in a
nursing home, are Medicaid patients, which again cuts down the
feasibility of bringing in outside help, because in New Jersey
Medicaid does not pay for social workers and this type of thing.

We contacted Medicaid and we contacted the welfare department
for assistance from their social workers. They are a lot of wonderful people who do a lot of good work, but their response was, "If
we try to involve this woman's family and counsel her family, then
we are logically going to have to counsel every other family of
every other welfare patient that we have, and that's a pretty big
job," so we basically took it over ourselves. Again, I do have a
background in counseling. We did work very hard getting this
patient's family involved, because our feeling was the longer they

withdrew from her, the worse it was going to be to face her when
they had to, and the worse it was going to be to face their own
probability of developing the disease. It's very easy just to put
someone somewhere and that's it. We did try very hard to involve
this family, and we did get a certain amount of involvement, but it
kept slipping away. We spent a great deal of time with that.

We did get her extremely involved with her religious activities.
She was a very religious woman, and volunteers from the church would
come in and take her to services and to picnics and to all sorts
of things. However, her depression did progress, as the Huntington's depression does continue. We were not able, among other
things, to be involved with a neurological center because, again,
she is a Medicaid patient; it doesn't pay, and the family funds
had been depleted many years ago, so there was very little we could
do. We finally did send her to a neurological center, in Livingston,
New Jersey, where she underwent one neurological examination in
March or April of this year.

Her daughter-in-law, incidentally, was the only member of the
family who could be involved with her. She took her shopping, and
things like this. The neurologist recommended immediate hospitalization for treatment of the disease. When the daughter-in-law came
back, we spent a great deal of time discussing this. But somewhere between the nursing home and home a great deal was lost in
the translation and the family was given the message that "Everything is fine with Mama; she will remain in the nursing home.
Things are great." Immediately after this we did have a psychiatric
consultation because we felt that the depression was becoming
dangerous. Here's where Mrs. Guthrie came into play. I went to
the home and spent several hours with the family, exploring alternatives and so on, which they accepted beautifully, and the next
morning came at us with lawyers and court orders to cease and
desist and all sorts of things, because they were beyond the ability
to control this emotional thing which said, "Wow! Mom isn't just
a sick patient in a nursing home. Mom has something that is not
doing well."

As a result of my experience with this patient and family,
the nursing home administration and I have come to a few conclusions, one of which is, before we accept a Huntington's patient,
we are going to have to have assurance from other agencies in our
area that there will be continued counseling of the patient and

the family so that we are not left alone with this patient, and
that when the time comes that this patient cannot be confined in
our facility we are not left alone to deal with this disruptive,
highly traumatic thing for both the patient and the family. The
patient ended up being transported to a neuropsychiatric unit by
a welfare worker whom she had never met in her life, which is a
very cold, horrible thing to have happen.

Another thing that we are very concerned about is that there
be continuing counseling of the youngsters in this family over
the years, a continuing relationship with a counselor so that they
can have basic crisis counseling as things go on. Her 13-year-old
daughter calls us occasionally because there's no one in a crisis
area that she knows. There must be a crisis center dealing with
these youngsters and dealing with the tremendous emotional up-
heavals that they have.

The other thing is that we do feel that basically a
Huntington's patient is out of place in a normal nursing home.
There must be centers where these people can be cared for, with
recreational and social programs which are geared to their age
group so that they're not totally isolated with a group of elderly
people with absolutely no contacts in their own groups.

GUTHRIE: A very important testimony. I feel very strongly
about it. By the way, what was Medicaid paying you for that
patient?

SAINBURG: Medicaid had evaluated her Intermediate Care,
Level B, which pays $24.15 per day for everything. This includes
board and room and any counseling and anything that had to be
done for this patient.

GUTHRIE: I understand that this represented a great hardship
to you.

SAINBURG: Our costs are basically $30 to $31 a day to maintain
a patient in a nursing home. This, again, is true of all Medicaid
patients. However, the biggest thing, notwithstanding the cost or
the loss of money to us, is the fact that this was a tremendously
misplaced patient, that she was totally out of the area that she
should have been in.

GUTHRIE: From what you know of people in the nursing home
industry throughout the country, do you think they would have
similar stories to tell?

SAINBURG: I think they would have. Again, as I said, I
talked to nursing home administrators from various areas of the
country, and the average age of the nursing home patient is somewhere in the 80's. It seems to me that if I, at my age, were
thrown into a place with a bunch of 80-, 90-, and 100-year-old
people to spend my life there--"This is it. This is where you're
going to live the rest of your life. These are your social contacts. These are your friends. Enjoy!"--I think it would be a
very horrible thing to face.

N. WEXLER: I am assuming that your nursing home is in some
way typical of most, that you have terrazzo floors and sharp edges
on furniture and--it's not?

SAINBURG: No. When people ask me about my nursing home, I
say, "There are three kinds of nursing homes: The very modern
institutional type, the older noninstitutional type, and Hartwyck"
[laughter]. We do not have that type of thing. We have linoleum
tile floors. We have eliminated square or rough corners. We have
eliminated this because your geriatric patient also is in great
danger when you have this type of thing around them. Basically,
your facilities are good for a Huntington's patient as far as
physical facilities are concerned, but your patients aren't.

N. WEXLER: The question clearly isn't relevant to your
place. But many nursing homes seem to have legal difficulties
because the patients want to remain mobile and the conditions are
hazardous. Their choice is to risk being sued by the families if
the patient breaks a bone, or to strap the patient in a wheelchair.

SAINBURG: Again, this is not the type of thing that we do.
Because of our smallness, we are able to: (1) be extremely cautious
of all our patients; and (2) our administrators are very cognizant
of these things and they do have two larger nursing homes which,
again, have the same type of precautions that we have in our
nursing home: people are not strapped in; people are not tranquil-
ized, unless it's to protect them from running, for instance, or

something like that. Basically, it's the type of environment that
Huntington's patients could exist in physically, but not emotionally.

TESTIMONY OF
JOSEPH TAUBMAN, ESQ.
NEW YORK, NEW YORK

TAUBMAN: My name is Joseph Taubman. I am a member of the
New York Bar and counsel, virtually since its inception, of the
Committee to Combat Huntington's Disease. I've been involved
since 1958 as attorney for the Guthrie Children's trust funds,
and in that capacity we were concerned with what happened to
Woody Guthrie until his death from Huntington's disease.

There are a number of areas in which legal problems have
arisen I'd like to bring attention to. Here is a clipping from
the Sunday St. Louis Post-Dispatch called "Brain Isn't Sent For
Study: VA Sued." Unfortunately, I don't have the date--it's
not given--but it was sent to me on September 13, 1976.

Your Executive Director is familiar with the problems and
confusions involved with sending brain tissue on the death of a
Huntington's disease patient. I find the fact most disturbing.
It's like a small cloud on the horizon that will get bigger and
bigger. I'm talking about malpractice. For this reason there
may or may not be technical liability. Apparently, judging from
the newspaper account, the widow had requested that the tissue
be sent to a particular hospital. It was not sent; hence, the
suit. If this is it, there is trouble, trouble for this reason.
Juries are generally used in malpractice suits. They are sympathetic to people who are in trouble. While I am neither pro-
plaintiff nor prodefendant, I am concerned for this reason.

I was in St. Louis on the occasion of a meeting of the board
of trustees in March 1976. I spoke to the doctor who was involved
with it. (I was not involved with this litigation.) I requested
a copy of the complaint so that I could at least get the particulars. I am still waiting; I don't have it. I do not believe it
will be forthcoming. One reason, just as Huntington's patients
are concerned about coming out of the closet, in malpractice the
less said the better. This is from the point of view of the medical profession. And so we have a situation where, in terms of
being able to meet the situation, we have no facts. Because of

what I consider the flimsiness of the damage possibility--legal
damage, I'm talking about, arising from any possible liability--
opposed to the problems of encouraging the doctors and the scientific community to expend their time in research and not have it
inhibited by situations like this, I consider it a most unhappy
situation, and I think the Commission should take note of it.
Unfortunately, the medical profession hasn't had much success in
putting a damper on other malpractice suits. Here with Huntington's disease, again, two persons suing for malpractice are minus-
cule compared to the damage that may be done to research in prevention or cure of Huntington's disease.

The second item I want to cover is discrimination. I have a
copy of the article--unfortunately, it's not dated--but a forwarding
letter indicated a Sunday edition of the St. Louis Post-Dispatch.
With the permission of the sender and the recipient, I'd like to
offer this, but this is a garbled copy. Basically, it deals with
the mix of the various laws relating to Huntington's disease
patients getting into nursing homes and the discrimination in
relation to it.

The proposal was that a class action suit be brought to
prevent such discrimination. I think the proposal is excellent,
whether it can in fact be realized. This was submitted to the
CCHD to bring the class action. I have recommended approval of
it, but whether it can be implemented--and here's another factor
that I will mention in a few moments. It seems to me the technique
of getting at the guts of some of the areas where the medical
problems, the care problems in particular, and the legal problems
come together, or should I say clash, a proper case can be made of
a general nature. I don't mean that Miss A had a problem of insurance with a particular company, but I'm talking about a general
problem such as this. The whole area can be exposed to sunlight,
so to speak.

The third area for the Commission to take note is perhaps to
come to some definition of standards and criteria for genetic counseling. I mention that because--and this was purely hearsay--I
know of one instance where a person allegedly held himself or herself out as a genetic counselor. Based upon my knowledge of the
background of that person, I questioned their qualification. It
seems to me that a report from the Commission should take note of
the presence of any, if any, legal standards presently in being

as to that. Offhand, I don't know of any in the State of New York,
for example. I may be wrong, but I don't know of any licensing requirements or any particular standards or criteria for holding one-
self out as a genetic counselor.

The fourth area is generally privacy and confidentiality. I
think, in the main, good marks can come to the fact that there is an
awareness of this area. However, in connection with any studies
that may be proposed by the Commission, efforts should be made to
balance the two aspects of privacy and confidentiality with the
encouragement of those who have the information to come forth and
produce it with appropriate safeguards.

The fifth area is one that I think will take a great deal of
exploration. It's there. We pass it all the time, and only the
afflicted and their families are painfully aware of it. It put it
under the category of "domestic relations." They call it divorce.
I refer to the fact that in a very real sense we are Neanderthal
about our knowledge and treatment, in the legal sense, of H.D.
families, and they can extend this to afflicted and kindred
diseases. I've practiced law for more than 30 years, and yet I
can say that the attention of the Bar is not given to those who
are minorities; in a sense, H.D. people are minorities. The laws
of divorce are not directed to them.

It seems to me that the only way, apart from noting it in your
report, that you're going to get any long-range results is by
calling a conference of related health organizations. I don't mean
limited to Huntington's disease at all, but those who have problems
with the complete destruction of family life. Then, after study
of these problems in such a conference, come out with an overview
to be able, by reason of the fact that this represents a coalition
of substantial number, to go to the American Bar Association and
other Bar associations and say, "These are problems." You're
looking in a distorted mirror at the problems because the ones who
can get something done are the lawyers and Bar associations. I
don't think it will come initially from Congress or the State leg-
islatures, as such. The kind of thing I'm referring to is what
happened to the Uniform Donor Card Act. Here the problems are
much more complex, much more in need of unraveling and analysis
and recommendations.

The next category I call "Who/Legal." This is a troublesome area, because who will deliver the legal services that are required in the numerous instances of discrimination of all kinds against persons and the families with H.D. (or Huntington's disease)? Let me run through various categories who might do something.

Public Interest Firms: Yes and no. Let's face it. The health, or should I say disease, has no glamour. There are hundreds of lawyers and volunteer lawyers for the arts, literally hundreds. Many of them may not have the knowledge and background to do much, but it is glamorous. There are lawyers involved with particular causes, whether in other public interest battles, whether the consumer advocacy, or what have you. Those, in a sense, are glamorous. But who can be involved on a consistent basis in behalf of poor people who are afflicted?

In terms of public interest organizations, perhaps the Commission might suggest and recommend that there be at least one public interest firm in the United States devoted to the area of neurological and genetic disorders so that they can pay attention specifically to these areas, to bring on a class action of the kinds I've indicated. I strongly suspect that no organization presently involved with Huntington's disease has the funds to actually go ahead and carry on a legal battle of this magnitude all the way down the line.

The second category is Legal Aid Society: I suspect that there it's a matter of getting an individual who is sufficiently committed. Legal Aid people are fine, but this is one of hundreds of different types of legal problems that they get, and they thrust their emphasis against discrimination in relation to H.D., and it will not get any particular attention.

The third category comes under the fancy Latin phrase "pro bona publico," which means "for the public good," those members of the Bar in private practice who generally contribute some of their time to really good causes. I submit that in general this is not, in contemplation of pro bona publico, a particularly worthy cause because it doesn't have the glamour of other causes, and so you're not likely to get much support from a pro bona publico basis. Perhaps in the Commission report you might consider some H.D.

ombudsman, someone with a legal background who can correlate the
different aspects of problems in relation to Huntington's disease
or perhaps, if that's too narrow, neurological and genetic
diseases. "Ombudsman" is a Scandinavian term meaning, in effect,
"public defender." Applying that concept, we don't have it here.
It may be in a few states. In New York you have a public administrator. We have one now who is concerned with unknown heirs, which
really don't exist, but if they took a fraction of their interest
in this kind of thing, it would be much more productive. But,
again, there is no existing machinery or mechanism for it.

Finally, I refer to the category of intelligence. By "intelligence," I mean knowledge and inclination. There is no machinery for
really organizing information of a legal nature as to what the
problems are. It just doesn't exist. The instance, for example,
that I spoke about: domestic relations. I've been associated for
many, many years with Huntington's disease in one category or
another, and yet the thrust of this came from Dr. Arthur Falek in
Atlanta, Georgia, at a meeting of the trustees. In one of the
groups we had, in terms of a game-problem type of solution, there
was a doctor who felt the problem and brought it into focus. We
don't have the machinery yet for bringing these problems into focus.
I suspect that perhaps what is required is for the doctors and
lawyers to talk to each other a little more, and not through
malpractice suits.

GUTHRIE: Thank you very much.

TESTIMONY OF
AUDREY HEIMLER, M.S.
GENETIC COUNSELOR
LONG ISLAND JEWISH HILLSIDE MEDICAL CENTER

HEIMLER: I'm Audrey Heimler, genetic counselor at Long Island
Jewish Hillside Medical Center. My first professional experience
as a genetic counselor was with H.D. families at Creedmoor Institute. I counseled approximately 30 to 40 families in collaboration
with Drs. John Whittier and Charles Korenyi before going on to
work in a genetics clinic where the patients represent a wide range
of genetic diseases, including patients with H.D. The problems in
families with H.D. impress me still as more difficult than in any
other single disorder.

All individuals at risk for H.D. worry that they will
eventually develop the symptoms. The second universal concern is
about reproduction. Most patients have the need for verbal cathar-
sis, explanation of the genetic mode of transmission, and understanding the clinical features of H.D. Issues discussed in genetic
counseling include whether to marry, whether to inform their
marriage partner of the risk, pregnancy, adoption, artificial
insemination, contraception, sterilization, how to inform family
members, social stigma, career choices, and insurance problems.
Other practical considerations include planning and management for
the H.D. patient, when to hospitalize and how to arrange this, how
to compensate for the inability of a spouse or parent to function
adequately, when and how to inform children of the genetic risk,
and how to evaluate and deal with the child's response to this
information as well as the child's response to the affected parent.

It is not unusual for the genetic counselor to meet with an
at-risk individual several times before the barriers of denial and
hostility are surrendered so that the underlying concerns can
begin to emerge. Because the concern over the disease encroaches
upon many aspects of the lives of even those who never develop
symptoms, ongoing supportive counseling is required and some at-
risk patients need referral to a psychologist or psychiatrist.

It is imperative that relatives of H.D. patients have the
opportunity to make an informed decision regarding marriage and
reproduction. At the present time, physicians are prevented by
the existing laws from approaching at-risk relatives of their
parents. Patients must assume responsibility for informing other
family members, but often are resistant to this suggestion or meet
with little success, even outright abuse, when they attempt to
discharge this obligation. The same applies to efforts to obtain
medical records for possible H.D. patients in order to confirm
the genetic transmission of the disease.

Unlike most genetic disorders, where the counselee is either
the affected individual or the parents of the patient, for H.D.
the counselee is more often an at-risk symptom-free individual or
the spouse, single parent, sib, or grown-up child of an affected
individual. For each patient, there are numerous relatives who
could benefit from genetic counseling. The number of persons

requiring genetic counseling for H.D. is not insignificant, and the
time and personnel required for this task is considerable.

The person providing genetic counseling should be an individual
with formal training on the graduate level in genetics and counseling, in addition to training in other disciplines, in some cases.
This person should have the following prerequisites:

1. Knowledge of autosomal dominant transmission.

2. Knowledge of the clinical and biochemical features
   of H.D.

3. Psychological counseling skills.

4. Ability to obtain and record a detailed family history
   for the identification of at-risk relatives.

5. Adequate time for long-term counseling of the patient
   and other concerned members of the family.

6. Knowledge of community resources for the H.D. family.

At the present time, the number of individuals trained to
provide genetic counseling is inadequate to the need. I respectfully submit the following recommendations:

1. Genetic counselors should be funded to work with H.D.
families. I agree with others who have spoken before me that
ideally the service could be performed in a neurogenetic clinic.
It seems to me that it would be practical to consider only a
limited number of neurogenetic clinics throughout the United States,
so that geographically patients who are located all throughout the
country or the world would need to have access closer to their
homes. Not all would be residing near a large medical center
where such a service would be available so that certainly the
referring physician should consider referring the patient to a
medical center where there is a genetic service.

Where referral of H.D. patients to a specialized clinic
or medical center is not possible for genetic counseling on an
ongoing basis, regional satellite genetic clinics should be established for the diagnosis and counseling of genetic disorders,

staffed by physicians and allied health professionals under the supervision of the nearest medical genetic unit. With Federal subsidization, these services could be provided on a sliding scale.

2. The training of health professionals who work with families with H.D. should include the prerequisites listed above, with particular emphasis on the training required to counsel children and adolescents in H.D. families when this is requested by the parents. At the present time, parents who are counseled are generally instructed on how they could help their children, but a single parent who is not affected is not always able to do this.

3. Consideration should be given to an alternative to the present legal restrictions regarding confidentiality which restrict the ability of the physician to contact at-risk family members. I, too, am concerned for the privacy of individuals in H.D. families, but I'm also concerned for the individual who goes on to reproduce without knowledge of his or her risk.

4. Medical insurance companies, including Medicaid, must be directed to include coverage for genetic counseling even when the individual is symptom free. In preparing this report, I made several calls to medical insurance companies in the city of New York to determine whether or not benefits would be available for genetic counseling if an individual had no symptoms, no diagnosis. I talked with several very confused individuals and nobody seemed to feel the coverage would be available without a diagnosis.

5. A central registry of individuals with H.D. should be considered to permit verification of the diagnosis in individuals with symptoms, and, of course, consideration for confidentiality.

6. Research efforts should continue to seek the underlying defect which will, in turn, make carrier detection, prenatal diagnosis, and treatment available. But carrier detection without treatment to prevent irreversible central nervous system damage would not be beneficial, in my opinion.

With increased availability of accurate, compassionate genetic counseling, the all-pervading psychosocial concerns that exist within H.D. families could be ameliorated and the incidence of the disease reduced, at least within families where this is the desired alternative.

McKHANN: That's a very nice statement. You may have written the Commission's report for them. Let me raise one point with you, if I could. You make the statement, "carrier detection without treatment to prevent irreversible central nervous system damage would not be beneficial." I agree with what you're saying, but it seems possible to me that that may be a necessary interim step on the way to understanding the basic disease mechanism. I think one of your predecessors brought up the point that this kind of information could be obtained and not necessarily provided to the individual.

HEIMLER: This is done during research on other genetic diseases also, where prenatal diagnosis becomes available, for instance, in an autosomal disorder. It's important to be able to tell the difference between a healthy carrier of the disorder, which can be true in some genetic diseases, or between that fetus and the fetus who will actually have the disease. In other words, you wouldn't want to abort a fetus who would be clinically free of signs along with those who would have the disease.

During the stage where the research is in a learning stage, let's say, patients who are cooperating understand that they are cooperating for research, but not for diagnosis. I think perhaps this is necessary for Huntington's disease also in order to learn. With Huntington's disease, long-term followup of patients would be needed before you could verify whether the individual identified prenatally or early in life will eventually develop the disease, whether that 50-50--how it will fall for each individual tested. It will be a long time between the development of tests and the verification of the diagnosis made at that point, and you know this has to be considered for the people who are tested and waiting for results.

TESTIMONY OF
DAWN HATTER

HATTER: My name is Dawn Hatter. I am 12 years old, and I am in the National Huntington's Disease Association. When I first

found out about H.D. I was in the third grade. At that time, I
really didn't know much about it because I was too young. When
I'd have my friends over and stuff, the other kids would say that
my mother was drunk and that, "How come your mother is always
losing her balance?" The only thing that I could say was, "She is
not." I couldn't understand much because I didn't understand that
much at that time.

When she got worse she started to get mean and would always
hit me and my brother. Once she tried to take an overdose of
nerve pills. Before she went to the hospital she was always
falling and hurting herslef. She broke her wrist and was falling
up and down the stairs, off chairs, and burning herself on cigarettes and the stove.

When she went into Central Islip Hospital she would come for
the weekends, and in the beginning she was okay. But she cried
when she had to go back. Then she got bad and she would come home
and start to say the doctors were coming to get her or the doctors
were here, and to get them out of here.

Then she went to the nursing home, and she was good. But
then she kept fighting with all the other people, the patients,
the nurses, and then she said she had to go back to C.I. Hospital.
When she came home from the nursing home, she would wave to all
the people in the cars. When my father would say, "Stop," she
would tell him she would not. When I went to see her in the
nursing home, I would say, "Hi, mom," and she would say, "Who are
you?" She always had bruises on her legs, arms, feet, hands and
head.

When she was living at home, my brother and I had a lot more
chores to do. I had to help cook, clean, wash, and help take care
of her because she would always sleep. My father had to work
harder and longer to pay the bills and to get more money for the
doctors, drug stores, and nursing home. He also had to pay for
the housekeepers to come and take care of the house, but then he
found out that they were drinking so he had to fire them and leave
us alone, to go to work. I would go shopping with my father to
buy the food for our house. I had just wished that somebody
could help.

Now I have to worry about me and my brother, who is 16, getting it and my aunt and uncle who have it and all the rest of the adults and kids at risk. If we had enough money to give to research, then maybe they can find a cure for it before we are old enough to get it. I feel that I have no time to worry, just to help raise money for the people who have it. Everybody can help if they try. My mother was only 33 years old when she died in 1975 of Huntington's disease.

GUTHRIE: I'll ask you a question, Dawn. Do you know about what research is going on?

HATTER: Well, yes and no, but I don't really understand it.

GUTHRIE: But you do know that there is a lot of money being spent for research? And you do know that a lot of people care or they wouldn't be here, right? I would hope that you would feel good knowing that people like you, all the people here, and all the people who aren't here that we know about are doing a great deal, and we're going to do more so that you don't have to worry about the future. We do want you to keep helping and trying in the way that you're doing and to feel good because you're helping. Do you know how many people there are who could help and don't help? A lot of them, aren't there. That's unfortunate, because they don't know that with their help we could do more. I want you to feel good, and I thank you for coming.

TESTIMONY OF
JESSICA DAVIS, M.D.

DAVIS: Thank you. It's a great privilege to have been asked to come and speak with you. I am a pediatrician who is interested in the care of the handicapped individual and also deals with their families in terms of human development; and lastly, I am a medical geneticist. I think that some of the speakers, at least the ones that I heard, have already touched on all of the essential points, but I would just like to respond to some of these I heard today and kind of tell you my thoughts on what's needed.

I run a genetics program which has just been designated as a regional center. We provide services in Nassau County, see patients from Queens, and we have some patients occasionally from far distant parts. In addition, as of November 1 we will be starting

a large satellite program in another county which has had no
genetic services up until the present time.

We've seen an awful lot of individuals and families over the
years, both at North Shore and Einstein, and certainly at the home
base, which is New York Hospital, Cornell University. All kinds of
things, really, are needed. I can't stress enough the need for
education. I think this is the message that comes through at
every single organizational meeting, regional meeting that I
attend. One cannot do enough, even if this means going out late
at night, talking to professional groups, speaking to individual
health providers. I'm not just stressing education for the lay
public. Education for individuals at risk and individuals who are
known to have the problem, education for my colleagues in all
branches of medicine, the young physicians, physicians in training
as well as the older individuals who are working in an academic
setting or out in the field in practice of one sort or another:
This really has to be done.

At the same time, education is needed for all health care
providers. This means social service, nursing. Even the aides
in the hospital are interested and concerned and often times are
the best people to deal with the patients and their families and
really give us physicians some clues as to what's going on.
People need to know, and this probably should happen on an annual
basis because knowledge is very fast moving in our field and
people have to be updated constantly.

You have to know about the disorder. You have to know what's
available. You have to know about programs in your geographic
area and how to reach individuals who have the capability of providing either complete or incomplete services, but at least good
services. These individuals have to be identified. They are identified at the moment through booklets put out through your organi-
zation--I have a whole file of these letters and scientific docu-
ments--but also through the March of Dimes National Foundation,
the university program where anybody could phone and instantly get
a number through the computer as to who might help them in their
area, the National Genetics Foundation and its local chapters. I
think that has to be emphasized, how you can get information if you
think you are at risk.

I also feel that we need some guidelines. These should be developed on a national basis; probably on an international basis. I'm really not into that as yet, though. In my discussions with my colleagues in genetics, I think we are talking about the real probability of a national genetics program. I think the needs and special problems of Huntington's disease ought to be fit into an overall plan. I think we need some protocols. I don't think these really exist in terms of what kinds of information we're all getting: some places, it's really excellent; other places, it's fair; some places, it's just poor.

What could one do in terms of additional studies? Are there things one can do that might involve contacting colleagues in other parts of the country? I think this kind of protocol has to be circulated amongst medical geneticists, neurologists, psychiatrists, and people in rehabilitation medicine who often-times are really not involved in learning about genetics or genetic problems.

I think Mr. Taubman talked about confidentiality, invasion of individual privacy, et cetera. I, too, am concerned about this, and I'm also concerned with the registry problem. Obviously, one really needs data in order to be helpful in the long run, but it has to be collected with some kinds of guidelines. Again, a proto-col is needed there and some control of this data and how it's used. I think that really comes under the reaches of the Federal Government and perhaps Federal guidelines for state governments to follow, I don't know. I think maybe that's important.

I feel we also need some guidelines on how the families are told about this particular problem. There is no monitoring (I mean national basis now) of genetic counseling. There was one attempt. I think it's been long standing. They've done some work with data collection now, looking to see what's really going on on a daily basis in each genetics counseling clinic on the eastern seaboard. I think more of that needs to be done and per-haps guidelines for what constitutes good genetic counseling. Certainly, the American Society of Neurogenetics has a committee for this purpose, and I think they should, too, be involved in drawing up these protocols.

Another problem I want to address myself to is in terms of funding and finances and psychologic, and I'm going to try to

expand on that. I would like to tell you that, at least in New
York City, the Task Force on Medical Genetics, which is kind of an
ad hoc group that likes to meet and talk, has committed funding
for genetic services. I am chairperson of that committee. We are
now in the process of serious discussion with Blue Cross/Blue
Shield and are trying to get funding for all genetic services. I
have listed just about every task and have also included a fee
schedule for genetic counseling. We're just at the talking part.

We are now reviewing fee schedules from out of the city, and
hopefully some kind of decision will be reached in the next few
months. This will be first. I think one of the things that we're
stressing is that with each new test or service that becomes available with respect to genetic problems, there is some mechanism so
that years don't have to go by for families that are not with
hospital services. For those of you who don't know what services
cost, I'll just throw a few figures out for you: counseling sessions in the city, from $50 to $75 per session or two sessions,
depending upon how generous people are with their time, and then I
think most specify four or five or six sessions. They just get
locked into that one fee. That is basically what one would try to
collect or could collect if this were available. In terms of lab
fees, some of our studies run as high as $300; others, as low as
$15. Anything that would expedite cheap, simple tests that could
be available at the university and are reliable is the route that
I think we should go. Those kinds of things should be and could
be included.

What I would really like to stress the need for is dollars
for research. I'm a clinician. I work very closely and have
spent all my life with people doing basic research in neurologic
sciences, and I feel that this must not be neglected. Everything
that we've been able to accomplish in clinical labs has really
depended on our close collaboration and on their basic discoveries.
I think what would help us now is a huge rush of technology made
available by colleagues who have spent many hours at their micro-
scopes and in their laboratories, and I feel they really need
support. I think there should also be a group to speak for the
people in Atlanta who are drawing up some quality control guidelines
for a variety of genetic disorders.

Lastly, the legal questions are very difficult for me. I'm
not an attorney. I happen to be married to one. We have a very

good talking relationship, and that's the best way to settle
disputes between doctors and lawyers. He has been extremely
helpful as a resource in terms of helping me with my problems,
so I felt that the suggestion of someone with expertise rather
than my picking my spouse's brains every evening would be terribly
helpful for the genetic questions. Of particular recent importance
to us, however, is the issue of adoption. I'd just like to tell
you about one of our recent sessions with four families who have
adopted children who are at risk. Each was unaware of the history
of Huntington's disease at the time of adoption, so we now have
four families who have children who are at risk with this disorder
whom we have now been able to document through our efforts at
getting records. We don't really know what to do. There are a
lot of problems that arise, problems of what we do with this information about the children. When is this disclosed? How is it
going to be disclosed?

We have siblings in all of these families who are not blood
relatives but who do have the responsibility for caring for these
very young children. All the children who are adopted happen to
be the youngest children in the families.

The question is raised about financial burden to the state
clinic, and also what the responsibility is for the social
agencies in the future now that this disorder has really sort of
come to light. How does one plan for the health needs of an individual financially, spiritually, et cetera, particularly with
parents who are now getting along in years and---

N. WEXLER: I'm not sure if I should ask you or your husband
or Mr. Taubman, but what are the problems in getting tissues for
research, particularly brain tissue? The autopsy rate has been
declining radically across the country. There are approximately
one-fourth to one-third running autopsies now because the threat
of malpractice suits is so high. After opening the cranium and
finding a different disease, the doctor would be in trouble, so
they opt not to do autopsies, which means that we can't get that
tissue for research. Do you have any suggestions as to how we
might get around that problem?

DAVIS: First of all, I think everybody looks at malpractice
actively. We have not had this problem. The reason we have not

had this problem is that we have really gotten the education of
the physician and family and really tried to explain, particularly
with your degenerative processes, why it is necessary to have
accurate information. I think that it just takes effort and it
takes that personal kind of contact and the kind of contact situation of physician to physician and family person to physician in
a calm atmosphere to try to get this discussed.

I think one of the things that we've been talking about is
preserving tissues and putting them in a center and issuing interstate regulations, to which most of us just kind of say, "Well, we
know they're there, but we're really not..." When it comes to
transporting tissues to Canada, which we all do because there is
tremendous research going on in genetics and good people up there,
then we'll get into some sticky thing with Customs. We have to
get some license, and I don't know if those people know that, so
they need some information. This could go to heads of departments;
it can be discussed with clinical pathologists and is something
that could be brought to the physician and discussed again. I
think this needs more work.

TESTIMONY OF
VERA M. BURKE
DIRECTOR, COMMUNITY HOMEMAKERS' SERVICES
JEWISH FAMILY SERVICES
PRESENTED BY IRENE KELLY

KELLY: Vera M. Burke, Director of Community Homemakers'
Services of Jewish Family Service of New York City, was unable to
attend but has written a brief paper about homemaker care. My
name is Irene Kelly, and I'm from Rush Presbyterian-St. Luke's
Hospital in Chicago.

"The current awareness in Congress, in the newspapers, and
elsewhere of the need for in-home health services, including homemakers and home health aides as an alternative to nursing home care,
underscores the urgency of developing these in-home services for
the care of the chronically ill patient, whatever be the diagnostic
category.

"Quality home health services should be an integral part of a
continuum of health care available nationwide. But in the absense
of such a nationwide program, voluntary agencies have a responsibility

to establish quality home care programs to serve as a model for the development of a nationwide program under public auspices. A person suffering from a chronic illness such as Huntington's chorea, muscular dystrophy, multiple sclerosis, amyotrophic lateral sclerosis, et cetera, and living on a fixed income, cannot pay for the kind of home help that is necessary to enable him or her to remain in his or her own home; and yet to place such a patient in an institution is to deprive him or her of the opportunity to remain in his or her own home as long as it is medically possible.

"According to the Cost of Living Index, a family of four living in New York City requires a minimum of $12,000 for a moderate standard of living; yet to be eligible for Medicaid that same family income may not exceed $5,000 a year. It behooves us, therefore, to take a look at a family having one member with a chronic illness. Such a person requiring in-home care is unable to meet the cost of such care and may be forced to go into an institutional setting, costing the community more in terms of actual dollars and cents and an immeasurable amount of emotional costs that cannot be equated in terms of dollars.

"Chronic illness in the family presents special problems in adaptation to family members, and these problems are especially disturbing in their effect if the ill person is the mother of young or adolescent children. We know that children suffer from separation from the mother and maternal support whenever she has to be hospitalized for any reason; but chronic illness, so difficult for adults to understand, places an even greater burden upon the children because its mystery is even more difficult for them to comprehend and to cope with. Because of the high cost of providing in-home services to families with patients with a chronic illness, voluntary agencies cannot fulfill the enormous need that exists in the community but can set up programs to serve as models for national health programs to follow in establishing appropriate services in the home. We feel that there are many ways whereby a concerned community can take action. Among them are:

"1. To help bring about national and statewide legislation that would fund the development of homemaker/home health aide programs in every community, and broaden eligibility requirements for public financing on more realistic financial criteria.

"2. To provide under existing Medicare and Medicaid programs funds for training and supervising homemakers and home health aides so as to meet standards as defined by the National Council for Homemaker/Home Health Aide Services.

"3. To assure supervision by either a social worker or a nurse of the homemaker/home health aide so as to coordinate the helper's duties with the patient's needs, medical or psychiatric recommendations, and the use of help as it affects other family members.

"4. To develop in the community sources of communication between agencies, hospitals, and medical people so that all would be aware of the available community resources and utilize them to the optimum."

GUTHRIE: Another aspect of care, in terms of sending somebody out to the home, which is very important. Thank you very much.

McKHANN: I think we've had a long session. Is there anyone who would like to appear before us? [No response.] Then I think we'll consider the meeting adjourned. Thank you for coming.

New York, New York   September 22, 1976

ROSLYN ALPERT
LIVINGSTON, NEW JERSEY   AUGUST 29, 1976

        In answer to your request for information on the
experiences and problems of H.D. families, I will attempt
to document our family's story.

        My grandmother (maternal) died in 1932 (approximately)
in Overbrook Hospital. She was admitted with a diagnosis
of having had a nervous breakdown. We realize, now, that
many diseases and disorders were given the collective name
"nervous breakdown," because medical personnel were unaware
of the real cause. My father's recall of her symptoms
coincides with my mother's, and with what we now know to be
symptomatic of H.D.

        My mother had always been a "nervous" person, but when
she was in her early forties, we began to realize that her
condition was something more. She began to have choreic
movements, lapses of memory, and loss of balance and sense
of touch. Our family doctor diagnosed her condition as
Parkinson's Disease, but because of her progressive debilitation and lack of relief of symptoms, we took her to a
neurologist, who diagnosed her affliction as Huntington's
Disease.

        My mother's condition progressively worsened. She
would fall out of bed at night and be knocked unconscious;
she would drop things and not be aware of it until she saw
them on the floor. My father could not leave her alone, so
he hired a practical nurse as a companion for her while he
was at work. However, the symptomatic change of character
for H.D. victims caused much friction, and he was unable to
keep companions for her.

        The next step was a nursing home. Unfortunately,
because H.D. and its symptoms have been somewhat obscured,
nursing home operators and their personnel (and many doctors
and other medical people) know very little about H.D. and
treat the victim as a mental patient, offering little or no
physical therapy. My mother's mind was untouched, but even
now, I still shudder at the feelings of restriction and
rejection she must have felt at her treatment and lack of
physical assistance.   She had been a most placid, kind,

sensitive person, but with the reaction to her treatment and personality change, she became hostile and agressive, and a move was necessitated--to Overbrook Hospital, where her mother had died. The connotation of the name and awareness that it was a mental institution was horribly demoralizing to all of us, including my mother.

She received superior care and treatment at the hospital, because all personnel were professional. However, even here, there was unawareness of the proper treatment and therapy for H.D. victims. Her condition worsened progressively, and she became unable to speak, although we could tell from her eyes that she knew what we were talking about. Her jaw and throat muscles became affected and she ate and drank with much difficulty. She became agitated because of the problem and her involuntary movements increased. The nurses were afraid she would injure herself, because she had lost so much weight (her digestive system was no longer absorbing the food she ingested), so they tied her hands to the sides of the bed during and after eating time. On the day of her death, she had a great deal of difficulty, became extremely agitated, and while the nurse left the room with her dishes after feeding her, the gauze bands loosened and she slipped in-between the mattress and the side of the bed. The pressure on her chest kept her from breathing and she died.

I couldn't begin to describe the terrible physical and mental anguish that accompanied our visits to the nursing home and hospital. To see a loved one deteriorate, with no way to help and no place to go for proper care, is a tragedy no one should have to experience.

My husband and I had two children when we became aware of the genetic consequences of H.D. He wanted more children, so we went to see Dr. Flicker, the neurologist who diagnosed my mother's condition. Instead of referring us to a genetic counselling service, of which there are so few, he said he saw no symptoms in me, and to go ahead and have more children if we wanted them. So, now, I am at risk, with four children, and so is my brother, with three.

My mother's first cousin has since come down with H.D. in his early seventies, and has deteriorated very rapidly. My aunt, my mother's sister, has developed choreic movements, and although her family physician has diagnosed her condition as Parkinson's Disease, we feel that she may also be an H.D. victim.

    If this lengthy narrative has any meaning it is to
impress upon the reader and listener the desperate need for
a national program of education, instruction for doctors,
nurses, and other medical personnel (we in N.H.D.A. are
constantly educating doctors, etc. who know little or nothing
about H.D., whereas we, who are in afflicted families, have
learned by necessity), trained physical therapists, knowledgeable genetic counselors who are easily available, and above
all, hospitals and nursing homes where patients who can no
longer be cared for at home can be sent with the comforting
knowledge that their affliction is understood and being
treated properly. The primary needs, and ones which are
impossible without federal assistance, are discovery of the
cause of H.D., tests, especially including prenatal, for
victims of the disease, and methods of treatment and cure.

New York, New York   September 22, 1976

ROBERT W. BARTLETT
CAMP HILL, PENNSYLVANIA   MAY 26, 1977

        This is my statement concerning the effect of Huntington's
disease on my family.

        I am not a writer and, on this subject, I am filled with
sorrows. Therefore, please be patient with my ramblings. I
will make a sincere try at getting my point across to you.

        My wife Romaine and I have been married for 28 years. Dur-
ing our courtship, I saw that her father was very ill. Staggered
gait, slurred speech, poor coordination, etc. When the subject of his health came up I was told he had multiple sclerosis.
The family doctor said so; one or two other doctors said so.
After we were married and my father-in-law's health began to
deteriorate even more, we took him to Pittsburgh for more diagnoses. Several new diseases were discussed. The final diagnosis
of three or four doctors was a vague reference to multiple sclerosis or Parkinson's and even one veiled hint at locomotor ataxia
(syphilis). Unsatisfied, we went to Philadelphia Children's
Hospital where, after 2 weeks of study, it was finally called
Huntington's chorea. Very hush-hush. No one wanted to talk
about it. No one seemed to know what to do about it either.
(This was in the early '50s.) We returned to our home in Harrisburg, Pennsylvania, and set out to find if there was a doctor
in the city who knew anything about H.D. We found one: a
Dr. Dennison, since deceased. He looked at my father-in-law
and stated that it was a "textbook case." On leaving his
office, he looked straight into my wife's face and said, "My
dear, you have GOT to get it!" That statement seems very blunt
but it was the first time anyone had the guts to face reality.

        By this time, our first child was 2½ years old. Needless
to say, he was our only child!

        So much for background.

        My wife first showed signs of problems about 1967. Meno-
pause seemed to coincide with the onset of H.D. There was
some depression and a definite loss of initiative and energy.
No stagger, no slurred speech. Fretful, unnecessary worries
became frequent. When discussed, she blamed everything on
menopause. However, we noticed that just one can of beer

would cause a slight speech problem and a balance problem.
In these early stages, she dropped things more than a normal
person would: dishes, combs, etc.

It should be said about here that my wife's father
died a very slow and horrible death, with all the grotesque
H.D. symptoms. He was well cared for in the Dauphin County
Home but H.D. made a complete gnarled, grunting vegetable
of him in the final 2 years. During his 8 final years of
hospitalization, my wife visited him every week. The H.D.
symptoms had a profound effect on her, I am sure, and must
have given her cause to think when she began to have problems.
However, she never spoke to me about them.

Now, back to the story.

Slowly, my wife's "depression" became more severe. She
lost interest in more and more activities. She gave up her
work in my studio (bookkeeping, typing, errands, etc.). She
said she could not think clearly enough to work with figures.
Handwriting began to show marked deterioration. She continued
to withdraw from everyday life more and more. She went to a
psychiatrist for 7½ years, had hospitalizations for "depression" and about 30 shock treatments. In my opinion, this
psychiatrist did us very big disservice. When my wife failed
to make the normal response to his treatments, he should have
sought other avenues of diagnosis and treatment.

Finally, when it was obvious to me that the psychiatrist
was not helping, I sought the services of a trusted family doctor. He had my wife hospitalized for 3 days and a team of
several doctors explored for everything...and came up with H.D.
Neither my wife nor her "shrink" would accept this diagnosis.

My wife Romaine continued to become more ill. Her worries
became all-consuming. She lost her sense of humor, lost interest in books and newspapers, said her attention span was too
short and she couldn't retain what she was reading. Housework
became "overwhelming." Her energy level was extremely low.
She slept 14 hours a night. Another unusual ramification I
noticed was a fear of water, bathing, etc. She began to get
very careless about her personal hygiene. She was just too
tired to care. We tried to discuss matters, but she was unable
to accept H.D., so our discussions ended. One day in summer
1976 she was more uptight than usual and wanted to see a psychiatrist immediately. Hers was out of town, so I took her to

the local Crisis Intervention Center (Camp Hill, Pennsylvania).
They calmed her, and her "shrink" later prescribed some pretty
strong tranquilizers. This kept a lid on things. Symptoms
continued to increase in severity so I, alone, confronted her
psychiatrist about H.D. and facing FACTS! He said OK. I
said, "How about an H.D. research place somewhere?" He said,
"Fine." I mentioned three that I had heard of. He said, "Fine,"
but gave no help at all. He said he would forward Romaine's
medical records to whomever I chose to send her to. He did
nothing to help me. He was poorly informed or just plain lazy.

I asked three women from the local Committee to Combat
Huntington's Disease to come by to counsel us. My wife received
them but did not enter the conversation. The ladies were most
helpful, especially with literature from the New York office
which lists places that one may take a patient for help.
After 3 solid days of phoning every place I could find in the
east, I got a Dr. Neophitides at the National Institutes of
Health. He was marvelous! Truthful! Frank! Informed!
And dedicated. I got my Congressman, William Goodling, to
help to have Romaine admitted to NIH and quickly. NIH said
yes and we took her to Dr. Neophitides on November 8, 1976.
He did whatever tests and research he could on her, and she
returned home after 6 days.

Neophitides needed a full family history, so he asked
if our 24-year-old son could come to Bethesda for his research
work. Our son Kevin went and was given a spinal tap and other
tests which the researchers need. NIH said Kevin was too young
to make a diagnosis of possible H.D. He shows no signs of it
thus far, but Neophitides said it would be a good idea if
Kevin remained childless. He stated that no cure is at hand
and the only way known to strike back at H.D. is to go childless.

My wife is now in the Cumberland County Nursing Home,
Carlisle, Pennsylvania. She is receiving very sympathetic
care from good doctors and great, well-trained social workers.
The nursing help is kind to her and she seems to be relieved
of the responsibilities of home.

The financial effects of H.D. on this family have been
monstrous. For one 3-year period, Romaine's prescriptions
cost over $100 per month. Psychiatry is costly! Blue Cross
and Blue Shield took care of the four hospitalizations.

The emotional effects on the family are devastating! My son now must question every time he fumbles or drops something...every time his tongue gets tied...every time he thinks of a family of his own.

My recommendations as to steps which could be taken to help H.D. families are as follows:

1. Through publicity to all segments of the population, try to track down every living H.D. patient. Give them the facts and encourage them to submit to sterilization, NOW! Especially alert our doctors. They see it before anyone else, but our experience showed doctors to be rather uninformed and careless.

2. Give the Neophitides of the country all the help and money that you can so that their research can move faster. A dedicated research man like Dr. Neophitides is one of our country's most valuable assets. Try to get them what they need!

3. Encourage frankness about H.D. My wife's relatives still only mention H.D. in hushed tones and only to other family members. It's time to get H.D. out into the light! If potential victims have seen H.D. in their family, the way we did, getting sterilized would be a cause for rejoicing! Unlike cancer, H.D. can be stopped! Once people know the facts, they will choose to stop it!

4. Financially, we should classify H.D. as a "catastrophic illness." Generally, it runs its course in 15 to 20 years; this is a long time. We, during our worst hours, found very adequate help from the Visiting Nurse Association and Homemakers, Inc. Both were good and fees were minimal.

I cannot think of anything more that I want to say at this time. However, all the facets and facts of the effect of H.D. on our family could fill a book. Please feel free to call on us if we can help you to make your decisions.

New York, New York   September 22, 1976

JULIA D. BRADY FOR
JUNE D. DUNN
WILMINGTON, DELAWARE   MAY 17, 1977

RESPONSE TO QUESTIONNAIRE DISTRIBUTED BY CCHD, MICHIGAN CHAPTER

1.   About my family and relatives: How many have died with
     H.D.?   Three known.

     How many are afflicted now? Two.

     How many are "at risk?" Thirty.

     This disease is not in my family but I am writing for a
     / / Male   / / Female Friend.

2.   Was the afflicted patient diagnosed in a doctor's office,
     in a hospital or in a nursing home? Hospital clinic
     (outpatient).

     What problems had to be met? The doctors had misdiagnosed
     my mother's condition for a couple years. The family history
     had been lied about by many members for a long time.
     Finally, when the truth was known about her father and
     brothers (H.D.), they knew what she had.

3.   After the diagnosis:

Did different living arrangements have to be made?

Yes. Her condition was rapidly getting worse. She was
unable to maintain herself or her home. She went to live
with a sister and her sister always denied her H.D. and
the fact that it was in the family.

Were there any financial troubles?

Yes, many. For the last 2½ years she has been totally
dependent on me for her care. She hasn't got any income
other than Social Security ($131) and VA ($155) out of
this her food and medication and portions of uncovered
medical cost are paid for. She cannot pay for a nursing
home and we don't want her to have to resort to a mental
institution. Her father and brothers and a sister with
H.D. all spent the rest of their lives in mental institutions.

Was there an employment problem?

She is not only physically disabled, H.D. has severe effects
on her personality and thinking. Rehabilitation or
employment is not possible.

How were your requests for assistance received or
refused?

Rough; I had to go to bat for her and it took a long
time to claim benefits. No sooner did we qualify for
Social Security and they took away her Medicaid check and
hospital coverage. Now she's right back where we started.

Was there difficulty with an insurance problem or
disability payments?

Her insurance payments were recently waived because of her
disability, but she cannot increase her present policy or
purchase any more. Her present policy pays only at death;
there is no disability coverage.

4. How has the presence (or threat) of Huntington's disease
    affected your social life?

    Drastically. Friends and family, neighbors, etc. don't
    understand it at all. Many people think that she drinks
    because she can't walk or talk properly. This is very
    sad.

    How many children do you have, and what are their ages?

    MALE __One_____   FEMALE __Two_____

    Has there been extra stress placed on your children?

    I am her daughter, and taking care of her is a full-time
    job. I cannot afford outside help. She lost her visit-
    ing nurse when they stopped her Medicaid. My brother and
    sister have children and work and cannot help.

    Do your children know they are "at risk?"

    Her children know.

5. In the future, I would certainly appreciate and HOPE for:
    (check:)

    /x/ More and better research.

    /x/ Better public understanding of our problem.

    /x/ Better and less expensive nursing care for H.D.
         patients.

    /x/ RELIEF from financial burdens. "Amen and Amen!"

    OTHER:

New York, New York   September 22, 1976

VERA M. BURKE   SEPTEMBER, 1976
NEW YORK, NEW YORK

The current awareness in Congress, in the newspapers and elsewhere of

the need for in-home health services including homemakers and home health aides

as an alternative to nursing home care, underscores the urgency of developing

these in-home services for the care of the chronically ill patient--whatever be

the diagnostic category.

Quality home health services should be an integral part of a continuum

of health care available nationwide, but in the absence of such a nationwide

program voluntary agencies have a responsibility to establish quality homecare

programs to serve as a model for the development of a nationwide program under

public auspices. A person suffering from a chronic illness such as Huntington's

Chorea, Muscular Dystrophy, Multiple Sclerosis, Amiotrophic Lateral Sclerosis,

etc. and living on a fixed income cannot pay for the kind of home help that is

necessary to enable him or her to remain in his or her own home, and yet to place

such a patient in an institution is to deprive him or her of the opportunity to

remain in his or her own home as long as it is medically possible.

According to the cost of living index a family of four living in New

York City requires a minimum of $12,000 for a moderate standard of living, yet

to be eligible for medicaid that same family income may not exceed $5,000 a year.

It behooves us therefore to take a look at a family having one member with a

chronic illness. Such a person requiring in-home care is unable to meet the cost

of such care and may be forced to go into an institutional setting costing the

community more in terms of actual dollars and cents and an immeasurable amount of

emotional costs that cannot be equated in terms of dollars.

Chronic illness in the family presents special problems in adaptation to family members and these problems are especially disturbing in their effect if the ill person is the mother of young or adolescent children. We know that children suffer from separation from the mother and maternal support whenever she has to be hospitalized for any reason, but chronic illness so difficult for adults to understand places an even greater burden upon the children because its mystery is even more difficult for them to comprehend and to cope with. Because of the high cost of providing in-home services in families with patients with a chronic illness voluntary agencies cannot fulfill the enormous need that exists in the community but can set up programs to serve as models for national health programs to follow in establishing appropriate services in the home. We feel that there are many ways whereby a concerned community can take action among them are:

(1) To help bring about national and statewide legislation that would fund the development of homemaker, home-health aide programs in every community, and broaden the eligibility requirements for public financing on more realistic financial criteria.

(2) To provide under existing medicare and medicaid programs funds for training and supervising homemakers and home-health aides so as to meet standards as defined by the National Council for Homemaker Home Health-Aide Services.

(3) To assure supervision by either a social worker or a nurse of the Homemaker Home Health Aide so as to coordinate the helpers' duties with the patient's needs. Medical or psychiatric recommendations and the use of the help as it affects other family members.

(4) To develop in the community sources of communication between agencies, hospitals and medical people so that all would be aware of the available community resources and utilize them to the optimum.

New York, New York   September 22, 1976

MRS. CHARLES F. BURNER
MORGANTOWN, WV

                                          SEPTEMBER 13, 1976

     I am writing of my experience with Huntington's Chorea in
hopes of adding to any help that can be given to folks in my
position.

     My husband and I were married in 1929, just an average
married couple. My husband was 19 years old. I was 17 years
old. We had 3 sons and 1 daughter. They were a healthy,
normal, well adjusted family with the usual ups and down that
go with growing up.

     All the boys were athletes, playing baseball, football,
and basketball in high school. The daughter played in the
high school band.

     My husband's grandfather was just an old man that
visited his father's home. He had, what we were told, was
St. Vitus Dance. He would sit on the porch not saying anything to anyone. He had a shaking, jerking condition. He
died January 1, 1933 at the age of 76 years.

     Until about 6 years ago we had no idea that it was
Huntington's Chorea nor the heartaches and problems that are
associated with it.

     My husband's father also had H.D. He died in 1933 at
the age of 76 years.

     My husband was a dozer or heavy-equipment operator
for a coal firm, a farmer, and a good worker. Then in 1962
at the age of 52 years old his physician told him he could
work no more and retired him. He just didn't seem capable
of any activity nor business transactions, any planning of
everyday things that came up.

     I was 50 years old at the time, had no experience for
any kind of public work. I'd just kept house and raised
my family. I did get a good job, managed to keep us off
public welfare, but it took a lot of patience, planning, and
understanding to keep my husband as content and healthy,
physically as I could. His mental attitude was very bad.

He kept appointments with his physician every 3 mos. for as long as he lived. Each time he was given a thorough examination, chest x-ray, cardiograms, his blood pressure checked, etc.

Then about 3 years before his death, he grew very violent. In order for it to be safe to keep him at home I persuaded him to see a physiologist. It was just taking a chance but the times he was in a livable mood he would have been very unhappy any place but at home. Also the families would not have understood the entire situation. So he was admitted to the hospital for 3 weeks and given physiotherapy treatments which were very, very helpful. He was able to return home in much better spirits. On July 5th, 1975, he had a sudden heart attack, lived only a few minutes. He was 65 years old.

His physician had told me 5 years before it could happen that way.

Our oldest son, age 45 years seem very healthy and shows no signs of H.D. He has 2 daughters and 2 grandsons.

Our second son was educated, had a master's degree, taught in high school, was a football and basketball coach, was married and the father of 1 daughter and 1 son. Then he began to have a twitching around his mouth, he grew very nervous and had an upset stomach most of the time. I knew what was happening. It was just a matter of time. Then he resigned his coaching position and complained almost constantly. He said he just couldn't explain to us just how he felt. He started seeing a physician, was given tests and told he had H.D. He had helped me a number of times with his father and was well aware of how it was affecting his sister who was very bad with it. He just couldn't face what he knew he was coming to and on December 30, 1974, at the age of 42 he committed suicide. He shot himself with a 22-rifle.

About five years ago, our third child, a daughter, started showing signs, to me, of jerking, nervousness and a neglect of her 8 children. I asked her if she noticed herself and would she see a doctor. She said she hadn't noticed but she would see a doctor.

Then, and only then were we told what Huntington's Chorea really was, that it was hereditary, and that it was a 90% chance of her children having it. She got very bad, could hardly walk, lost weight, was very unsteady, lost control of her speech. You could hardly make out what she was

saying. She couldn't cook, wash dishes or any kind of work.
She did see a physician regularly and did take very strong
medication.

After her husband admitted her to a mental institution
she lived 3 days. She passed away on October 2, 1975. She
had a very bad bruise on one side of her head. I have
no way of knowing for sure what really happened. But I wrote
to Vital Statistics for a death certificate. It said she
had lived 2 hours after her accident. I am presuming she
fell out of bed or fell somehow.

Our fourth child, a son, died in a tragic automobile
accident when he was 33 years old. In 1971. He has 2
daughters and 1 son.

In my searching, I have found H.D. came into the
Burner family from a great, great grandmother, Kerr. She
died in 1907 at the age of 78. One of the families, at the
present time have 6 out of the 9 members that have H.D.
Another has 4 out of 9 members.

So you see that anything that could be done would be a
benefit to the next generation. The families could be
educated about it and not find out the hard way as I did.

Somehow they should see what to expect when having a
family and how to cope with the many, many problems of H.D.

Since I've already lost 3 members of my family within
a 9-month period, it is too late to be of any help to me
personally. But I have 15 grandchildren, 6 great grandchildren, some almost certain to have H.D.

So anything that could be done may help them and millions
of other grandchildren.

All of my family was treated at W.Va. Medical Center
at Morgantown and I feel everything was done for them that
could be.

New York, New York   September 22, 1976

MARY C. CASANOVA
HAVERTOWN, PA   SEPTEMBER 8, 1976

My husband has Huntington's Disease.
I am Vice President of the local chapter of CCHD, and have been
involved with Huntington's for several years, so am not only aware
of my own problems, but also of many other people's.

Our first problem was getting the disease diagnosed. My husband
went to several General Practioners, trying to find out what his
problem was. They would usually give him medication for his
nerves or if his blood pressure would be a bit high, give him medication for that. His personality changes did not seem to indicate
anything to them. Finally, my husband felt so concerned with the
way he was feeling and acting, that he went to a Psychiatrist who
immediately made an appointment with a Neurologist for him. It
took about five months for the Neurologist to definetly diagnose
it as Huntington's. Therefore, I feel that if the General Medical
Practioners were better informed about this disease, it would be
a great help.

We have two children, and the chances of them having Huntington's
disease is very very high. When my Husband's disease was finally
diagnosed, my Daughter's wedding was two weeks away. Fortunatly,
her Fiance was very understanding, and was willing to face whatever problems would arise. They seem to be handeling things
ver y well. They have been married six years now. My son, who
is 22, seems to have a harder time facing the problem, but is doing
better than at first. Talking with others and knowing my own
children's problems, I feel that some help in this realm would be
helpful.

New York, New York   September 22, 1976

My husband has been diagnosed for six and a half years, and, of
course, has been getting progressively worse. His speech is so poor
that most of the time I cannot understand what he is trying to tell
me. He stumbles and falls a great deal of the time now. To swallow
is very hard for him, so that he is unable to get many different foods
down. He is very anti-social and has been since the onset of the
disease when the symptoms started appearing. These problems make it
very hard for either of us to enjoy any type of recreation or social
functions.

I must bathe him, help him dress and have to help him when he eats
as it is very hard for him to handle his utensils. We have steps
to go up and down and this is getting very hard for him. I must work
in order to live and feel that perhaps within the next year, he will
probably have to be placed in some kind of nursing facility. This
is one of our big problems - WHERE CAN THESE LOVED ONES GO? - The
cost of a nursing home is so high, and mental hospitals certainly
are not the place for them.

We also need a great deal of help for the Doctors who are doing
research to relieve the symptoms and hopefully wipe out this horrible
disease completely.

New York, New York   September 22, 1976

MR. JOSEPH CHECCHIO
SCOTCH PLAINS, NJ

                                            SEPTEMBER 13, 1976

    Please, please help. Our (children) married daughter
and husband are very much in love and happy, but there
is an aura of sadness in the obvious way they openly show
their affection.

    When they returned from their honeymoon (7 years ago),
they learned of John's mother's disease. H.D. My daughter
is a nurse and knows all of the ramifications and suffering
involved.

    She cried (only once) because she dreads the idea of her
husband's 50-50 chance of such a fate.

    I cried because they should have beautiful babies.

    They say nothing about this and the silence is deafen-
ing to us here at home. Her brothers are also saddened
because of this.

    We have a grandchild (my son's) and it is heartbreaking
to see the love and controlled envy when we get together.

    Please help us help them. My friends have all noticed
how much our family is affected by this. So many ways they
try to show us some understanding.

New York, New York   September 22, 1976

ROSE CHECCHIO   AUGUST 8, 1976
SCOTCH PLAINS, NEW JERSEY

        I feel the need to do more research is very important.
For a person who finds out after 25 years of age that his
parent has H.D. is a terrible shock.

        If people could know before they marry or have a test to
relieve them of the fear of propagating such a disease it
would be a real victory over such disease that's existed so
long and yet so little is _known_ about.

        Our family is sadder and feel very helpless because our
son-in-law's mother has H.D. We visit her and love her and
try to show concern and still not be obvious because she's so
alert. However, communication is hopeless and therefore our
visits are infrequent. Terrible because we would love to be
able to enjoy some of life's goodness with her and her family.

        Please help us.

New York, New York   September 22, 1976

CLAYTON FAMILY
ROSLYN, PENNSYLVANIA   MAY 16, 1977

RESPONSE TO QUESTIONNAIRE DISTRIBUTED BY CCHD, MICHIGAN CHAPTER

1. About my family and relatives: How many have died with
    H.D.? One, believed to be first case.

    How many are afflicted now?   One.

    How many are "at risk?"   Three.

    This disease is not in my family but I am writing for a
    /7 Male   /7 Female Friend.

2. Was the afflicted patient diagnosed in a doctor's office,
    in a hospital or in a nursing home?   In a hospital.

    What problems had to be met? He became almost helpless,
    and was at the point when he could not walk more than
    10 feet without falling. He doused himself with gaso-
    line and set himself on fire and died 5 days later (at
    Cozier Burn Center) at age 44.

3.   After the diagnosis:

Did different living arrangements have to be made?
His wife worked nights and the children took care of
him when she worked.

Were there any financial troubles?

No.

Was there an employment problem?

Yes.

How were your requests for assistance received or
refused?

We have never asked for assistance.

Was there difficulty with an insurance problem or
disability payments?

No.

4. How has the presence (or threat) of Huntington's disease affected your social life?

    Before the suicide of our first H.D. victim, friends and relatives stopped visiting because they feared the disease.

    Has there been extra stress placed on your children?

    Yes.

    How many children do you have, and what are their ages?

    MALE <u>25 (H.D. victim), 24</u>   FEMALE <u>20 and 16</u>

    Do your children know they are "at risk?"

    Yes.

5. In the future, I would certainly appreciate and HOPE for: (check:)

    /x/ More and better research.

    /x/ Better public understanding of our problem.

    /x/ Better and less expensive nursing care for H.D. patients.

    /x/ RELIEF from financial burdens.

    OTHER:

New York, New York   September 22, 1976

BETTY COFONE
MOUNT FREEDOM, NEW JERSEY   NOVEMBER 7, 1976

    When my mother died in April, 1960 I had taken care of her for 15
years. In March of 1968, at 44 years of age, I was diagnosed as having
Huntington's disease. At about the same time my sister (7 years my
junior) was also diagnosed. A brother 9 years younger than I has shown
signs for two years now, while a brother 14 years younger has no symptoms
as yet. Between us we have 11 **children** and 3 grandchildren, all of whom
will be at risk for having H.D. and living with the ax that has hung over my
head all my life.

    One of the greatest heartaches is the necessity of increasing de-
pendence on other people. By this time I am unable to do much of anything
for myself, and going out almost anywhere has becoming too taxing.
Since I was a teenager, I have prided myself on being financially self
sufficient; now I am a financial, not to mention the emotional, drain on
my family. My **medicines** alone this year have been $1,040.00 plus at
least $300.00 in doctor's bills. At this point to keep a part-time house-
keeper costs $1,820.00 per year, and very soon I will require full-time
help which will be more than twice as much!

    My great fear now is that although my husband earns a decent
salary, if I live two years or longer in a nursing home it will completely
deplete his salary and the home we own will also have to be sacrificed.

    We need your help.

New York, New York   September 22, 1976

MRS. WILLIAM DEUTSCH
ERIE, PENNSYLVANIA   OCTOBER 12, 1974

                                            October 29, 1974

        On October 12, 1974 I sent copies of this [the following]
letter I have enclosed to Senator Kennedy, Senator Javits,
Senator Schweiker of Pennsylvania, and also Congressman Vigor-
ito of Pennsylvania.

        I was having quite a time to know what to write so I just
sat down and wrote what came to my mind about Huntington's
disease. Hope it is what you wanted.

        I also received a letter from Dick Clark and I am sending
a copy to him.

        Many thanks for all you have done for the Disease.

                                            October 12, 1974

        I come from a family who had Huntington's disease for
many years. All I can remember about my grandmother is her
being tied in a rocking chair so she wouldn't fall out on the
floor. At that time there was no other place to go and if
there had been, I am sure there was no money to get help or
care. I can never remember talking to her because she
couldn't talk or eat because her body was jerking all over at
all times. She finally died in the Poor House in a stall on
the floor. She had five children who all got the disease and
were dead by the age 50-55 years.

        My father started getting the disease when he was about
40. After a few years, my father was in bed and would jerk
all over and we had to stay up all night and watch him so he
wouldn't fall out of bed. He also couldn't eat or talk. He
would try to tell us something but we couldn't understand anything he was saying. We didn't know if he wanted to eat or
maybe even a glass of water. He couldn't even tell us when he
had to go to the bathroom and that was a problem with my
grandmother. We had to put him in an institution as there
again, there was no money for help or care. He died in about
six months from a heart attack.

                            5—268

New York, New York   September 22, 1976

I was thankful he didn't linger on like my grandmother.

My brother at this time is in a nursing home in Denver, Colorado, with this same disease. He lost his job from the disease at about 45 years old. At work he had a piece-work job and they would be after him all the time to produce more work. He was not able to do more because when you first get the disease it slows your movements. He had taken medicine for a few years. It helped for awhile but he had to leave his job after 18 years of service. He didn't qualify for a pension because he had to have two more years of service. He lived in Phoenix, Arizona, with my mother and was arrested several times for being drunk and he didn't even drink. He staggered so bad from the disease that my mother was afraid to let him out on the streets anymore. She had to put him in the Veteran's Hospital because she was no longer able to take care of him. They sent him to a nursing home. He now can't talk or write to us.

Please support and contact members of the Conference Committee on Huntington's disease. Thank you.

September 11, 1976

P.S. to letter of October, 1974

Here it is two years have passed and we still have worries from Huntington's disease. John is still in a nursing home in Denver, Colorado. My mother who receives $132.00 a month from Social Security is not able to pay for him being at the nursing home. I believe the nursing home gets some aid from Colorado State. The Veterans are John's guardian and he was sent there through them. My mother is living in Phoenix, Arizona, for health reasons and John had gone there to live after he was no longer able to work. John had wanted to come back to Erie and live with me but I have to work and am not able to leave my job to take care of him. My husband and I both work today to make ends meet.

Thank you for being interested and caring.

New York, New York   September 22, 1976

JOAN H. DIMMICK
ROCHESTER, NEW YORK   FEBRUARY 15, 1977

     This letter is to be used as testimony for the Congressional
investigation of those families afflicted with Huntington's
Disease. (HD)

     My mother-in-law and my husband each had HD. My mother-
in-law died of HD in 1946. My husband's illness, after visiting
several specialist, was diagnosed in 1960. At this time, I
was told it was terminal with no hope. In November, 1967, after
struggling with HD for eight years, he succumbed to this illness.

     I am very concerned about the future of my three children
and their spouses and my grandchildren, of which I am expecting
my first in June of this year. I realize they are all
"at risk".

     I urge you to do all that is possible to help not only
my family, but also all families that are afflicted with HD.

New York, New York   September 22, 1976

MARIE DOBROWOLSKI
SCRANTON, PENNSYLVANIA   MAY 17, 1977

RESPONSE TO QUESTIONNAIRE DISTRIBUTED BY CCHD, MICHIGAN CHAPTER

1.   About my family and relatives: How many have died with
     H.D.?   Three.

     How many are afflicted now?   Two.

     How many are "at risk?" Seven.

     This disease is not in my family but I am writing for a
     /_/ Male   /_/ Female Friend.

2.   Was the afflicted patient diagnosed in a doctor's office,
     in a hospital or in a nursing home? In a hospital.

     What problems had to be met? Obvious ones, but mostly
     having the family adjust to the illness and its conse-
     quences.

3.   After the diagnosis:

Did different living arrangements have to be made?

Not immediately, but after the illness progressed, my
mother had to be moved to a nursing home, for we were
unable to care for her.

Were there any financial troubles?

Certainly. A long-term illness of this type has a
fantastic financial burden.

Was there an employment problem?

No, my mother has not been employed for several years
before the diagnosis.

How were your requests for assistance received or
refused?

I had great difficulty proving Mother was disabled in
the earlier stages while she was not too bad. I found
people very uninformed of H.D.

Was there difficulty with an insurance problem or
disability payments?

I had terrible difficulty with obtaining Social Security
disability payments.

4.   How has the presence (or threat) of Huntington's disease
     affected your social life?

     Since I am young and only "at risk," it hasn't affected
     me too much, except for the fact that sometimes I feel
     there are so many things I want to do and am afraid there
     is only a short time.

     Do your brothers and sisters know they are at risk?

     Yes, we do.

     How many brothers and sisters do you have and what are
     their ages?

     MALE One, age 15   FEMALE   One, age 29, myself
                                          age 19

     Has there been extra stress placed on your brother and
     sister? Yes, especially with my sister, who has
     three children. She is very concerned for their future.

5.   In the future, I would certainly appreciate and HOPE for:
     (check:)

     /X/ More and better research.

     /X/ Better public understanding of our problem.

     /X/ Better and less expensive nursing care for H.D.
          patients.

     /X/ RELIEF from financial burdens.

     OTHER:

New York, New York   September 22, 1976

RICHARD D. EPIFANIO
BROOKLYN, NEW YORK   SEPTEMBER 14, 1976

        The following testimony is based both on my experiences
as a relative of a diagnosed Huntington's patient and as a
person at risk to Huntington's.

        Approximately six years ago my mother was diagnosed as
having Huntington's. At that time we met with her doctors to
discuss the diagnosis. Myself and other family members found
it difficult to understand why it was so hard to diagnose
Huntington's, although a number of tests were performed. It
seemed that the doctor involved placed more weight on family
history than on the tests which had been performed.

        Thereafter, based on what I felt was a questionable diag-
nosis, we were all told that we should be aware of the consequences of this disease and the probable odds of it being
passed on. We were also advised that the way to stop the
disease was to give serious thought to not having families of
our own. We were not advised of the existence of any Huntington's organizations or of any sources of further information.

        The doctor who made the diagnosis was a neurologist, how-
ever, he admitted that he had very little knowledge of the
disease.   He started my mother on some medication, which was
later discontinued since it caused her to suffer some stomach
upset.

        For the next few years, there was little change in my
mother's condition. At no time did we ever receive any word
regarding sources of information regarding Huntington's.
Approximately three years ago my wife heard a radio spot
regarding Huntington's and CCHD.

        Through CCHD we were at least able to get some informa-
tion. However, it appears that this organization, probably
due to lack of funds and volunteers, has difficulty in meeting
the needs of those affected by Huntington's.

        As you know, there are no real means for diagnosing Hunt-
ington's before the physical symptoms appear. However, even
if such a test is developed, whereby people learn at an early
age that they have Huntington's, it will be necessary to have

programs which will enable them to live a somewhat normal
existence, while being aware of their fate.

Early detection obviously has its good points and bad
points. Many would probably take the position that they would
rather not know ahead of time, if they are going to develop
Huntington's. Since there is no method available it does,
however, make it very difficult to decide whether or not to
have a family, or to formulate future plans.

Since I believe that early diagnosis is important I think
that it should be given serious consideration. However, it is
just as important to work on a method of control and of course
a cure for Huntington's.

It has been my experience in the past few years that
there is definitely a lack of both professional assistance
and information available to those affected by Huntington's
especially outside of the larger metropolitan areas. By
professional assistance, I refer not only to diagnosis and
treatment but also to meaningful counseling to both patients
and the family members, whether or not they are at risk.

Finally, I believe that it is important that the public
and the government be made aware of the anxiety that is felt
by those affected by Huntington's. In my case I am concerned
regarding the well being of my mother, brothers, sisters,
children and, of course, myself!

We are encouraged that the Commission has been formed,
and truly hope that something concrete will result from its
investigation.

New York, New York   September 22, 1976

MARY ETTENHOFER
PIPERSVILLE, PENNSYLVANIA   MAY 22, 1977

RESPONSE TO QUESTIONNAIRE DISTRIBUTED BY CCHD, MICHIGAN CHAPTER

1.   About my family and relatives: How many have died with
     H.D.?   Three.

     How many are afflicted now? None.

     How many are "at risk?" Twenty-five or more.

     This disease is not in my family but I am writing for a
     /_7 Male   /_7 Female Friend.

2.   Was the afflicted patient diagnosed in a doctor's office,
     in a hospital or in a nursing home? In a hospital.

     What problems had to be met? The patient was unable to
     care for self and had alieniated all friends and family
     due to emotional changes.

3.   After the diagnosis:

Did different living arrangements have to be made?
Protective and custodial care were obtained at the
nearest state hospital.

Were there any financial troubles?
The patient was entirely without funds, so Social
Security provided the only financial source.

Was there an employment problem?

The patient was unemployed for several years before
diagnosis.

How were your requests for assistance received or
refused?

I was unable to obtain additional help from anyone,
and was personally unable to give financial assistance
myself.

Was there difficulty with an insurance problem or
disability payments?

Social Security payments were no problem. There was
no insurance or disability available.

4. How has the presence (or threat) of Huntington's disease affected your social life?

    Tremendously. I live in constant fear of it. This manifests itself in depression, anger, hostility--all the while knowing the only way to handle it is calm acceptance.

    Has there been extra stress placed on your children?

    Yes, they visited the grandmother while she was hospitalized and are fearful that I may become as she was.

    How many children do you have, and what are their ages?

    MALE____One_____   FEMALE____One_____

    Do your children know they are "at risk?"

    They know I am at risk and they are not--they are adopted.

5. In the future, I would certainly appreciate and HOPE for: (check:)

    /x/ More and better research.

    /x/ Better public understanding of our problem.

    /x/ Better and less expensive nursing care for H.D. patients.

    /x/ RELIEF from financial burdens.

    OTHER:

New York, New York   September 22, 1976

ROBIN FADEN
NEW YORK CITY, NEW YORK   OCTOBER 13, 1976

    Enclosed is my written testimony. There is so much to
say, I found it difficult to write it all on paper.

    I would like to testify verbally before the Commission.
Please send me further information.

    I feel it is important for physicians and the public to
be educated about H.D.

    We must work towards this and many other problems con-
cerning H.D.

    My problem with my mother is still unsolved. We don't
know where to turn. I would appreciate help with this matter.

    My mother was admitted into a Queens hospital six years
ago for tests to determine what her illness was. She was
extremely nervous, couldn't sit without her legs always moving
and twitching and worst of all, she seemed to be in a fog.

    The hospital immediately gave her shock treatments.
After these treatments she seemed much worse and the hospital
prescribed heavy tranquilizers. They said she had St. Vitus
dance and sent her home on tranquilizers. The pills did not
help and my mother became deeply depressed. She took an overdose of the pills. My father called an ambulance just in
time to save her life. She was brought to Elmhurst Hospital
and put in the psychiatric ward for observation. She was kept
in a locked room with two other patients. The ward itself was
locked and we would have to wait for an aid to open the door
when we visited her. My mother was very upset and unhappy in
this ward. She did not belong there. This was obvious by
watching how the other patients behaved. She would sit and
talk with me and tell me her feelings. Her mind seemed sharp
and clear, it was her body that wouldn't respond to her com-
mands. This can be depressing for anyone. This hospital also
gave her large amounts of tranquilizers. They didn't know
what was wrong with her but wanted her to take tranquilizers.
She was sent home with the pills and my father and I were
still searching for a doctor with an answer.

After many doctors and no answers we brought my mother to Mt. Sinai. She was admitted to the neurology ward, where they performed many long and painful tests on her. She had lost a lot of weight and had large dark circles under her eyes. She complained of severe headaches from the tests. What bothered me the most was the fact that she seemed to have lost her will. She had given up and was tired. Tired of the hospitals, the pills, the doctors and not knowing anything. We all waited for the results of the tests. It took three weeks before they told us it was Huntington's Disease. They also didn't know very much about it. The doctors were basically unhelpful and seemed to be secretive. We received most of our feedback from the nurses and they were really uninformed.

A psychiatrist was sent in to talk to my mother to thwart her depression. We found out that depression is very common with H.D.

We were told that there wasn't any cure, treatment or medication and we should take her to a warm climate. We were under the impression that she wan't going to live long. She was sent home without hope and more pills.

My father had no alternative but to close down his business although he had spent much of his savings. He decided to take her to Florida, since that was the only advice we had received from the doctors.

I was with them at the airport and felt very hurt by everyone staring at her. I overheard people remarking on her drunken condition.

A year after my parents had gone to Florida I went to Mt. Sinai Genetics Clinic and asked about the disease. An appointment was set up for me with a panel of doctors. I was told I had a 50% chance of inheriting H.D. They knew of no cure, no tests that were being done to determine if I would get H.D. Nothing. This was the first I'd found out about inheriting H.D. and the doctors were very cold and pompous. A childrens doctor from the clinic told me of CCHD. I wanted to know why we weren't told of CCHD when the disease was diagnosed. At that time we were not told much of anything. I feel the family should be informed of this organization.

My mother is now sixty-three years old. Since she has been in Florida she has gotten much worse. She weighs about 75 pounds and her body is black and blue from falling all the time. Her mind still functions but she is not always rational. Her speech is badly slurred. Her arms and legs are in constant motion. She has not been out of the house in three years. Sometimes she refuses to wash her hair for a year.

Her day is spent lying on the couch with the television on channel seven. She couldn't tell you what is going on on the TV but she becomes very upset when the channel is changed. Her meals must be cooked and cut up for her. She washes and dresses herself with great difficulty. You must have iron nerves to spend the day with her. She has been violent towards my father many times, striking out at him with her nails and a few times with a kitchen knife she picked up. Anything that could be used dangerously in the house must be hid. Sometimes she remembers things from thirty years ago. She'll tell you, very clearly about them.

Last October my father had to go into the hospital for surgery. I had to watch my mother as well as take care of him.

I tried to find out how to get her into a hospital for professional care. The hospitals will not admit her without a private doctor. She has not been out of the house in years. She refuses to go out or to see a doctor. I tried to explain this to the hospitals but they weren't helpful. The doctors there don't make house calls. I spoke to the social service department and they couldn't help me either. I went to the police and filled out a grievance report. They said to call them when she becomes violent and they could take her to the hospital on the Bakers Act. Only with that, if they enter and she isn't violent they could not help. My mother always calms down and becomes quiet when someone strange enters the house.

I spent a week and a half trying desperately to find a solution. My father didn't want to go home, back to a living hell. I couldn't stay much longer. I was emotionally and mentally exhausted. I had to get back to work also. It seemed in the whole State of Florida, there wasn't any help, any answer for our problem.

We couldn't afford a nursing home because she isn't sixty five and my father lives off of his Social Security checks. The CCHD chapter couldn't help me either.

The only way we could get her into a hospital is to legally commit her and she would be put in a psychiatric ward. This is not what we want, but what is the alternative? My mother is ill, not mentally ill.

New York, New York   September 22, 1976

My father is still taking care of her, because I couldn't
find help when I was there. I'm afraid his health and his
mental strength are being totally exhausted.

While I was in Florida taking care of my parents, I
watched my Aunt also go through much pain. Her husband (my
mother's brother) was put in a nursing home. He has H.D.
also. His mind is like a small child's and he's quiet most of
the time. The opposite of my mother.

There are a few other brothers of my mothers that died of
H.D. as well as her mother. And I don't know how much more is
buried deep down.

Growing up with an H.D. parent

When I was fifteen I developed an ulcer. Everyone was
surprised. The doctor wanted to know what was so upsetting in
my young life to bring about this tension. Growing up with a
parent that has H.D. is very difficult. But when you don't
know it, it is very upsetting, confusing and mentally disturbing.

My mother was very nervous and each year she became more
nervous. She was a fanatic cleaner and I wasn't permitted to
sit on half the furniture in the living room. She was always
yelling. She would scream about anything. It would always
become a negative situation. As I got older she became worse.
She went off into screaming fits, similar to what she does
now. She would corner me, pull my hair and bang my head
against the wall. You couldn't reason with her. My father
had to pull her away.

I stayed with friends much of the time because I was so
scared of her behavior. I had no idea she was ill.

When I was 17 I left home. I could not stand being in
the same household with her. Her constant fits had my stomach
in fits and I lived with the fear of coming home to her, not
knowing what she would do next. I left with a severe bleeding
ulcer and I was on tranquilizers.

New York, New York   September 22, 1976

JUNE DE FILIPPIS
BAYVILLE, NEW JERSEY   SEPTEMBER 4, 1976

        Here is my story for the Commission for the Control
of Huntington's Disease:

        My mother (a Huntington's disease victim) and I lived
alone after my father died. I noticed, several years after
my father died, personality changes in my mother. I wanted
to take her to a doctor. She said no. Being "the baby" of
the family at age 19, I told my older brother and sister
that I thought something was wrong with my mother. My
brother seldom saw my mother but he did come then. He
decided, it was that my mother and I just had too many
fights and that's why she was acting strangely.

        And so two years went by and I got married and my
mother went to live with my sister and her children. I saw
my mother several times the first four months of my marriage
and each time I could see her failing. But she wouldn't go
to a doctor.

        My husband, then in the Air Force, got sent to
California and I went with him. After I was there five
months, I got a call from my brother asking me to fly home
to New York, that my mother was sick and it would do her good
to see me. I flew home to find out that my mother and
sister had been fighting. My sister said my mother was
doing very odd things at times and she wanted my mother out
of the house. My mother knew, too, she herself was acting
strangely and she signed herself into Suffolk Psychiatric
Hospital.

        So, I came home to find my mother, a once active and
efficient registered nurse, as a patient in a mental ward.
All they did for her there was keep her so sedated, that she
would sleep sitting up. Her hands were black and blue from
needles and her mind wandered terribly. I found out that
she had been to different doctors and that she did indeed
have Huntington's disease. She did not have the quick movements of the limbs though. However, once the diagnosis was
made, that was it. Only a tranquilizer was prescribed,
which did not help.

                            5—283

She stayed in the hospital two weeks and then went to
live with my brother in Brooklyn. He took her to more doctors
and nothing was found to be wrong with her so the general
opinion again was Huntington's disease. (Her mother and sister
died from Huntington's disease). But again, no treatment, no
medication, no counseling, no nothing. Just a diagnosis "we
believe your mother has Huntington's chorea." Period.

My husband and I came back home after he got out of the
Air Force. We lived in Jersey because that's where he teaches.
I would go once a week to see my mother. She definitely needed
help now. My brother had gone to Maryland and left my mother
in a two family house where the landlady was very nice, but
how much could she do for my mother.

So I started taking my mother to doctors. I had a seven-
month-old baby girl that I had to always take with me because
I had no one to watch her. There were also arguments between
my husband and I as to what to do for my mother. I wanted my
mother to come live with us but I doubted I could take care of
her and the baby--plus keep a marriage going smooth. My trips
to doctors offered no help.

Finally, my mother was so distraught I took her home with
me. Her coordination and thinking ability were poor and she
was very belligerent at times. So unlike her personality in
healthier years.

I called my brother and I said I can't handle her so we
decided to put her in a nursing home. I started calling nursing homes asking if they were able to take care of someone with
Huntington's chorea. I always spoke to the Director of Nurses.
Most of them did not know what Huntington's chorea was. I was
amazed that they hadn't even heard of it. After many calls, a
home in Elizabeth, New Jersey had an opening and was responsive to the Huntington's chorea name at least. My mother entered the home against her will. It tore my heart the day my
brother and I admitted her and then after a visit in the room
left her there.

The doctor assigned to her checked her over and he, too,
agreed she had Huntington's disease. But again the only treatment is a traquilizer. She was often belligerent when I visited her. It made it very hard. I felt like I just wanted to
scream and shake her and make her like she used to be, but I
couldn't. This was the way it was. This was reality and
there was no changing it.

My husband and I had our second child. It became
harder to visit her since there was no family to watch my
children. My weekly visits to her dropped to two a month.
Then I had an operation and couldn't get to see her for
about 2 months. As my brother still lived in Maryland and
my sister in Long Island, my mother had no visitors. By the
time I got to see her, she was very depressed. I felt so
helpless. What could I do for this woman who had given me
everything. It's so frustrating. How can there be an
illness that has no treatment or medication to go with it?
It's not fair.

Anyway, we moved and I moved my mother to a nursing
home closer to our new house. Her new doctor took a real
interest in her and ran several tests including a brain
scan. He tried to disprove the Huntington's diagnosis but
couldn't. He, too, after running tests agreed it was Huntington's disease. I asked him "What can be done for
her" --He said "nothing--we can just keep her as comfortable
as possible." She presently takes a tranquilizer and mood
lifter. Her coordination and speech are bad. She can no
longer eat with a fork. She uses a spoon and very clumsily
feeds herself.

I now have three children whom I take with me to see
her. Her face does shine when she sees her grandchildren.
She still wishes she could be home. I honestly don't know
what to say to her. When she was in Suffolk Psychiatric,
she did realize she had Huntington's disease. I didn't know
what to say to her then either. When she said to me--"I
know I have chorea." What do you say?

All I can do now is bring her what she needs and remember how she used to be. I also usually feel quite
helpless. Then I look at my three children and wonder. Did
I do the right thing in bringing them into the world. I
pray they do not get Huntington's disease. I dread having
to tell them about it when they are older. Will they hate
me for giving them life knowing their possible fate. So
many things go through your mind. I don't have much to do
with my brother or sister, but I wait and wonder if I'll
hear that they have symptoms of Huntington's disease. They
are 13 and 10 years older than me. And then I think--"well,
my mother has it so one of us has to get it and if my
brother and sister don't show any sign, then it must be me
who will get it." But again, there is nothing.

It's a sad situation but one that I hope and pray can be helped. I don't talk to anyone about it. Only two of my friends know about the Huntington's disease. I can't talk and tell other people I know about it.

I feel that they'll feel differently toward me and my family. Perhaps I'm wrong. Maybe someday I'll be able to tell people openly that I'm at risk with Huntington's disease, but now I can't.

I hope the Commission for the Control of Huntington's Disease can help in establishing a humane and decent way to take care of Huntington's disease people.

Suggestions

1. Push research to find cause, treatment, tests to determine if one will get Huntington's disease.

2. Enlighten doctors on Huntington's disease, what medicine is best.

3. Encourage doctors to talk to Huntington's victims' family so they know how to help.

4. Have nurses in nursing homes read or attend a class on Huntington's disease.

5. Make people in general more aware that Huntington's disease exists.

New York, New York   September 22, 1976

MRS. SAM EDELSON
BROOKLYN, NY

                                      AUGUST 23, 1976

        It is most encouraging to learn that the government is
finally trying to do something about Huntington's Disease.

        My mother had Huntington's Disease, but at the time
no one seemed to know anything about this disease and was
told she had a very bad nervous disorder. We were a family
of seven children and being so ignorant of this condition,
we could not understand her deterioration, her most peculiar
behavior and most people thought she was mentally unbalanced.
At this time there was no one to explain what we, as her
children, were facing. She died at the age of 57--an old
broken woman.

        My eldest brother when he was about late thirties or
early forties started to show the same symptoms--an uneven
gait, slight tremor of the hand, etc. At that time he was
already married and the father of two children. He lived in
Welch, W.Va., at the time and since this was a very small
town, his wife started taking him to various hospitals and
clinics. Even then, there was very little known about his
condition and most doctors were more or less guessing and
groping. My sister-in-law, ignorant of his condition, tried
to keep it a secret from us in NY and told her children very
little about her various visits to the numerous doctors she
took my brother.

        Right after this, the next brother started his middle years
and also showed the same symptoms. He however had an additional problem. He had cancer and when a colostomy was performed and he could not handle his own toilette, he committed
suicide.

        In the meantime, my older brother was going down fast,
and this brilliant handsome man was now reduced to a mere
vegetable having to have everything done for him, and I mean
everything. My sister-in-law would not hear of putting him
in a hospital, but kept him at home and took care of him.
By this time, a little more was being found out, but none of
this information was being passed on to the younger members
of the family, and so when my older sister started to have
the tremors, speak in a slurry manner, walk in the same manner
my mother did, we became alarmed. Still no enlightenment.
However, I wrote to my sister-in-law begging for some

information and she finally informed me that the Mayo Clinic
had told her that they thought my brother had Huntington's
Chorea. I immediately wrote to Mayo and they told me to take
her to a local doctor and they also sent me a pamphlet telling
me the history of Huntington's and how it was passed from
parent to child. I was then married and mother of two
daughters, my other sisters were also married with children.

It was then that our terror began. Everytime I dropped a
dish, tripped, or slurred a word I thought, "this is the
beginning." Fortunately for me, I have passed the "danger
years" and am not afflicted with this dreadful disease. The
four youngest children in the family are okay, but the story
doesn't end here.

My sister who had Huntington's also committed suicide
when she was convinced that she was a victim. She left a
note saying she couldn't do to her family what our mother had
done to us. We had the most miserable childhood because of
a sick mother who couldn't be helped at all. We suffered with
her from the earliest afflictions. This sister has a
daughter who lives in constant dread of the future. She is
still young enough to be stricken, God forbid.

Still the curse goes on for my eldest brother's daughter
is now going through the agony of Huntington's Disease.
Fortunately for me, she lives in Maine and I don't have to
witness daily the deterioriation of one of my loved ones.

I thank God every day that I and my daughters were spared
and live with hope that in my life time I will see some sort
of treatment and cure for Huntington's Disease.

Please see that every effort is made to wipe out this
dreadful disease and many people will bless you forever.

New York, New York   September 22, 1976

MRS. JAMES FITZPATRICK
ROSELLE, NEW JERSEY   SEPTEMBER 7, 1976

    As a child I remember always running and hiding when my
father came in the house. I never knew what would happen--I
knew he didn't work like other fathers, he couldn't walk
straight, his arms were always swinging in some direction
never knowing where. I remember children saying he was drunk,
but I knew there was no liquor around and no one ever saw him
in a tavern. I remember walking to school every day and finding I couldn't walk straight; the harder I tried, the worse it
got. Mother always seemed to be crying and always getting us
out of the way; he was always yelling at one of us and scaring
us.

    I remember my father in a hospital but not knowing why,
then changing from one hospital to another--Graystone, Mar-
boro--everyone said they were for the insane. Mother said it
was the only hospital that would take him since we had no
money. I remember every time we went to the hospital he cried
and begged us to take him out of there, but there was no way
we could take care of him and go to school too, and Mother was
trying to support six children. I remember having a nervous
breakdown when I was about thirteen and lost a whole year of
school.

    When my father died, we still didn't know what it was and
why, but it's easy to forget your problems when they're not
around and we were told he is finally at peace; we didn't
think about it until my brother started to show signs of
things we wanted to forget.

    He was the nicest fellow you wanted to meet. He was in
the Air Force overseas, fighting planes in Okinawa; he came
home, married, had four children, then started to show signs
of the same thing daddy had. His wife read, called and made
all kinds of inquiries, and found out that he had Huntington's
disease and that his four sisters (one had died earlier) could
get it and also his four children.

    He was let go of his job and all the bad memories came
back, plus knowing we all now had children and they too had a
50-50 chance of getting it, if we got it.

I don't know how hard it was and still is for his family, only living in the same house can tell all, but I can look back and remember my horrible childhood and now it's back again. He is in a Soldiers Home, can do nothing for himself, he has no control over anything--he has to wear diapers, be fed baby food, be lifted in and out of bed, his speech is getting worse day by day--we can hardly understand him. His only pleasure is to be taken for a walk around the grounds in a wheelchair but only if the day is nice and only if it's warm and also it's only on Saturday or Sunday.

He was given a television set but he can't hold his head up long enough to see. And all his children look at what could happen to them; so far none of his sisters show any sign of the disease--no definite sign anyway--but who knows, you live with the thought that any time it could be you. There are many cases where mother and daughter come down with it about the same time; the only requisite is adulthood and one of your parents had it or died before showing signs of it.

We don't have a big organization behind us; all monies are from sales of different objects--yearly raffle and yearly dues from a very small group of people.

Our needs are great for someone to help, will you be the one?

New York, New York   September 22, 1976

KERRY J. FREEMAN
ROCHESTER, NEW YORK   MARCH 7, 1977

The purpose of this letter is to plead with you to
provide financial support for research to combat
Huntington's Disease. In your Commission rests the
hope and prayers of all of us who live in the shadow
of Huntington's Disease.

I have watched the despair Huntington's has brought
to my husband's family. His father has suffered from
H.D. for fifteen years, while his mother has borne the
burden of trying to hold the remnants of a family together on a small secretary's salary. I pray that our
family will not suffer the same fate, but we live in
the ever present fear that it may.

Bob, my husband, is a brilliant young man who is
currently employed by Xerox. His lifelong dream,
though is to be a congressman from New Hampshire.
Whether he has a chance to fulfill his dream may very
well depend on the research your commission has
the opportunity to support.

Playing at my feet is Jennifer, our beautiful, healthy
five month old daughter. Our decision to have her was
based on the hope that in the near future research
will find a cure for Huntington's so that she can live
free from the fear of that genetic disease. In your
power lies the hope of her future.

I pray that you will have compassion as you make decisions
to support research on behalf of our family and the
thousands who must also live with the shadow of H.D.
over their lives.

May God bless you and your important work.

New York, New York   September 22, 1976

JANET GRIEPP
ROCHESTER, NEW YORK   SEPTEMBER 14, 1976

My husband, Carl's, H.D. was diagnosed in 1968. His trade was pipefitting 1946-April 1974. By March 1969 the quality of his work was affected noticeably. Carl is a calm, pleasant person, and he accepts his H.D. well. Daily exercises aid his balance and coordination. I have taken mood elevators, attended several group therapy classes and belonged to Recovery, Inc. for two years. Recovery helped me gain a fair control over my angry temper.

Dr. Bruce Singh, psychiatrist, began seeing me late in 1975. In three monthly visits, he helped me understand my feelings. I felt that my family neither cared nor understood. I find Carl's mental problems hardest to cope with. Dr. Singh equated accepting Carl's H.D. with accepting his death. He said it was reasonable that I have difficulty. He said stress situations like this cause you to grow, or you are overcome by them.

At one point, Dr. Singh offered me a suggestion for easing my tension at mealtime. Carl stood idly by, only an arm's length away. This frustrated me, but I kept silent. Dr. Singh wanted me to make lists of all the items needed to set table for the different types of meals. Carl could set table using the appropriate list, and gain satisfaction while I could remain calm. I did not act on this idea. When the children were around, they helped. Carl began sitting in his easy chair until called for meals.

Once I told Dr. Singh that Carl couldn't correctly select even one grocery item. After learning the circumstances of the episode, Dr. Singh explained that at this stage, Carl had good recall of the past, and the most recent experience. His problem area is in taking an accumulation of facts and drawing the proper conclusion.

This past April after surgery, I needed a great deal more help from Dr. Singh. Our situation seemed insurmountable to me, and I felt of no use to anyone. I found my merit system was obsolete. The more upset I was over H.D., the more work I did. Dr. Singh stressed that I was a person of worth if I did absolutely no physical work.

At another session when Dr. Singh asked how I was handling my feelings about Carl, I complained that he sat in a chair when not urged to be active. He was stern, Dr. Singh called this the same problem that he had given me the remedy for several months earlier. He asked me why I had not implemented his suggestion of lists of things Carl could do, when his idleness was so frustrating to me. At this point he merely waited in silence for my answer. I could only say that it seemed easier to do it by myself. He answered, "Carl can help if you supply the iniative, and you refuse to do this." Carl and I tried the lists for several days, and he would only partially read them. Carl did accept the lists as a show of both Dr. Singh's and my confidence in his ability to be helpful. He has since kept on doing the parts he can remember and then asking what else is needed. Dr. Singh did accomplish his mission for both of us.

Dr. Singh was able to help me work through this more acute stage of anxiety from April through the present time because of the groundwork he laid earlier, when my situation was less troublesome to me. It is for this reason that I feel psychiatric counseling should always be available to families with H.D. It is necessary to maintain the mental health of the H.D. patient's partner so that society does not end up with a whole family to care for.

New York, New York

September 22, 1976

ELSIE M. HAND
SWEDESBORO, NEW JERSEY

MAY 25, 1977

RESPONSE TO QUESTIONNAIRE DISTRIBUTED BY CCHD, MICHIGAN CHAPTER

1.   About my family and relatives: How many have died with
     H.D.? Three--husband's mother, grandmother, one brother
     who committed suicide.

     How many are afflicted now? Three we know of. Brothers
     and sister's husband.

     How many are "at risk?" Three--my son's four grandchil-
     dren.

     This disease is not in my family but I am writing for a
     / / Male   / / Female Friend.

2.   Was the afflicted patient diagnosed in a doctor's office,
     in a hospital or in a nursing home?   Hospital.

     What problems had to be met? Taking care of my husband.
     Helping with the loneliness and money problems.

3.   After the diagnosis:

Did different living arrangements have to be made?

No. I take care of my husband alone. Seems my children
come home less and less. They make like it will go away.

Were there any financial troubles?

Yes. There are plenty financial problems. I take him
to the clinic. Dr. Leopold and Dr. Mancall are his
doctors in Philadelphia.

Was there an employment problem?
Yes. He had to stop work, also driving car.

How were your requests for assistance received or
refused?

Poorly. Couldn't get any for 4 or 5 months, then got
S.S.I. until disability came through the following month.

Was there difficulty with an insurance problem or
disability payments?

No. Only that we were without funds for the 6 months
waiting for disability. Children had to help.

4.   How has the presence (or threat) of Huntington's disease
      affected your social life?

      No one comes to the house. My children only come when
      it's an emergency. It's so very lonely for both.

      Has there been extra stress placed on your children?

      Yes. My 39-year-old son doesn't seem to grasp. They are
      going to have their first child next month. One went to
      California so he wouldn't have to see it.
      How many children do you have, and what are their ages?
      MALE Three--39, 27, 41   FEMALE None.
      I have four grandchildren and a new one next month.

      Do your children know they are "at risk?"
      Yes.

5.   In the future, I would certainly appreciate and HOPE for:
      (check:)

      /x/ More and better research.

      /x/ Better public understanding of our problem.

      /x/ Better and less expensive nursing care for H.D.
           patients.

      /x/ RELIEF from financial burdens.

      OTHER:

New York, New York   September 22, 1976

MRS. LILLIAN HARRISON
TEANECK, NJ

                                      SEPTEMBER 2, 1976

    My husband who passed away in 1965 at the age of 71 was
a victim of Huntington's Disease and I wish to relate to
you the hardships and problems I was confronted with during
his illness. I am 76 years old, semi-retired and in fairly
good health.

    We were married for 37 years and I have a son, age 45,
married with two children, a daughter, age 38, married with
three children. My husband was an artist, a highly emotional
personality, an intellectual with a sound view of life, also
had a fine tenor voice and studied music for a time.

    He functioned very well until the age of about 55. I
noticed slight movements of his feet, etc., but when he
would read or paint he was quite normal. In fact, when he
was involved in his art work there was no sign of motion
or abnormality. In 1950, when he was about 57, I went into
business, opened an art shop, hoping that he would be able
to carry on with me for a time.

    His condition slowly got worse. I had to employ a
practical nurse to stay with him during the time I was at
the shop. He did pass his time reading and painting as much
as possible. His condition became so bad that nurses refused
to attend him. Nursing homes were out of my reach financially,
and I was unable to nurse him, due to lack of knowledge,
physical inability, and had to run my business for daily
living. Inasmuch as he was a veteran of the first World
War, I was advised to contact the mayor of Teaneck for help
to have him admitted to the Veterans hospital. Through his
kindness and manipulation, my husband was shortly admitted
to the hospital in Lyons, N.J., although there was a waiting
list a mile long. He was given excellent care. He was there
several years.

    I wish to emphatically stress the fact that patients
with Huntington's and related diseases have no where to turn
for treatment and help, and the government is responsible
to these thousands of families.

    I had a sister with Huntington's Disease who was later
admitted to Creedmor Hospital in L.I. under the care of

New York, New York   September 22, 1976

Dr. Whittier. This hospital was shut down due to lack
of funds. We must have special hospitals for these patients.

New York, New York   September 22, 1976

MS. JOAN HORANSKY
BROOKLYN, NY

                                            SEPTEMBER 12, 1976

       I am 21 yrs. old. I have a sister (24), a brother (15),
and 2 step-sisters (15 & 19). The five of us are at-risk
with Huntington's Disease. My mother died of HD 2-1/2 years
ago. She was sick for 13 years and in the hospital for 9
years. My mother had a brother who died of HD 6 years ago.
His wife married my father after he and my mother were
hospitalized (when I was 12-1/2 years old) and my two cousins
became my step-sisters.

       I don't really remember my mother when she was well.
I have very few pleasant memories of time spent with her
when she was well. When she started getting sick, no one
knew what was wrong with her (she didn't tell my father about
the disease--he found out by threatening my mother's
father to take me, my brother and my sister and leave my
mother. My grandfathr told him about HD.) My parents got
into a lot of fights and my mother lost control of herself--
my sister used to come in with scratches on her arms from
fights with my mother.

       In third grade (when I was about 9 years old) my family
started going to Jewish Family Service once a week. We had
a man and a woman talk to us. I don't remember everything
we discussed but we did discuss my mother's illness. I
was told that she had an unknown disease of the nervous system. I was shown that when she had her hand on a table, her
fingers moved up and down involuntarily. We got a housekeeper, Mrs. Myers, who stayed with us for four years. She
came from 8:30 A.M.-5:00 P.M. on weekdays. She was a very
kind and warm person and I grew to love her (and cried when
she left--I couldn't understand why she couldn't marry my
father, or come with us when my father did remarry). My
mother was still home for a little while when Mrs. Myers
came, but was put in the hospital shortly after this. At
first my mother came home for weekends or one day each
weekend and we would visit her at the hospital (my father
would bring her down in a wheelchair).

       During the time that Mrs. Myers stayed with us, my
father started dating my aunt. He spent a lot of his time
with her. He would wake up, go to her house, go to work,

go to work, go back to her house, come to our house for
dinner, then (sometimes) go back to her house. He worked
full time and taught one or two nights a week. He also
worked on Saturdays sometimes. My sister was taking acting
lessons on Saturday and wasn't home too much. I was left
with the responsibility of taking care of my brother (I was
10 - 12 years old and he was 4 - 6 years old). I learned
to cook and watch out for him at a fairly young age. I
also had to take him on the bus sometimes. I grew up pretty
fast.

I remember the day my father told me that he was
divorcing my mother and my aunt was divorcing my uncle,
and my aunt and my father were getting married (we were going
shopping for school clothes). He said that my mother and
uncle agreed to this since it was the best thing for us
(the children). We all went to the wedding (minus my
mother and uncle), and to this day I wonder what would have
happened if, when the judge asked if anyone objected to
this marriage, I said I objected to it (I was only 12-1/2
years old but I did object to it). I started going to
Jewish Family Service by myself, but only went twice. The
social worker was constantly saying "A penny for your
thoughts" because I didn't talk too much.

We moved into my aunt's neighborhood, which I resented
because I had a lot of friends where we lived. We moved
into a 2-family apartment and then a house. There were
many adjustment problems in the house--my older sister
moved out at 16-1/2 yrs. old and moved to California at
18 yrs. old. Everyone else has had their share of problems.

My mother and uncle were at Brooklyn State Hospital and
we would take them out once a week to eat or talk. They
couldn't eat by themselves too well and they both smoked
cigarettes and burned themselves. It was hard seeing them
this way. My uncle died and my two step-sisters and my
aunt (step-mother) stopped going to the hospital with us.

About the time I turned 16 (the age to go into the
wards of the hospital) my father told us that my mother
was getting too sick for him to bring her down (he would
bring her down in a wheelchair and my brother and I would
talk to her--my sister was in California). The first time
I went to visit her on the ward was very upsetting. It was
a ward for women with neurological diseases and it seemed
like a mental ward. Many women just sat around like vege-
tables, staring at the TV, or nothing. Other women would be

in their beds and others walked around and talked to themselves (or acting weird). It was a horrible experience.

The summer I was 17 years old, my parents told me about my mother and HD. I guess I always thought that it might run in the family since my mother and uncle had it, but I always put it in the back of my mind because it was too upsetting. Now I was confronted with it. I called my friend but she didn't know what to say. I always felt a little different than my friends in junior high and high school because all of my friends came from families with two healthy, "real" parents and a brother or sister. I was always too embarrassed about my family to tell people about it unless I was really close to them. The first time I went to visit my mother after I knew about HD was hard for me and my father--it was just the two of us visiting her. I looked at her, thinking that that could be me in 10 or 15 years--it was a very frightening experience. My mother was slowly but surely getting sicker and sicker and becoming less and less aware of our presence when we visited her. We brought her cookies and ice cream.

At about this time, I started seeing the family psychiatrist, Stephen Hempster. I still see him occasionally. He knew my whole family and the situation, so I didn't have to go into the whole thing--he understood. I was also talking to my guidance counselors and one teacher, in high school, about the situation. They were helpful.

I was getting along with my parents okay, but not great. For some reason my step-mother has never really trusted me and through the years, I've become a little more distant. We were becoming a little closer, but it's changed. She knew about HD and had children anyway (and it was mostly her idea to have children). She has a huge guilt complex and worked for CCHD and now NHDA incessantly--working off part of her guilt. She's a little too obsessed with the whole thing--that's all she and my father talk about. My younger brother and step-sister, both 15, don't know about the disease. My parents told them that they're working for retarded children. I went to a few meetings of the New York City chapter's CCHD--it helped a little.

I was deciding to go to an out-of-town college. I couldn't stay at home anymore. But I was feeling guilty because my father would have to visit my mother alone--he told me not to worry about it. I go to college about 1 - 2 hours away from my parents' house. When I came in from

school, I'd visit her sometimes. It was always hard. (When
she first went into the hospital we would visit her every
week. That changed to every other week and then every three
weeks--it was just too hard to see her.)

My brothr was Bar-Mitzvahed and my mother wasn't able
to come--it was upsetting not to have her there. I was
also thinking of going abroad for a semester. Again, I felt
very guilty. I was also afraid that she would die while I
was abroad.

My mother died a month after my brother's Bar Mitzvah
and four months before I was leaving for Paris. I was sad,
relieved, guilty, angry and generally upset when my mother
died. All of these people came to her funeral --all so sad
to see that she died. But none of them went to visit her
all those years when she was alive. It was just my father
and I. I also felt afraid--afraid that that would be me (in
the coffin) 10 or 15 years from now. I expected her to die
and I "lived through it" so many times, that I didn't believe it was really happening. I felt guilty because I was
happy that I wouldn't have to go to the hospital and visit
her any more. The last few times there, she barely realized
that we were there, let alone who we were. All I kept
thinking was, "This could be me."

Living with the disease is a very difficult thing to do.
The uncertainty of my future is upsetting. (I went to a
wedding of someone on my mother's side and my aunt-step-mother
was pointing out all the people at-risk with HD!) I think of
getting married sometimes, but I wouldn't want anyone to go
through what I went through as a child. I don't remember
getting too much attention, love, or affection when I was
younger--not too much recognition of my problems. If I got
HD, my children would have to go through what I went through
(or a modified version of it) and would have to worry about
being at-risk with HD. My husband might want to remarry,
but would feel obligated to visit me, no matter how hard it
may be. That's a hard thing to think of imposing on someone,
even if he is willing. I couldn't bear it. Sometimes when
I'm really nervous and my fingers move involuntarily, I put
them flat down of a surface to make sure it's just nerves
and not the onset of HD. I sell raffles for HD sometimes,
and I feel like I'm selling a part of myself. If someone
comes over and asks what HD is, I have trouble verbalizing
it. I have to give them a pamphlet with a description of it.
Even if there was a predictive test, I'm not sure I'd want
it done. I don't know what I'd do if I found out if I was
going to get HD in 10 years. Until there's a cure for the
disease, there is no real solution to the problem.

New York, New York   September 22, 1976

MRS. S. C. KUPERMAN
SPRING VALLEY, NEW YORK   MARCH 14, 1977

     In view of the enormous suffering Huntington's disease
can inflict on individual victims, their families, and future
generations, I urge your Commission to make every effort to
combat and cure it.

New York, New York   September 22, 1976

ANNE LACHENMAYER
SOUTHEASTERN PENNSYLVANIA   JANUARY 10, 1977

        I am writing to you to explain how I am affected by Hun-
ington's disease. My mother died from it in 1966 at age 60 after
ten years of progressive deterioration. I was spared living
with my mother during that time but my family and I would visit
my parents frequently. Sometimes I wonder how my father lived
through it. He's a patient man with a sense of humor which no
doubt pulled him through. He also has faith in God and a deep
sense of responsibility and duty. He kept my mother home the
whole time except for the last five weeks of her life which she
spent in a private nursing home. Up to that time, he always had
a housekeeper.

        I know the expense must have been great. Thank goodness
he only had my brother at home (who graduated from college in
1964). My father is an accountant and has put all three of us
through college.

        My mother never talked about her mother to me as I was
growing up. When my mother's symptoms were beginning to appear,
some relatives made comments that she acted like her mother.
After a few years of wondering what was wrong with my mother, my
father took her to a hospital for a week where she was diagnosed
as a Huntington's chorea patient. I remember my father acted as
though it was a death sentence right then, but I had no idea what
that meant at that time. I knew three of her brothers had spent
the last years of their lives in hospitals, but it really started
to sink in when I visited another brother (at home) with the
same symptoms as Mother's. This uncle I had known before. My
mother's family consisted of five boys and four girls. Four of
the boys and my mother inherited the disease. Luckily my uncles
didn't have children except for one who had two. I am going to
contact them now about CCHD to see if they are affected. CCHD
has given me the courage to talk about it and some hope to give
them if they need it.

        My sister (who has two boys) and my brother (who has two
boys) are aware of CCHD although not as involved as I. I try to
keep them informed of what I learn. I am the eldest in our
family--age 48, my sister is 46 and my brother 34. My mother
was about 50 when she started, so it is on our minds (in the

New York, New York   September 22, 1976

back, at least). I have six children, ages 25 to 14. I also
have a granddaughter and one on the way. I'm hoping I won't
get the disease as I'm optimistic, but I'm also realistic and
I have too many lives at stake not to do all I can for CCHD.

After Mother died, I thought well, now I can forget it,
but through the efforts of Marjorie Guthrie and CCHD, I have
begun to feel differently. I want to fight the disease, not
just sit by passively and in fear--waiting. Now I'm not
waiting. I'm learning, supporting and trying to reach as many
people as I can with the message of CCHD. If it should be too
late for me, I know at least it won't be for my children. I
also think I'll be better able to handle the disease than my
mother.

New York, New York   September 22, 1976

MRS. GRACE MARCONI
BARPHACE, NY

    I will make this as concise as possible. My story be-
gins with marriage in 1950. At this time our family had no
knowledge of Huntington's Disease. In 1963, five children
later, my mother-in-law began personality changes, depression, and a mental state which drove her husband out of the
home and almost out of his mind.

    At this time, my husband Angelo Marconi was imprisoned
for manslaughter and could not understand what was happening.
Having only one sister who also has the disease, and a father
who did not understand, everything was left to me. By the
time he returned, he was able to visit his mother in Creedmor State Hospital who was reduced to a babbling mad woman.

    In 1970, Angelo was diagnosed as having H.D. and from
that day until this he is impossible to live with.

    He cannot face what is happening to him and insists
on punishing his children and myself. In 1973 he was admitted to Pilgrim State Hospital to await the same
horrible fate as his mother.

    My oldest daughter, Frances, was diagnosed in 1975.
What is her fate. Must it be the same as all the others in
this day and age? She is 24 years old, cannot look forward
to having a child or any kind of decent life with her husband.
Must we someday visit her amidst drug addicts, alcoholics,
perverts of every description, and an endless number of
other unfortunates only because there are no hospitals or
centers where any one is experienced with H.D.

    My husband does not receive proper attention. They
give him a mild tranquilizer and a vitamin pill. He walks
around the grounds all morning telephoning everyone, plead-
ing to be taken home.

    I am told that he must be allowed to walk freely on the
grounds. It is called "therapy." Is it also therapy when
he hops into a cab and arrives home to terrify the younger
children? Then he is taken back by police screaming. Have
you any idea of the trauma to these children and their

New York, New York   September 22, 1976

friends when they witness this?

It would take a book of encyclopedia size to write my
personal stories of suffering, anxiety, poverty and despera-
tion. But would anyone care?   I am on welfare. I have
signed over my home in order to have food on the table. We
have no furniture and feel stripped of pride, dignity--
not to mention my own health and state of mind.

I now have 6 children, ages 24, 23, 20, 19, 15 and 9.
Where are they going to receive help? What encouragement
can you give them besides looking forward to years of
deterioration in a horrible mental institution which they
don't belong and then sudden death.

Please! Please! do something now.

New York, New York   September 22, 1976

JOAN H. MARKS
SARAH LAWRENCE COLLEGE   SEPTEMBER 10, 1976

                The Need for Genetic Counseling Services

        In 1969 Sarah Lawrence College, Bronxville, New York established
the first training program in the nation in Human Genetics at the
masters level in order to meet the perceived need for increased
clinical services in genetics. Since 1969 Sarah Lawrence College has
graduated 78 women who serve primarily as genetic counselors on
interdisciplinary clinical genetics teams in 12 states and 2 foreign
countries (Canada and Israel). Based on the experiences of these
graduates serving around the country, it is our opinion that the
present clinical services in this country are available to an infinitesimal
number of the citizens who could benefit from genetic counseling. The
technology which has been achieved in alleviating or managing genetic
disease in the past few years, much of which has been funded by federal
support, is of questionable value unless the citizenry is in a position
to receive these benefits.

        At present, these health workers, whose title is Genetic Associate,
serve primarily in academic health centers where the population served
is almost exclusively white middle class. The reasons for this limited
access are complicated but certainly due to some extent to the lack of
attention and funding which has been afforded clinical genetics. Funds
are not currently available to serve properly the established population
in need of counseling services and staff support often comes from
research funds. Funding is generally not provided for public education
to apprise the populace of the availability of genetic services in a
given community. Despite the development of prenatal diagnosis to
screen pregnant women over 37 years of age for a Down's syndrome fetus,
for example, the need to avail themselves of this test remains a
carefully guarded secret except for the 5% of the pregnant women now
utilizing this screening mechanism. Thorough pre-amniocentesis counseling
is a crucial component of this newest technique yet it is not routinely
available even at the few centers performing the major numbers of the
tests.

        In our nation, which is ostensibly committed to providing the
highest quality of life to its people, approximately 15 million
Americans are estimated to be afflicted with genetic diseases and the

majority of this number are unaware that thier disease is genetic in
origin or that it may be transmitted to other members of their family.
Much could be done to prevent the transmission of these genetic conditions
if genetic services were properly funded. In addition to affecting
the incidence of genetic disease, the development of comprehensive
genetic services would allow for humane treatment of patients and
families whose lack of counseling has left them burdened with
enormous personal guilt for afflicting their progeny with a disease
whose cause they do not understand. Huntington's Disease families,
who often live a major portion of their lives in terror of developing
the illness, represent an extreme example of a group whose access
to the health system has been shockingly blocked, partly out of
inefficiency but certainly because of nearly total lack of genetic
counseling services.

Now that awareness of the psychological and medical needs of this
Huntington's Disease population exists and that health professionals
are available to serve these needs, it is essential that comprehensive
programs be designed and funded to serve these patients. A national
network of genetic services should be organized and provision made
to train and support adequate numbers of geneticists, Genetic Associates,
and public health specialists.

New York, New York   September 22, 1976

RONALD J. MAUGEN
POMPTON LAKES, NJ
                                      SEPTEMBER 6, 1976

    Do you know what it is like to wake up in the middle of
the night and find your wife crying? Why? Because of H.D.
and how it is affecting you.

    How many times have you seen a drunk stagger down the
street and you just miss hitting him with your car? Do you
curse him or do you stop and wonder to yourself if he has a
muscular disorder such as H.D.? It's cute when a normal
person drinks a little too much and starts to slur his words.
He can sleep it off and return to normalcy. What about an
H.D. victim? Can he sleep it off and be normal again? Never!!
And we need your help.

    My uncle recently passed away because of H.D. My
father has been disabled for the past 10 years because of
H.D. Have you ever had someone close to you degenerate at
such a slow pace and know there isn't any help at all. There
isn't even a way to arrest this dreadful disease.

    I don't plan on going into great detail about H.D.
because you should know most of the particulars. However
I would like to make a few points.

    If you were an H.D. victim how is this going to affect
your children? For example, how are they going to marry?
How can your son or daughter ask someone to give up their
human right to mother or father a child? Do you think it is
easy? You probably will never know because you aren't affected.

    When I courted my wife a few years with me meant more
than anything in the world. But try and live with it. It is
there every day of your life. Plans have to be made well
beyond your means in order to compensate for if and when
that dreadful day comes. For example, is it right for me to
deprive my wife of natural motherhood? Some of us just
aren't strong enough to accept artificial insemination. Do
you know what it is for my wife to see my father and then
visualize me in ten years? Have you ever seen a man eat
enough for 6 people and still lose weight? This is how my
father is and again it's because of H.D.

5—310

New York, New York   September 22, 1976

    What have you done for us? Absolutely nothing as com-
pared to what you could have done. You increase our taxes
and let us take care of ourselves.

    How would your wife cope with the situation of losing
your financial support and not being able to support your
home and family?

    Go on welfare? That's the biggest joke going and you
know it. Get off your fat tails and allocate us money for
research. United we stand; divided we fall. With our
system of government the small people are always falling
because our government believes in arms races or space
races. Sure the population will always grow but is this what
we want; a decadent society?

    Jerry Lewis just raised 23 million dollars for muscular
dystrophy. Why should he do this on his own? What in
heaven's name are you people doing in Congress for us?

    Just remember this: we put you there and we the people
created the government. You are in Congress to represent
us so how about doing it for a change.

    Thank you for your time and consideration.

New York, New York   September 22, 1976

HELEN MC DOWELL
GENEVA, NY
                                          JULY 26, 1976

        I have been on CCHD mailing list for a little over a
year when my son was diagnosed as having H.D. I was so
shocked as I never had heard of the disease. His father died
at the age of 55 of a cerebral hemorrhage after having several things the matter with him, which were all blamed on
alcoholism. I can't blame anyone as we had no money for
doctors and I had two children to raise.

        My son is only 43 and I am the only one he has to care
for him and he seems to slowly becoming worse. We have a
fine hospital here (Geneva, N.Y.) but as this is a city of
only about 16,000 the doctor who is treating my son is not
familiar with the disease either as there is only one other
case documented in the hospital here.

        The neurologist who diagnosed it as H.D. is in Rochester
about 55 miles away. It might as well be 500 miles due to
the transportation.

        What I wish to know is what kind of place he will have
to be put in if something happens to me (I am 68). I wish
to make some arrangements ahead of time. I am managing
all right now as thank God I have good health. I have a
daughter also but she is much younger than my son and has
two small children and a husband to care for and I don't want
the burden to fall on her.

        Where is the nearest facility where an H.D. patient can
be placed? There is a nice nursing home connected to our
hospital but it is always full and are mostly old people.

        The nearest cities to us are: Rochester, Syracuse and
Elmira. We are just about the same distance from all of
them. I just wondered if you could tell me where to get a
little advice about this as it would relieve my mind to know
where he could be sent if something happens to me. I want
to care for him as long as I can.

        Also, I would like to know if Medicaid would help with
finances as my son gets $337.00 per month and I don't think
that would be enough for a nursing home.

New York, New York   September 22, 1976

      I know you are a very busy and wonderful woman, and God
bless you for the wonderful things you are doing.

New York, New York   September 22, 1976

VIVIAN McKENZIE
PATERSON, NEW JERSEY   SEPTEMBER 7, 1976

    I have known of Huntington's disease for only a short
time, but I have seen what it can do to an individual and a
wonderful family.

    You can only imagine the fear these people have encoun-
tered. Every little illness with symptoms associated with
Huntington's disease they are in constant fear that Huntington's
has claimed another victim.

    The worst part is that it can drag on for years and years.
I have only known of the disease for about three years and this
is because of a friend of mine on the job. Her husband is one
of its victims.

    On meeting him for the first time, I knew that something
was wrong. He had a sort of twitching movement but he could hold
his own. On inquiring about his illness I found out that this
was an hereditary disease and what was more frightening was that
there was no cure.

    During several conversations with this friend I found that
this type of disease deals with the brain cells. Mr. Sirota
would come quite often and have a break with his wife and each
time we could see that it was getting a little worse.

    Finally he couldn't keep his balance enough to walk down
the street because he was in danger of falling or getting hit by
a car. I saw this and I was afraid for him.

    Then I found out that his children and grandchildren were
in danger of inheriting this disease. It was like seeing a beautiful little flower crushed under foot hearing this. I had met
her grandchildren by this time and I was so sorry for them.
There was nothing that anyone could do and it gave me sort of
a hurt feeling.

    This organization needs help. There are a lot of ways
that money can be raised and I know that quite a few ways have
been tried. But research costs millions of dollars. We need
help.

New York, New York   September 22, 1976

    I know that we live one day at a time and many things can
happen in a day, but to live constantly in fear is a lot different.

    This disease has not claimed any victims in my household,
but I personally would like research done in this field.

    This disease is a menace to our society. It can claim a
victim with little unnoticeable symptoms. For example, in talking
to Mrs. Sirota, I found that he had a personality change first.
Now nine times out of ten, we would put this change to the fact
that someone is changing the span of life or he's getting moody.
You would never think it could be a disease.

    We are asking for help and that is what we feel is right.
Please issue funds to organizations for the control of Huntington's.

    This would mean a lot to a man that may not make it, but
he will get satisfaction in knowing that maybe something can be
done for his children and grandchildren.

New York, New York   September 22, 1976

MRS. H. MILLS
PHILADELPHIA, PENNSYLVANIA   MAY 17, 1977

RESPONSE TO QUESTIONNAIRE DISTRIBUTED BY CCHD, MICHIGAN CHAPTER

1.   About my family and relatives: How many have died with
      H.D.?   One.

      How many are afflicted now?

      How many are "at risk?" Two.

      This disease is not in my family but I am writing for a
      /_7 Male   /_7 Female   Friend.

2.   Was the afflicted patient diagnosed in a doctor's office,
      in a hospital or in a nursing home? Hospital tests sent
      to doctor.

      What problems had to be met? The sick man had to agree
      and sign himself into a mental hospital.

3.   After the diagnosis:

Did different living arrangements have to be made?

Yes. Eight years of around-the-clock care.

Were there any financial troubles?

No, only because of pension and medical coverage plus savings.

Was there an employment problem?

Retired.

How were your requests for assistance received or refused?

We did not have to ask.

Was there difficulty with an insurance problem or disability payments?

No, retirement pension.

4. How has the presence (or threat) of Huntington's disease affected your social life?

    Couldn't leave the house for 8 years.

    Has there been extra stress placed on your children?

    Yes, always concerned.

    How many children do you have, and what are their ages?

    MALE___One, 44_____   FEMALE___One, 47_____

    Do your children know they are "at risk?"

    Yes.

5. In the future, I would certainly appreciate and HOPE for: (check:)

    /x/ More and better research.

    /x/ Better public understanding of our problem.

    /x/ Better and less expensive nursing care for H.D. patients.

    /x/ RELIEF from financial burdens.

    OTHER:

    If my husband had not signed papers of admittance for mental hospital I would be dead now as he almost killed me once.

New York, New York   September 22, 1976

EUNICE MISTRON
CHATHAM, NEW JERSEY   SEPTEMBER 10, 1976

My father and aunt were victims of Huntington's Disease.
At age 39 my father started showing symptoms which in his
case were personality changes rather than physical and
subsequently made my mother miserable along with the rest
of the family with his accusations of infidelity. During
this time he kept her awake nights with this diatribe
which I, as the eldest child, heard from the age of 9.
Meanwhile he was fathering children (until there were 5)
which he wouldn't support or feed which dictated that my
mother was working full or part time between pregnancies
just to keep the family fed.

When my mother tried to seek help from various agencies,
private, public or religious, they each told her to go
to the other. The family doctor wanted as little to do
with the problem as possible although my father would not
see the doctor either. The priest said "see a physician."
When a psychiatrist was finally consulted, he made a
diagnosis of "male menapause" then finally paranoid schizophrenia.
Not one doctor or psychiatrist ever once mentioned Huntington's
although my mother informed all of them in medical histories
that my father's sister died as a result of Huntington's
Disease. It was not detected in my paternal grandparents
because they both died at or before 40 as well as my two
uncles who may have had the condition since one died as a
result of a fall from a scaffold and the other was a
suicide victim. After my junior year of high school my
father spent almost 6 months in a state mental hospital,
my youngest sister was born, I was working and going to
school and my hopes of going to college were dashed.
Under these circumstances I felt I had to contribute something
to the wellbeing of the family by going to work. All this
time my mother was extremely strong and competent.

Between the ages of 47 to 52 when he was disabled, my father
was in and out of Marlboro State Hospital and his employer
was rapidly becoming disenchated with his performance.

He had been a mattress finisher but no longer had the manual
dexterity to move a broom across the floor (he had been
relegated to janitorial duties) nor the concentration to
finish a task. When he was permanently disabled at 52,
he then vegetated at home bothering my mother all the time
with his accusations. Within a few years as the mind
deteriorated, he began reaching out into the community
offending young girls. Around this time my mother was
desperately trying to get a social worker, the police,
and the family court to recognize that although this man
was to be released from the mental hospital he was no means
cured which was what she was told each time he was released
in her charge. Finally she was working full time to support
herself and her children, and she couldn't stay at home
maintaining a guard over him so one time she refused his
acceptance into the home environment. He was placed in a
shelter nursing home maintained by the state where his
condition at last exhibited the typical Huntington's
rolling gait. Now there was no doubt that my father had
Huntington's Disease. The real diagnosis took only 18 years.
Unfortunately there is very lttle that can be done to stem
the daily destruction of the affected Huntington's gene.

The scientific community has come a long way in genetics.
Optimistically one day defective genes will be replaced
with normal ones. But someting must be done in the meantime
to detect H.D. and alleviate the debilitating symptoms with
a control drug. Diagnosticians and health professionals
should be better educated on how to determine if one has H.D.
We should have mental health centers and social service
centers more aware of the needs of these people. To go further
we should have a national medical disaster insurance for
the chronically ill. A comprehensive bill would help the
families who become the unwilling victims of Huntington's
Disease. Shelter nursing homes that cater to the special
needs of an H.D. person would be a wonderful idea.
Too often many of them don't eat because they can't feed
themselves.

Hopefully the commission will interview many people and
come up with many sound ideas. We've waited such a long
time for intelligent help. I would be happy to appear
before the commission should I be called.

New York, New York   September 22, 1976

MARTHA MORROW
ROCHESTER, NEW YORK   SEPTEMBER 10, 1976

PHYSICAL THERAPY USED WITH HUNTINGTON'S AFFLICTED

Although PT is not usually accredited to be an integral
or helpful approach in the management of H.D. patients, the
following case is reported of a patient who appears to have
benefited by a realistically planned and supervised PT program.
In H.D. there is persistent, repetitive and abnormal, involuntary movements and posturing. This could conceivably result in
asymmetry of opposing muscle groups, disuse atrophy of infre-
quently used muscle groups and gait unbalance. Patient has not
taken any medication for control of his choreic movements. PT
has represented the primary therapeutic approach in the patient's
management of his movement disorder.

It should be noted that one very important effect of a
supervised physical therapy program has been the motivation to
continue trying to move functionally. It is indeed difficult
to continue to be active when ability to function is slowly but
surely lessening each year.

Miss Martha Morrow, physical therapist, first saw Carl
Griepp February, 1974. Although H.D. afflicted, diagnosed 1968,
he worked a 40-hour week as a pipefitter. He dragged his right
foot, particularly the toe. He toed in enough to stumble at
times. He arched his shoulders back in order to balance. He
also tired enough in a fifteen-minute walk outdoors to list off
course.

Miss Morrow put Carl on a series of exercises which he
began doing 5 to 10 times daily. He had to be supported by
putting his hands on the shoulders of a person walking in front
of him for exercises Nos. 1, 2, and 3. Gradually the number of
exercises and their duration was increased. A part of the motivation for Carl came from a chart of the exercises which was re-
corded daily and which was evaluated by Miss Morrow when he had
his next appointment. Carl learned to execute the balance
exercises without holding on to another. In spite of this,
muscle spasms in his back became a problem. His last day of
work was April 19, 1974. Miss Morrow gave Carl more extensive
exercises in order to aid him with balance and coordination, as
well as to fill his day. Today, September, 1976, he follows

exercises No. 1 through 9, plays the organ, reads, walks a
little, bicycles about five miles leisurely, and cares for
his own personal needs. He shows increased involuntary motion,
can no longer clip his nails, sits idle when not urged along,
but he is still able to walk unaided.

HUNTINGTON'S DISEASE PATIENT'S EXERCISE REGIMEN
INCLUDING PURPOSE

1. Fifty steps walking on heels - strengthen muscle in
   front of leg below knee (weak anterior tibials).

2. Fifty steps walking on toes - main calf muscle was
   weak (poor balance and neglected gastrox).

3. Fifty steps knees raised high (weak hip flexors).

4. Twenty steps toes out - to correct toeing in (asymmetry
   of opposing muscles).

5. (a) Fifty steps 10" apart and aimed perfectly
       straight.

   (b) Fifty steps feet 8" apart and walking in place
       (two strips of tape can be put under a throw
       rug).

   (c) Two parallel strips of tape placed the length
       of driveway 10" apart (balance).

   Carl uses (a) but all accomplish correct foot placement (hip abductors and external rotators).

6. Play organ or use typewriter (prevent increasing
   finger flexion contracture, maintain hand and
   shoulder strength).

7. (a) Twenty-five pelvic tilts (Increase strength
   (b) Twenty-five sit-ups   of stomach muscles
                                   and balance trunk on
                                   legs better.)

8. Twenty-five regular push-ups until May, 1976. Carl
   now does 25 push-ups from a kneeling position (arms,
   shoulders and upper back are strengthened either way).

9. Twenty-five butterfly like motions lying on floor.
    Early in 1976 Carl began to hold elbow at shoulder
    height when putting food to mouth. A call to Miss
    Morrow resulted in this new exercise. Arms extended
    overhead and drawn rapidly to hips and return and in
    contact with floor throughout (arm adduction).

Bicycling is excellent for both balance and coordination
of legs. This Carl had done on his job. He carried supplies
in a basket on the bicycle.

In winter walking and exercycle are substituted for bicycling. If it is too slippery underfoot, shopping plazas can be
utilized. Walk approximately one mile (strengthen leg and
postural muscles).

Despite this, Carl is no longer walking briskly, but his
posture did improve, peak and is now worsening. His balance
improved and seems at present to be holding quite well.

Miss Morrow wished that it be noted that these results
with Carl are dependent upon the fact that he climaxed his working years nearly simultaneously with the start of physical therapy.

SUMMARY

Our purpose has been to maintain strength and flexibility
in all muscle groups as long as possible and to the greatest
degree possible. In a disease like Huntington's disease, certain
nerves and their associated muscle groups are affected sooner
than others. This tends to make the patient substitute other
motions, especially where balance is concerned, and neglect muscles which are actually capable of functional activity. Then,
as with any unused muscle, the muscle strength slowly drops--
unnecessarily--to below functional level.

When the physical therapist observes the H.D. afflicted,
look for:

1. Things causing lack of balance;

2. Asymmetry of opposing muscle groups;

3. Muscles that are not being used, or not used
    maximally.

New York, New York   September 22, 1976

MRS. MAXINE MURA
WAYNE, NJ   SEPTEMBER 7, 1976

    I am writing this letter because my father has H.D. It
took many years of going to different doctors for this
condition to be diagnosed. This in itself was extremely
frustrating. My father was always a very kind and mild man,
and all of a sudden he became very hard to live with. Of
course, this is one symptom of H.D. The doctors in NY
who diagnosed my father told my mother of the disease being
hereditary. You can imagine her feelings when he told her
that her children had a 50-50 chance of getting H.D. At that
time my sister was pregnant with her third child.

    My mother told us the name of the disease, but not all
the details. My sister sent away for information about H.D.
and then the whole family knew what they had to live with
the rest of their lives.

    My mother fought to get my father into the National
Institutes of Health in Bethesda. They confirmed the diagnosis.

    My father also has a brother and a sister who now have
H.D. At NIH they called a family conference to inform my
aunts, uncles, and cousins who were involved directly with
H.D. At the conference there was a social worker, doctors,
and some nurses who work with H.D. They told us that H.D.
is hereditary and that if one of your parents have it, you
have a 50-50 chance of getting it yourself. They also
told us that there are no tests to tell if you are going to
get it or no cure if you do get it. They also said if you
don't have children yet, they would advise you not to. This
conference was truly the most traumatic experience in my
life. All the people closest to me were being threatened
with a horrible disease. We all walked out of there feeling
completely helpless.

    My sister had three children at this time. They advised
that children should be told about H.D. at a very young age.
We spoke about this many times, whether to tell young children
that their mother might get the disease. It's more difficult
to tell them if their mother gets it. Then they have a
50-50 chance of getting it themselves.

5—324

I was engaged at this time and had to make a decision whether to have children or not. It's every girl's dream to have a baby and all of sudden I was advised not to have a child. I really couldn't cope with a childless future. A few months later, when I got married, we finally came to a decision to adopt. My husband wanted us to have our own child. I just couldn't knowing I would have to tell my child about H.D. and if I do get H.D., I don't want to pass it on to someone I love so much. I was fortunate enough to adopt a baby from Colombia, S.A.

Living with this disease in my family, I feel that the following is most urgently needed:

1. Funds for research so that a cure can eventually be found.

2. Nursing home facilities which are capable of handling H.D. patients.

3. Education for the medical field and the public about H.D.

4. Information about adoption for the people who do decide not to have children.

New York, New York   September 22, 1976

PATRICIA MURRAY
AVENEL, NEW JERSEY   SEPTEMBER 30, 1976

    Please allow me to add my support to the research being
done to combat the tragedy of Huntington's disease. The consequences of this dread illness are beyond measure for its victims and their families.

    Any research which can find a cure should be pursued to
the fullest extent. Funding should be provided for this worthwhile cause.

New York, New York   September 22, 1976

JACQUELINE JORDAN NIBLE
PHILADELPHIA, PA
                                            SEPTEMBER 12, 1976

        My name is Jacqueline Jordan Nible. I am trying to
remember the first time I heard HD. It was a long time ago.
I am 34 years old. My two sisters, ages 36 and 31,and two
brothers, ages 38 and 40, all have HD. My father had it;
he died in 1964. His sister had it, his mother had it, my
aunt's son had it, and a niece. My aunt's son and niece
died down in North Carolina in a hospital in Willington.
My two sisters are not in the hospital for good yet. My
two brothers are. So far I don't have it but I had a test
done in 1965 after my father died to see if I had HD and
the doctor said no, but for me to be tested again as I got
older. There are 18 grandchildren. I have five and one
grandson. My brothers and sisters have thirteen between
them. My one brother's son has been tested and he has HD.
He is around 15 years. I am without a husband and I am
trying to raise five kids alone; and with the threat of HD
on my back day in and day out it is hard. I tried to kill
myself two times. The last time was in January. I was five
months pregnant. I was in the hospital for four days, two
days in intensive care. The only thing keeping me from
trying again is that I have a three-month-old baby and it
would be rough on him. I know I should think about the
other kids but they can get through it without me. I hope
some day somewhere God will let HD vanish forever and my
family and everybody's loved ones all over the world can
rest and stop jerking and twisting and can talk just like
everybody else. There is not much I can do to help anyone
but if this letter helps, please use it. I don't have a
phone but you can write me and ask any questions about my
family. I will answer to the best I can. I am going to
New York on Friday. My two sisters and brother live in
Long Island. My sister, the one 38, is bad. She was in
the hospital. I called and she could hardly talk. Everybody thinks I am wrong because I don't go all the time.
First, I cannot afford it and then I cry so much my oldest
son tells me not to think about it. I don't know if I can
face all of them at once but this is the last time I will
get to go before school opens. I will appear if it will
help HD people and their families. Anyone who wants to
check my family out, I will give you a little information.

New York, New York   September 22, 1976

Nettie Jordan (grandmother) had H.D.   Of her three children,
Richard and Lucitte had H.D. while Kate did not. Lucitte
had two children Jettie Williams and Richard Bell. Both died
in the hospital from H.D. The doctor was George W. Paulson,
M.D., at the hospital in Willington, N.C. I spoke with the
doctor in 1965. My name was Jacqueline Jiminez then.

My father was Richard Jordan who died on December 24, 1964.
Of his five children--Richard, Jr.; Jerry; Joyce; and Grace
all have H.D. I am the only one free of the disease at this
time. Jerry's son who is 15 has H.D.

I hope you can understand it all because I don't think I can
write it again. This has been the hardest thing I could ever
do except when I put my brother in the PGH last May, the
same place my father died. His wife moved him to New York
a few months ago. Well, I will close for now and may God
help you in all you do.

New York, New York   September 22, 1976

PATRICK J. NOONAN
PHILADELPHIA, PENNSYLVANIA   APRIL 26, 1977

    I am an 18-year-old college freshman and an "at-risk"
person. The odds are 50/50 that I will contract Huntington's
disease. I am 18 and can contract H.D. at any time. The
average age for symptoms to begin to appear is 35. Knowing
this has strongly influenced my plans for the future.

    I am the eighth of 10 children and was only 5 or 6 when
my mother was admitted to a care home after her illness was
diagnosed as H.D. Because of my young age, my mother's leaving and her absence did not have a traumatic effect on me. I
knew that the possibility of myself contracting H.D. existed.
I know now that the possibility can become a reality at any
time. It frightens me and I wish a way could be discovered
to predict whether I or my brothers or sisters are going to be
victims of H.D. It is, however, slightly comforting to know
that this "rare disease" is becoming a subject of research by
more and more doctors and scientists.

    Standing at a place in my life where I am considering
the possibilities my life holds, I see the shadow of H.D.
falling on all areas. If I choose to marry, I have to consider the chance that I am a carrier, plus the real possibility
of a shortened lifespan. If I marry, I might choose to adopt
children rather than run the risk of passing on H.D. to children
of my own. I would also have to consider the need for obtaining financial stability, because it would take me 15 to 20 years
to die. In that interim my family would still need financial
support in addition to paying my medical bills. I think that
it would be helpful to have accurate and complete information
available through counseling, so that the best means might be
found to face the family's or the individual's problem. Remaining single would put an end to the transmission of the disease.
But if I remain single and don't contract H.D., then it is almost as if a life has been wasted. Another possibility would
be a religious vocation, where my life would still fall under
the threat of being drastically shortened by H.D. It doesn't
seem to matter which way I turn, H.D. seems to threaten all
aspects of my life, probably because it so closely touches me.

    In living my life up to this point, I have learned to
live with H.D. as an irrevocable fact of life. I am definitely
"at risk," and so are my brothers and sisters. I look at my
father, that granite wall that has been worn and weathered by
storms of pain and sorrow, and I see the effects that my
mother's contracting H.D., the years of raising a large family,
and the pain of seeing his wife slowly dying have caused. I
look at my mother, the patient, loving woman whose body is
showing the signs of H.D.'s steady onslaught, and I see a
woman who bore 10 children, then bore the pain of being separated from them, and who watched the reflection of pain and
loneliness in her husband's eyes. I hope and pray with all my
heart that a cure will be discovered. I guess a cure for H.D.
will be found, sometime. But for the present, all things possible must be done to help those who, directly or indirectly,
bear its burden.

New York, New York   September 22, 1976

GEORGE PANAGAKOS
BEECHURST, NY

My first personal contact with Huntington's Disease came
when my sister was stricken with it. It was not a sudden
thing. It started in her mid-fifties. She could not function properly at her job. Her cleanliness was at a low. Her
apartment was dirty and unkept. She became withdrawn. She
thought that people were talking about her and following her.
I took my sister to a general hospital to see a psychiatrist
who said she was crazy and to put her in the hospital for a
while. We had her released from there and took her to an aged
home where she had personal conflicts with other aged people.

We then took her to a neurologist who said she had
Huntington's disease and who then put her in a hospital for
studies. My sister had become very fidgety with movements of
arms and legs. Her walk was like a person under the influence
of alcohol. This neurologist had all the doctors on staff
coming to look at my sister because this illness is not too
well known. They gave her Dopa medication which did not help.

They released her after not being able to help her.
We were fortunate to get her into a nursing home. They have
to puree her food for her. Her coordination is bad. Her
clothes are soiled. They bathe her a couple of times a
week. She uses a walker to get around. She has periodic
falls.

I took my sister to Creedman Neurological Institute for
a work-up with Dr. Whittier who examined her and questioned
me and my sister as to the history of our family. I told
him that my father's sister had what they called St. Vitus
Dance. I found out that is what they called Huntington's
Disease in those days. She died from it. Her daughter,
my first cousin, was in a hospital many years with a mental
disorder they later said was Huntington's Disease. She died
a few months ago. My sister's name is Pauline and it is very
depressing when I visit her. Although her memory is still
good she gets these blank stares.

I am from a family of 8 children. My oldest brother
John who is in age right after my sister Pauline also came
down with Huntington's disease. He is 62 and also had the
illness in his mid-fifties. We first noticed his speech

became slurred and his walk became a little wobbly. Later
his hands lost some coordination and his feet would tremble.
John also has these vacant stares. His walk now is very unsteady and his head tilts.

He is also in a nursing home. They also cut up his food
for him.

I believe the disease is hereditary. They say it does
not skip a generation. My father died at 64 years of age with
no signs of Huntington's Disease. His sister and her daughter
died from it. It is possible that my father had he lived
longer, could have developed this illness because someone
had to pass it on to my oldest brother and sister.

We are hoping it does not hit any other member of our
family. They say we have a 50-50 chance of getting it. My
son is 26 and married four years. I had told him that if I
came down with Huntington's Disease he would also have a 50-50
chance of getting it.

What is needed now is an appropriation of funds that
will get into the right hands to help the suffering of all
Huntington's diseased people. The hands that will ultimately
find a cure or a medication that will help alleviate the
problems these people have.

If my letter has enlightened you in any way, I am
thankful. Thank you for reading it.

New York, New York   September 22, 1976

SHIRLEY PENNYPACKER
NEW CASTLE, DELAWARE   MAY 24, 1977

RESPONSE TO QUESTIONNAIRE DISTRIBUTED BY CCHD, MICHIGAN CHAPTER

1.   About my family and relatives: How many have died with
     H.D.?   Two.

     How many are afflicted now? Two.

     How many are "at risk?"   Five.

     This disease is not in my family but I am writing for a
     _   Male   /_7 Female   Friend.

2.   Was the afflicted patient diagnosed in a doctor's office,
     in a hospital or in a nursing home? He diagnosed the
     disease himself.

     What problems had to be met? No immediate problems yet,
     but our life has had to become very quiet and routine.

3.   After the diagnosis:

Did different living arrangements have to be made?

No. The patient is still working, but home life has
had to be stress-free. Patient has suddenly decided
he may not be sick.

Were there any financial troubles?

No yet. My husband only takes medication when he has
trouble sleeping. Unfortunately, I miss a lot of
rest. I'm not on medication.

Was there an employment problem?
No.

How were your requests for assistance received or
refused?

We have not requested any financial aid yet, but from
what we can find out, it is going to be a problem,
since Mr. P. is only 48.

Was there difficulty with an insurance problem or
disability payments?

No. My husband will be able to retire in 3 years but I
think payments will be very small. We have already closed
our blood bank membership, since he can no longer give.

4. How has the presence (or threat) of Huntington's disease
    affected your social life?
    Our social life is terminated. Most friends sympathize
    and call, but we don't party; pressure is too much.

    Has there been extra stress placed on your children?
    No. Their friends have been very understanding. They
    think Mr. P. is an alcoholic and they can understand
    that.

    How many children do you have, and what are their ages?

    MALE   Two, 23 and 18   FEMALE   One, 19.

    Do your children know they are "at risk?"
    Yes.

5. In the future, I would certainly appreciate and HOPE for:
    (check:)

    /x/ More and better research.

    /x/ Better public understanding of our problem.

    /x/ Better and less expensive nursing care for H.D.
         patients.

    /x/ RELIEF from financial burdens.

    OTHER:

PAPER SUBMITTED - PSYCHOLOGY
ROBERT B. POWERS
APRIL 12, 1975

Huntington's chorea, a disease which is believed to have an unusual origin to the United States, is characterized by conspicuous symptoms and an important phase which is not noticeable. If contact with the disease is made, the situation one finds himself in must be coped with, without resulting in permanent destruction through a desired release from reality. Huntington's breeds various psychiatric aspects, offers suggestions for social work, and presents two separate views on genetic counseling. Treatment is limited, physical therapy provides some hope, but more importantly, research sheds some light on the future.

In 1630, a man named George Pelham, who was a Puritan and a liberal, immigrated to Salem, Massachusetts from Bures, England. On board his ship were three men by the names of Wilkie Knapp, Nicholas Knapp, and Jeffrey Ferris who were known as "outrageous nonconformists." On the way over, Nicholas Knapp caused so much trouble he had to be put in irons. His behavior was later linked to Huntington's chorea. When they arrived, the other two were repeatedly arrested in Salem for what was listed as "deviant behavior." The famed "Groton Witch" was a descendant of one of the Knapps. Again, her erratic behavior was a result of the gene passed on to her by her ancestors. [1]

There was a great deal of work done by experts in trying to identify this disease. For three generations the Huntington family tried to locate the disease's existence in the human body. The grandson, George Huntington, succeeded in doing so and thus, the disease was named after him. He determined that this was the major cause of madness in some people. He also revealed that the disorder is not very common with only six and one-half out of every one hundred thousand people having the disease in their line. [2]

Huntington's chorea is an autosomal dominant which means that the defective gene is on a chromosome other than a sex chromosome and dominates its normal-partner gene (from the unaffected parent). [3] The disease is highly hereditary at a ratio of one to one for male to female. The risk of occurrence for the patient's sibling is fifty percent for each offspring if the parent is affected. In turn, the patient's children have a one in two chance of contacting the disease.[4] Even before the patient develops symptoms, he can pass this defect on to his children. In the case of twins, it would affect both in identical twins since their genetic patterns are exactly the same. If the twins are not identical, then it would affect either one or the other or both.[5] The age of detectability is usually between the ages of thirty-five and forty and very rarely found in children or adults over fifty.[6]

The first symptoms which one experiences having contacted the disease are usually clumsiness, nervous movement of the hands, and the lack of gracefulness.[7] These are followed by a carelessness in appearance, irritability, and the failure to keep promises and responsibilities.[8] As the disease gets progressively worse, the movements become more rapid and jerky[9] with a loss of memory and bodily functions.[10] Then the patient's speech becomes slurred, he becomes depressed, and finally, there is total incapacitation.[12] The disease has deteriorated the brain and central nervous system.[13]

Huntington's has been called "the most demonic of all diseases" because since after one contacts the disease, he or she has already reproduced. It is difficult to diagnose unless there is a family history of H. D. It resembles many other diseases and is often mistaken for one of them. That is why the family history plays an important role in the diagnosis process. An unusual thing about H. D. is that it never skips a generation, unlike other genetic disorders.[14] If one's grandparent had the disease, but his parent did not contact it, then he has nothing to worry about. The basic diagnosis process usually consists of an electroencephalogram, a pneumoencephalogram, and psychologic tests.[15]

"In the stage when most must struggle with the transition from youth to middle age," Ms. Wexler notes in her study, "the H. D. victim prepares himself for the passage from youth to death."[16]

HD hits in the prime of life. The victim usually becomes bitter because he does not possess the chance to live a fulfilled life. There is no hope left, which causes the victim to struggle against guilt, self-contempt, shame, and bitterness. The person is all wrapped up in the psychology of dying.[17]

The predominant fears are the loss of self-control and the loss of bodily functions. Each time the victim loses his memory or forgets

something, he sees the end in sight. In some, just knowledge of the fact
that they possess the disorder robs them of the will to live a life of
dignity. [18]

Clealiness becomes a problem when the patient loses control of
his bowel and bladder. The situation eventually becomes so bad that
the patient is forced to wear diapers. Belching and grunting noises are
not uncommon despite the fact the person is struggling to keep quiet.
Everything that has been trained in him at an early age becomes progressively undone. [19]

Elizabeth Kubler Ross cites five distinct stages in the progression
of Huntington's chorea. The first is denial. Some think that denial is a
part of the disease, but according to her it is not. The patient denies
because he does not want others to associate him with the disease. Circumstances occur when the patient is stripped of his job and hobbies,
and he is isolated from the community due to H. D. One person with H. D.
denied the disease, but he got medication to control his choreatoid movements and conducted his life normally until it got to the point where the
disease took over. [20] Sometimes, as in this case, denial can be used in
a partially productive manner, but for the most part, denial is harmful
to the person as it leads to the second stage.

Anger. This is mainly a form of resentment and envy due to the
fact that the victim is not normal like everybody else. Gradually, the
amount and intensity of the anger are weakened by the disease, but at
first the patient is very irritable and moody. The H. D. patient has
given up or was forced to give up his work and hobbies. All he does is
sit at home with no incentive, brooding over his illness. On occasion,
he goes out and is sometimes mistaken for drunk. This leads to harass-
ment of the patient and embarrassment for the patient's relatives. It is
extremely frustrating for both the victim and his family. [21]

Bargaining, the third stage, is nothing more than making pacts
of good behavior for the restoration of the victim's health. [22] It is the
stage when the victim appeals to his Supreme Being, doctor, or person
he feels can restore his health. He claims he will be good as just compensation for what he feels he will receive. It is all in his mind, and it
eventually leaves with the appearance of the fourth stage.

This stage is depression. First, the H.D. victim mourns his lost self and all his lost opportunities. Stemming from this are opposite and conflicting feelings about his affected parent and other affected siblings.[23] The individual does not know whether to hate or love the one responsible for his misfortune. He is totally confused and as a result becomes totally depressed.

The fifth stage is acceptance.[24] Until the patient reaches this stage, basically nothing can be done. If the person denies having H.D., why should I take the drug to control my choreatoid movements is the question he might propose. Nothing is accomplished through anger, bargaining or depression. But when the person faces up to what he has, then he can cope with it, which is a step in the right direction.

Now they are able to prolong the lifespan of an H.D. victim. What they must abstain from is prolonging useless years of inactivity and madness. What we must do is "include them among the living until the moments of their dying."[25]

One of the tragedies of dying is the separation from one's family at a time when support is probably needed most. Nobody wants to be reminded of their own mortality; therefore, we close all avenues of communication with the individual about to depart from this world at a time when that individual wishes to talk about his impending demise.[26]

The psychiatric aspect of H.D. deals mainly with children. A child with H.D. in his or her line, should learn at an age when he or she is mature enough to comprehend the complications it presents. It is a difficult first step for a parent to take in order to inform a child that his mother or father is go ng to die in ten to fifteen years. As Dr. John Whittier says:

> Reluctance to involve children is often rooted in the
> hope that the children can be protected from the neces-
> sity of making decisions while they are uncertain as to what
> the future may hold for them, or rooted in guilt for having
> children when they knew the gene for H.D. was in the
> family.

When informing a child, the parents must be truthful because children recognize an evasive answer and suspect something drastic.[27]

Although psychiatry plays an important role in the proper influence
and direction for the H. D. patient and his family, social work offers a
much more personal approach to the H. D. victim. Carole Hedges states:

> "...In the case of the H. D. victim there is an obvious
> need for physical care...But there is also a critical need to
> maintain human dignity and a need for communication and
> interaction with other systems: family, the institution,
> society as a whole. To provide merely physical care is to
> relegate the human being to a less than human status, and
> to ignore his potentials and abilities is to deny his humanity
> again."[28]

A major problem is the lack of visitation for the H. D. patients.
There are a number of reasons for the lack of visitation; a common one
being that the patient does not want to be a nuisance to his family, so
he cuts off all ties and requests that they do not hinder their own achievements because of him. The social worker must bridge the gap between the
patient and his family. The social worker must work with the patient
individually, the family minus the patient, and the patient and his family
together in order to try and bring communication back into the picture.[29]

In regard to being a hereditary disease, Huntington's chorea
presents two views on genetic counseling. The first one believes that
the genetic counselor should present all the information and options,
and then work with the family to arrive at decisions in planning a rational
future. On the contrary, the second is entirely against reproduction,
especially when the risk is so high.

In dealing with the first, Dr. Arthur Falek believes that special
attention should be given to H. D. families because of the futile feeling
the family receives due to the hopeless prognosis. He feels that the
genetic counselor must be aware of the emotional issues involved such
as existing fears and anxieties. Since the disease cannot be diagnosed
at an early age, young immediate family members must and will be concerned about their own future; therefore, the genetic counselor must
deal with all immediate members in the same manner. Those with the
risk of contacting H. D. seem to be concerned about limited time with full
capabilities. In response to this, Dr. Falek says:

It should be pointed out to such individuals that when
they deny themselves career accomplishments based on
the possibility that they may at some future date develop
the disorder, is to assume a conclusion which cannot be
determined with certainty utilizing sophisticated modern-day
medical achievements.

For the most part, he has a very positive approach to the whole thing
suggesting that it is up to the individual and his or her spouse if they
want children, not up to the genetic counselor. [30]

On the other hand, some genetic counselors believe that Huntington
individuals should refrain from procreation and adopt children or remain
childless. One of these counselors is Dr. John S. Pearson who has
said:

I feel that society has the right to see that he (the
individual) is provided with informed counsel and that
part of the information he brings to the counseling situation consists of a valid observation that people who
refrain from reproduction, whether they develop Huntington's disease or not, lead happier and more productive lives
on the whole than those who beget children but subsequently
do develop the disease.

He believes most people would be satisfied with forty years of
normal life, but that sixteen years of "pitiable deterioration" is too
high a price for anyone to pay when the chances are one in two. He
also points out that one has to be realistic about everything, and there
is no good assurance that science will find an answer. [31]

Although there is presently no cure for Huntington's chorea, some
medications are used as controls of various complications. For example,
some patients who were on the drug reserpine had complete control of
choreatoid movements; however, others did not. The drug D-ampheta-
mine can counteract drowsiness and mental retardation[32] with some
success, but for the most part, the only consistent improvement in
patients with H.D. has been through physical therapy.

The objective of physical therapy is to slow down the deterioration
process and roll-back the present symptoms in the patient. In turn, this
could lessen economic problems by decreasing or shortening the amount
of hospitalization required. [33]

Five H. D. patients were the subjects of a project to study the effects of physical therapy on mental alertness, motivation for change, and cooperation with the home and hospital. Two of these patients had minimal physical disability while the other three were moderately dis-abilitated. They were viewed in their homes for one-hour sessions twice a week for four weeks. The therapists stressed the importance of physi-cal exercise between the sessions and encouraged the patients to partici-pate in activities. Part of their program consisted of eating a well-balanced diet, eliminating smoking, and rising before nine o'clock in the morning. At the end of the four-week period the therapist gave them an exercise program that was to be carried out in his absence. [34]

In a prestudy questionnaire, observation revealed that each patient had a minimum of twelve hours a day he would spend in bed. When the patients did get up, all they would do for the rest of the day is watch television. Three appeared undernourished; all looked anemic, and all of them were weak and walked unsteadily. [35]

At the end of the four-week period, there was an overall improve-ment in the energy levels of the patients. Breathing patterns improved, skin color became much more healthy, two had gained weight, and they all achieved better balance. Two patients had graduated from grade two (need for minimal assistance) to grade six (totally independent). Initially, four of the five were confined to the home. At the end of eight sessions, four of five were visiting friends outside the home at least twice a week. In all of them there were improvements in attitude, less mental confusion and enhanced memory function. [36]

A follow-up was made six months after the last session. Three patients made increasing strides of improvement in the quality of their activities. Another's neurological disorder became so bad that he could no longer function. The last patient's son went back to school, so the patient no longer carried out the exercise program since his son was the instigator in the program. [37]

Carole Binswanger sums up physical therapy and the H. D. patient in the following statement:

There seemed to be many misconceptions the families
had regarding H.D. and what was the best way to care for
the patient. That exercise was not harmful for those with
neurological disorders was explained: that, in fact, weakness could be accelerated by a sedentary existence, and that
a neurological patient was no different from others in the population with exercise being an important factor in maintaining
good general health. The role of those responsible was further
stressed in relationship to their structuring activities and/or
exercises and encouraging the subject to participate in them;
to realize that although the patient may not be able to communicate as he used to, his ability to think and respond to situations
remains basically intact. It is important to avoid treating
the patient in a diminutive manner which frequently results
in passivity and withdrawal. And, finally, there was an
effort to demonstrate to the relatives of the proband what
can be achieved so that their future, also, could be viewed in
a more positive perspective. [38]

Although physical therapy apparently offers some hope, presently
there is not a cure or even a consistent control that will stop or limit
the deterioration of the brain and central nervous system caused by
Huntington's chorea. It has been suspected for years that H.D. was a
disturbance of the biochemistry of the brain. New sophisticated methods
are beginning to isolate the differences in the biochemistry between the
H.D. patients and normal people. The problem appears to lie with
the neurotransmitters, or chemicals which transmit messages from one
neuron to another. Some of these neurotransmitters send "go" messages,
others called inhibitory neurotransmitters send "stop" messages.
Scientists suspected that the H.D. victim lacked the normal amount of
inhibitory neurotransmitters since the victim is always on the "go."
This hunch proved true as brains examined after death revealed a significantly less amount of inhibitory neurotransmitters, which are known
as G.A.B.A. (gamma-aminobutyric acid) in the H.D. patient. Tests
also showed that the H.D. victim has ninety percent less of the enzyme
G.A.D. (glutamic acid decarboxylase) which helps make GABA in
the brain. A replacement therapy type of project is being investigated
where the H.D. patient would use G.A.B.A. as a diabetic uses insulin. [39]

About five years ago, my father desired a release from reality
and attempted to do away with his life. According to him, he was going
to lose his job, and he felt that everybody was against him. Neither

proved to be true, and fortunately his attempt was unsuccessful. He was
in and out of the Mental Health Unit of the Medical Center, Rochester,
due to the diagnosis that he had nothing more than "a lack of self-
confidence." My mother, not believing that the trouble stemmed from
a "lack of self-confidence" told the doctors that my father had Huntington's
chorea. Upon checking the results of various tests for H.D., the doctors
denied that he had it, for the test results had turned up negative. Finally,
the pneumoencephalogram test administered by the Oakland Veterans'
Administration Hospital diagnosed my father as having Huntington's chorea.
He has been in the Veterans' Administration Hospital ever since they told
him he had the disorder. At first, we thought nothing of it because he was
able to come home frequently. Now his trips are limited to the point where
he makes none at all. There is not a word in the dictionary that can adequately describe my feeling in the midst of this situation.

Recently, it occurred to me that I could be living a condemned life.
I possess a one in two chance of contacting the disorder, likewise so does
my brother. Are forty productive years of life too high a price to pay for
a possible fifteen to twenty years of "pitiable deterioration?" In my
opinion, most certainly not. I am extremely thankful that my mother and
father were not aware of the fact that the defective gene was present in
his genetic line, for if they were, I would not be in existence. To sacri-
fice my seventeen years of life thus far, is something I do not even desire
to attempt to conceive. I have been blessed with so much, that to have not
experienced these blessings would have been a tragic loss. The essence
of life lies in the quality, and not the quantity. It is my objective to live
each day to the fullest extent, so that I would have nothing to regret if I
am not around to live the next. In my opinion, living life with something
hanging over my head is far superior to not living life at all.

FOOTNOTES

1. Nancy Apgar, _Is My Baby Alright?_ (New York, 1967).

2. John Gilroy, M.D., and John Stirling Myer, M.D.,
    "Huntington's Chorea," _Medical Neurology_, (1969),
    pp. 160-161.

3. U.S. Dept. of Health, Education and Welfare, _Huntington's
    Disease (Huntington's Chorea)_ (Wash., D.C., 1974), p.16.

4. Daniel Bergsma, _Birth Defects Atlas and Compendium_, (Balti-
    more: Williams and Wilkins, 1973), p. 488.

5. H.E.W., p. 10.

6. Bergsma, p. 488.

7. Gilroy, p. 160.

8. William Cole, "Marjorie Guthrie's Fight Against Her Hus-
    band's Killer," _Good Housekeeping_, 176:64 (March 1973).

9. Gilroy, p. 160.

10. Cole, p. 65.

11. Gilroy, p. 160.

12. Cole, p. 65.

13. Apgar, p. 65.

14. Cole, p. 65.

15. Gilroy, p. 161.

16. Nancy Wexler, Ph.D., "Living Out the Dying: H.D., Grief,
    and Death," _H.D. Handbook for Health Professionals_ (Oct.
    1973).

17. _Ibid_.

18. _Ibid_.

19. Ibid.

20. Ibid., p. 14.

21. Ibid.

22. Ibid.

23. Ibid.

24. Ibid.

25. Ibid., p. 15.

26. Ibid.

27. John R. Whittier, "The Psychiatrist and Huntington's Disease," The American Journal of Psychiatry, 128:12 (June, 1972).

28. Carole Hedges, M.S.W., "Huntington's Disease Some Implications for Social Work," The American Journal of Psychiatry, 128:72 (June, 1972).

29. Ibid., p. 8.

30. Arthur Falek, Ph.D., "Issues and Ethics in Genetic Counseling with Huntington's Disease Families," The American Journal of Psychiatry, 128:72 (June, 1972).

31. John S. Pearson, Ph.D., "Family Support and Counseling in Huntington's Disease," H.D. Handbook for Health Professionals (Oct., 1973) p. 12.

32. Victor A. McKusick, M.D., Medical Genetics 1958-1960 (St. Louis, 1961) p. 83.

33. Carole Binswanger, M.D., "Physical Therapy Used to Extend the Creative Functional Lives of Patients with Huntington's Disease," H.D. Handbook for Health Professionals (Oct., 1973), p. 17.

34. Ibid.

35. Ibid.

36. _Ibid._, p. 18.

37. _Ibid._

38. _Ibid._

39. Nancy Wexler, "The GABA Project," (Michigan Committee to Combat Huntington's Disease), Unpublished letter.

Apgar, Nancy S., Is My Baby Alright? New York: Random House,
    1967.

Bergsma, Daniel, M.D., Birth Defects Atlas and Compendium,
    Baltimore: The Williams and Wilkins Company, 1973.

Binswanger, Carole, M.A., "Physical Therapy Used to Extend the
    Creative Functional Lives of Patients with Huntington's
    Disease," H.D. Handbook for Health Professionals.
    N.P., 1973.

Cole, William, "Marjorie Guthrie's Fight Against Her Husband's
    Killer," Good Housekeeping (March, 1973, 176) p. 64+.

Falek, Arthur, Ph.D., "Issues and Ethics in Genetic Counseling
    with Huntington's Disease Families," The American Journal
    of Psychiatry, June 1972, Vol. 128, Iss. 12.

Gilroy, John, M.D., F.R.C.P. and John Stirling Myer, M.D.,
    "Huntington's Chorea," Medical Neurology (1969), pp. 160-
    161.

Health, Education and Welfare, U.S. Dept. of. Huntington's
    Disease (Huntington's Chorea). Washington, D.C.: U.S.
    Government Printing Office, 1974.

Hedges, Carole, M.S.W., "Huntington's Disease Some Implications
    for Social Work," The American Journal of Psychiatry,
    June 1972, Vol. 128, Iss. 12.

McKusick, Victor A., M.D., Medical Genetics 1958-1960. St.
    Louis: The C.V. Mosby Company, 1961.

Pearson, John S., Ph.D., "Family Support and Counseling in
    Huntington's Disease," H.D. Handbook for Health Profes-
    sionals. N.P., 1973.

Wexler, Nancy, "The GABA Project," Unpublished letter.
    (Michigan CCHD).

Wexler, Nancy Sabin, Ph.D., "Living Out the Dying: H.D., Grief,
    and Death," H.D. Handbook for Health Professionals. N.P.,
    1973.

Whittier, John R., et al., "The Psychiatrist and Huntington's
    Disease," The American Journal of Psychiatry, June 1972,
    Vol. 128, Iss. 12.

New York, New York   September 22, 1976

BARBARA RUBIN
NEW YORK, NEW YORK   MARCH 21, 1977

Introduction:

The health problems of patients with neurological diseases are analogous with

those of the aged in our society. This is evidenced by physical and mental

deterioration in both groups when illness occurs. Such deterioration is

often exacerbated by secondary complications, the trauma of frequent rejection

by families, the excessive costs of good medical care, and eventual isolation

in institutions. It behooves health planners interested in geriatric and

neurological care to join in cooperative efforts for the establishment of

common goals to provide alternative models of preventive health care in lieu

of expensive institutional care. I can conceive of three programs which

might provide an integrated approach to the neurologically impaired individuals

as well as those of the aged. Community agencies which are not primarily

oriented toward health care, such as community centers, are appropriate

loci for programs which allow the individual to participate in social and

recreational programs, and at the same time receive some medical supervision.

These models provide a continuum of prevention and early detection of

disease to more intensive services for the physically impaired individuals.

They are designed to help an individual attain an optimal level of mental,

social and physical well-being; in essence they are life enhancing programs,

rather than life sustaining programs. The Associated YM-YWHAs of Greater

New York have developed some of these programs and are committed to the concept of an even larger health component within their senior citizen's

centers to meet the growing needs of the aged and infirm.

Preventive Health Care Program:

The provision of health services for the aged, especially those in the

inner city, has been impaired because of budgetary cutbacks in municipal

health services and the withdrawal of community services by voluntary hospitals

owing to fiscal constraints.   Therefore, incipient symptoms of disease often

go unnoticed until therapeutic intervention is ineffective.

To address this problem, a public health nurse working in conjunction with a

medical social worker can function as a health care team in a community based

agency.   By training and experience, such a team can develop a health

component suited to a non-medical setting such as a senior citizen center,

where many aged congregate for social and recreational purposes.   The

health care team can fulfill several important functions:

1. For many individuals who have neither the means for, nor have access to,

    regular physical examinations, early health screening and monitoring

    can prevent serious and complicated illness, e.g. hypertension, diabetes,

    glaucoma, cancer, hearing problems, nutritional deficiencies, anemia,

    kidney disease (uremia), neurological disease such as Parkinsonism,

    diseases of the teeth and mouth, etc.   Early case-finding, periodic

    screening and appropriate follow-up and referral are important functions

    of a Preventive Health Care Team.

2. Health counselling, based on an assessment of individual health needs, may be constructive. The team 1) identifies present and potential health problems 2) evaluates the person's physical and emotional condition 3) estimates the ability and readiness of the individual and his family to meet his health needs and 4) determines the urgency and complexity of a given situation and priority of action.

   After this assessment, the Preventive Health Care Team can enable the individual to seek the required medical care, support the family in the event of a crisis or the development of a chronic situation which requires long term supportive therapy.

3. Health education programs can be undertaken by the health care team. Such programs should help the individual understand and recognize early symptoms of disease and recognize the importance of general health maintenance, proper nutrition, the need for accident prevention and the importance of physical exercise and recreational activities.

Traditionally, the early settlement houses such as the Henry Street Settlement house, addressed themselves to the health needs of their constituents. Lillian Wald, the founder of the Henry Street Settlement house, was herself a public health nurse. The Associated Ys of Greater New York have already conducted Health Fairs and health education courses, but they also recognize the growing need for an on-going health component as an integral part of their services to them.

Day Care Centers for the Elderly or Neurologically Impaired Individual:
A Day Care Center can provide an alternative to institutionalization for
the frail, handicapped individual who is able to maintain himself at home
without the aid of skilled nursing. A Day Care Center may offer a wide
spectrum of services, from intensive restorative therapy to programs which
provide long-term health maintenance. A good example of the latter is the
Day Center for the Elderly (D.C.E.) of the Mosholu Community Center in the
Bronx, staffed jointly with Montefiore Hospital. This D.C.E. was initiated
in 1972 as a three year demonstration project under the Social and Rehabilitation Service of HEW, and is currently funded under Medicaid.

The Mosholu D.C.E. currently provides an alternative to nursing home care to
90 aged impaired individuals, enabling them to live independently in their own
community. The daily program includes activities to improve and maintain
their social and emotional well-being, health supervision and supportive
services, a meal and transportation.

The Day Care program is designed to prevent the unnecessary institutionalization of elderly, sick individuals. The causes of 'unnecessary
institutionalization' are complex, but two will be mentioned here. The
first is an inefficient and undiscriminating system of assigning
elderly persons to levels of institutional care. The City of New York has
no uniform evaluation procedure to assess the needs of persons who require
skilled institutional care. Essentially, an elderly person will be placed
at the level for which he, a relative or social worker has applied. In the

majority of cases, this is a more intense (and much more expensive) level

than the person actually needs, and often results in his unwarranted dependence

on institutional personnel. The second cause of unnecessary institutionalization

is the lack of sufficient community support for the elderly person. It is

not enough to provide scores of social agencies, each one specializing in a

particular service. Some elderly individuals, with deteriorating health, are

no longer completely independent, and need some assistance with housekeeping,

shopping, finances and personal care. A person whose medical condition

deteriorates, who can no longer do all the household chores and who becomes

increasingly depressed because of his isolation may be eventually overwhelmed

by the struggle to remain in the community. At that point he chooses to enter

an institution. Such an individual is in need of an agency which will help

him coordinate the network of services he requires. The Day Center for the

Elderly has developed into such an agency and serves a population with

multiple needs. The staff members and their independent duties are as follows:

A. Project Coordinator: A certified social worker is responsible for

    overall supervision of the Day Center program. This individual advises

    the project staff, and performs general administrative duties.

B. Clinical Social Worker: A certified social worker is responsible for

    supervision of social program staff, and facilitates in-service

    education, schedules patient attendance, provides liaison work between

    medical and social components of the program, and supervises the

    patient counselling programs.

C. <u>Public Health Nurse</u> and her assistant,(Licensed Practical Nurse):
The staff members are responsible for planning in-program medical
services, the daily monitoring of patients, the medical evaluation of
new applicants, the coordination of patients' health and medical care
(including contact with private physicians and families), and the
maintenance of medical records.

D. <u>Consulting Physician</u>: The Physician is responsible for the design
and implementation of the medical component of the program, medical
assessment of patients and for liaison between the D.C.E., Montefiore
and private physicians.

E. <u>Recreational Therapist</u>: This therapist designs and administers arts
and crafts programs tailored to the needs of the individual patient.

F. <u>Occupational Therapist</u>: This therapist is responsible for intake
evaluation, some rehabilitation work and patient training in the use
of prosthetic devices and assistance with exercises.

The medical regime is as follows:

1. <u>Monitoring of Vital Signs</u>- Patients with moderate to severe cardiac
conditions have their pulse and blood pressure taken by the nurses
when they attend the Day Center. The remaining members have their
vital signs monitored once a week, and everyone is weighed once a
month to detect any unusual change in weight. In the several instances
the nurse has detected the initial phase of congestive heart failure
in a number of patients. Hospitalization was then possible before the
acute symptoms of the failure emerged. The nurses always notify

the private physician of any significant changes in the patient's
condition so that he can review the case and recommend appropriate
action.

2. <u>Escort to Medical Appointments</u>-When a volunteer is not available, the
   nurse escorts members on visits to Montefiore Hospital. Often, the
   appointment has been made with the assistance and recommendation of
   nurse, who has discovered a particular problem. The nurses speak
   with the Physician at the time of the patient's visit, receives
   information relevant to the examination, and then discusses the problem
   with the patient. This is an important service since doctors may
   not have the time to give the patient a complete explanation of their
   medical problems. The nurses take the time to explain to the patient
   the nature of his problem, how his new medications (if any) should be
   taken, and any change in procedure (such as diet) which the doctor
   has recommended.

3. <u>Health and hygiene counselling</u>- Health and hygiene counselling by
   the nurse is arranged with individual patients upon their request
   or as deemed necessary by the staff. Health counselling includes
   discussing the patient's medical condition with him, helping him to
   understand any special diet, and checking that he is taking his
   medications. Often, in the case of confused individual, it is necessary
   to involve the patient's family or housekeeper in the process.

The community center as a setting for a D.C.E. offers the individual the opportunity of social interaction, mental stimulation provided by varied programs and activities, and finally offers him the opportunity to live in dignity within his own community among his family and friends.

Outreach Programs for Homebound Individuals:

For the homebound individual with chronic dysfunctions or temporary incapacity, an out-reach program originating from a community center can provide supportive services. These services can provide the link between an individual who is struggling to maintain himself in his own home and the community in which he lives.

An outreach program must be distinguished from a Home Care Agency. Medicare (Title XVIII of the Social Security Act) and medicaid provide reimbursible services for post-hospital convalescent care in the patient's home. Services may include; part-time nursing care, physical, occupational or speech therapy and part-time services of home health aides. To provide these services, a Home Health Agency must be approved by the State Department of Health. Health departments or hospitals are the most likely sponsors for Home Health Agencies. When funding, or a qualified sponsor is not available, a community center may perform a comparable, modified service for the home-bound individual.

These services may include:

1. Identification of the elderly or physically impaired individual who is temporarily or permanently homebound.

2. Assessment of the individual's psycho-social and medical needs by a social worker and a public health nurse.

3. Referral to appropriate agencies, depending on the need and availability of services. Frequently a homebound individual, in his isolation, has not availed himself of services for which he is entitled, e.g. medical, welfare, counselling or visiting nurse services.

4. After the identification and assessment of a homebound individual is made, and appropriate services mobilized in his behalf, the out-reach team, with the assistance of volunteers, or paraprofessionals, can perform on-going services for the homebound patient.

   a) The public health nurse can provide on-going monitoring and evaluation of the individual, thus providing the medical link between the patient and his physician. She can ensure that the prescribed medical regime is being followed and that the home environment is conducive for the person's health needs. She can also be alert to a change in condition or the presence of complications. A public health nurse does not do bedside nursing (as does the Visiting Nurse), but she can play an important role in the health management of a homebound individual.

   b) The social worker can act as the coordinator of the out-reach team, in addition to the tasks of assessment, referral and casework services to the patient and the family. The effects of chronic, incapacitating illness on an individual and his family can be burdensome, and for some, intolerable. A skilled social worker can work with the family to help alleviate these emotional, social and financial problems.

   c) Para-professionals can provide direct services such as light

      housekeeping chores, telephone reassurance, shopping, escort

      services and friendly visiting.

At the present time, the Associated YM-YWHAs have two outreach programs and one awaiting funding from the government. The projects are called "Helping Hand: Comprehensive Services to the Homebound Elderly", Project Extend (also for the elderly) and the Community Advocacy Program for the Elderly, a mental health outreach program for the socially isolated, emotionally frail individual. There is a need for far more outreach projects, but there are severe fiscal constraints which prevent the development of new programs.

Conclusions:

The three models require either liason with a medical facility for medical consultation or cooperative efforts in conducting annual or semi-annual health screening programs for the entire membership of the community center. These programs place a strong emphasis on preventive services.

Every effort should be made to minimize the incidence of potentially catastrophic illnesses, which necessitates extreme medical expenditures. For the individual in medically underserved areas, who frequently only seeks care in a crisis, preventive programs may be essential.

Federal funds are spent at all levels of care, from primary care to institutionalization. This may be the time to examine how the health dollar is actually spent and whether, indeed, preventive services should be increasingly emphasized, in an effort to reduce the cost to society of our present health system.

New York, New York   September 22, 1976

MRS. JOHN J. SCHNEPP
MERCHANTVILLE, NEW JERSEY   MAY 31, 1977

RESPONSE TO QUESTIONNAIRE DISTRIBUTED BY CCHD, MICHIGAN CHAPTER

1. About my family and relatives: How many have died with
    H.D.? One.

    How many are afflicted now? None.

    How many are "at risk?" Four.

    This disease is not in my family but I am writing for a
    /_7 Male   /_7 Female Friend.

2. Was the afflicted patient diagnosed in a doctor's office,
    in a hospital or in a nursing home? Doctor's office.

    Any problems in getting a diagnosis?

    What problems had to be met? Raising four children
    with Huntington's mother.

3.   After the diagnosis:

Did different living arrangements have to be made?

No.

Were there any financial troubles?

I don't know.

Was there an employment problem?

No.

How were your requests for assistance received or refused?

I don't know.

Was there difficulty with an insurance problem or disability payments?

I don't know.

4.   How has the presence (or threat) of Huntington's disease
     affected your social life?

     I was married before I realized the seriousness of it.
     I was pregnant when I found out.

     How many children do you have, and what are their
     ages?

          MALE_____   FEMALE One, aged 8

     Do your children know they are "at risk?"
     No.

5.   In the future, I would certainly appreciate and HOPE for:
     (check:)

     /X/ More and better research.

     /X/ Better public understanding of our problem.

     /X/ Better and less expensive nursing care for H.D.
          patients.

     /X/ RELIEF from financial burdens.

     OTHER:

New York, New York   September 22, 1976

MERRILL SCHUTZBANK
MORRISVILLE, PENNSYLVANIA   MAY 14, 1977

RESPONSE TO QUESTIONNAIRE
DELAWARE VALLEY CHAPTER, CCHD

About my immediate family and other relatives:

     How many have died with H.D.? Three.

     How many are afflicted now? One.

     How many are "at risk"? Many.

Was the afflicted patient diagnosed in a doctor's office,
in a hospital, or in a nursing home? All three.

What problems had to be met? Many.

Were there any financial problems? Yes.

How were your requests for assistance handled? Middle class
people don't get assistance.

How has the presence and/or threat of Huntington's disease
affected your social life? Many ways mentally.

Do your children know that they are at risk? No.

How many children do you have, and what are their ages?
One male, 11 years; two females, 13 and 16.

New York, New York   September 22, 1976

BRUCE SINGH, M.D.
THE UNIVERSITY OF ROCHESTER
SCHOOL OF MEDICINE AND DENTISTRY
STRONG MEMORIAL HOSPITAL   SEPTEMBER 14, 1976

      This submission to the Committee is made at the request of a
patient of mine, Mrs. Griepp, whose submission is also included.   I
am an internist and psychiatrist working in the Med-Psychiatric Liaison
Division at Strong Memorial Hospital.   Mrs. Griepp has been under my
care with one of the problems that is universal as far as the families of
Huntington's patient is concerned--namely, how to deal with and understand the progressive dementia in a loved one involving a change in both
intellectual capabilities and personality.

      The psychosocial problems of the families of Huntington's patient
have been widely recognized but have not been subject to scientific study.
Until a cure of the disease is found, there is going to be a need for expert
help with these families.   However, this help needs a scientific data base
on the behavioral aspects of the effect of the illness on the family.
Studies focussing on the way the family handles the disruption and its
impact on individual members are needed to assess better ways of inter-
vening to help such families.   This woman only came to my attention
because of her sense of a need to get help.   Many others, however, who
do not push themselves forward are also suffering and it may be possible
for help and research on these unfortunate people to go hand in hand.

New York, New York   September 22, 1976

ANNE SIROTA
PATERSON, NJ

                                            SEPTEMBER 13, 1976

        It isn't easy to write of one's feeling when everyone
you love most is or can become a victim of Huntington's
Disease.

        Huntington's Disease kills the brain cells of its
victim but also kills the spirit, hopes and dreams of each
of his family.

        Fifteen years ago, my husband developed a twitch of one
shoulder and his personality started to change. He was always
an even-tempered person; so I realized something was wrong;
we went to our family doctor, who said it's only nerves.
We had some problems at home and thought this was so. But,
Bill became worse. So I went to another doctor who said
the same thing. He suggested a psychiatrist, so we went
to a psychiatrist who bled us dry. Bill was getting worse.
He couldn't work--even walked off a job which wasn't Bill.
One day he fell on the street and was taken to a hospital.
The doctor asked me if he was an alcoholic. He X-rayed his
head, stitched him up and sent him home--the beginning of one
doctor after another, one fall after another, one hospital
visit after another. I heard of a specialist in New York.
He gave us a diagnosis of diseased nerve ends. All the
others said just "nerves." Medication, expensive office
visits, but no help. All this with trying to keep a job.

        Finally, I heard of a young neurologist who suggested
we hospitalize Bill to really test him. He was hospitalized
for three weeks, tested very carefully, and after ten years
and all our savings we were told this horrible news. My one
daughter had two children and was pregnant 7 months with her
third child. My second daughter, a school teacher, was planning
her wedding. How does a mother tell her children? It took
me two weeks, but it had to be told. Their reaction? Can
you imagine their feelings!! I feel fortunate that they
didn't pull away or have a nervous breakdown. I didn't
want to believe. So I contacted the National Institutes of
Health and they finally accepted my husband. They did try
to help, but Bill did have Huntington's--we had to face that
fact. Bill was willing to endure any test, any new medication, if he could spare his children any agony, but nothing

has helped. My husband is dying a slow tortuous death. I
am dying slowly with him and so are my two daughters (for
the grandchildren and for themselves and their husbands).

     My husband's sister and brother are also afflicted
and their families are also going through the same feelings.

     Please! Please help us. I will go anywhere or talk to
anyone if I can get help to fight this dread disease.

New York, New York   September 22, 1976

REGINA SMOLENS
NORRISTOWN, PENNSYLVANIA   MAY 14, 1977

RESPONSE TO QUESTIONNAIRE
DELAWARE VALLEY CHAPTER, CCHD

About my immediate family and other relatives:

    How many have died with H.D.? Four.

    How many are afflicted now? One brother (30 years).

    How many are at risk? Three.

Was the afflicted patient diagnosed in a doctor's office, in
a hospital, or in a nursing home? Patient was diagnosed in a
doctor's office.

What problems had to be met? No specific problems had to be
met. Our biggest problem was trying to live a normal life.
My brother at most times was depressed, withdrawn, moody,
and angry. Also he was unemployed and had no interest in
finding work.

After the diagnosis:

    Did different living arrangements have to be made? He
lived nine months in my home with my husband, three sons, and
father-in-law. It was dreadful. Finally, things got so bad
there was a mutual parting of the ways.

    Were there any financial problems? Yes, he received only
minimal assistance every two weeks from the State for about
a year, until Social Security disability payments started.
He is now confined to a state hospital so now his financial
problems have lessened.

    Were there any employment problems? Yes. He lost a
succession of jobs due to personality problems presented by
H.D.

Were there problems with insurance and/or disability payments? No problems other than a long wait.

How were your requests for assistance handled? OK.

How has the presence and/or threat of Huntington's disease affected your social life? When the patient was in my home, it was curtailed, but it is normal enough now.

Do your children know that they are at risk? Yes.

How many children do you have and what are their ages? Three sons, 12, 8, and 3 years.

Has there been extra stress placed on your children? Not yet.   They had difficulty when their uncle was living here but they seem okay now.

New York, New York   September 22, 1976

ROBERT D. TERRY, M.D.
ISABEL TELLEZ-NAGEL, M.D.
KHALID IQBAL, PH.D.
ALBERT EINSTEIN COLLEGE OF MEDICINE   SEPTEMBER 20, 1976

Huntington's Disease is a genetic disorder transmitted as a simple Mendelian dominant, expressing itself clinically through abnormal function of the nervous system. Two general functions of this organ system are obviously involved, one being in those mechanisms controlling coordinated movement, and the second regarding cognitive skills and general mentation. There are no well-defined symptoms indicating dysfunction of other organs, but subtle changes not expressed clinically may ultimately be found. The major pathologic alteration in the brain is a loss of neurons from the basal ganglia, especially the caudate nucleus which is known to be associated with motor control, and also from the cerebral cortex which is known to deal with higher functions including mentation.

Major research efforts currently under way in many laboratories involve neurotransmitters as to the enzymes which synthesize them, their catabolic products, and the substrate transmitter itself. A variety of very interesting data have evolved from this work, indicating deficiencies in major transmitter systems. These deficiencies, however, probably reflect the loss of nerve cells, and this loss of cells appears to us to be the major problem to be considered in Huntington's Disease. To put this question in another way, Why do certain neurons in the central nervous system disappear in Huntington's Disease?

While diseases of a heterozygote pattern usually relate to enzymatic abnormalities, those of the dominant pattern usually concern abnormalities of structural proteins. The implied aspects of research have barely been approached to date. Electron microscopic studies reveal some abnormalities of cellular membranes; these must be pursued very actively at extremely high resolution. This will require biopsy tissue from the brain of living patients. Fresh human autopsy material is extremely valuable, both for morphologic research and for biochemical analyses. The presumed deficiency or abnormality in structural proteins might well be concealed in the mass of complex tissue components which make up the brain. Therefore, preliminary isolation of nerve cells from potentially affected areas, that is cerebral cortex and basal ganglia, should precede extensive analysis for abnormalities of these proteins. Such studies involve cellular isolation and subsequent sub-fractionation of these cells, followed by separation of the various sub-cellular organelles. Each such fraction could then be analyzed for its major protein components, and each protein must be analyzed as to its peptide structure, amino acid content, and sequence, for comparison with analogous isolates from normal tissue. Funding must be increased so that these sorts of high resolution structural studies and extensive protein analyses can be accurately performed by investigators in well equipped laboratories.

Additional studies which might bear not only on the anatomical substructure of the symptoms, but might also be useful in determining the significance of specific transmitter deficiencies, involve the quantification of neurons in particular parts of the brain. This sort of cell counting is an essential study yet to be done.

Since this is a genetic disorder, it is quite probable that cells other than those of the brain might display certain abnormalities, and these must be explored. Roberts' fibroblast studies are of great interest, for example. However, since the primary target of the disease is the brain, there can ultimately be no substitution for the study of human brain cells, that is the neurons of the caudate and cortex especially. The implicit need for biopsy and autopsy tissue is obvious. There ought, therefore, to be a national tissue bank.

Our major point, in summary, is that there are significant avenues of relevant and promising research which must be pursued, and which are sorely lacking in funding support.

New York, New York   September 22, 1976

JAY H. TOLSON
·RADNOR, PENNSYLVANIA   MAY 20, 1977

RESPONSE TO QUESTIONNAIRE DISTRIBUTED BY CCHD, MICHIGAN CHAPTER

1.   About my family and relatives: How many have died with
     H.D.?   One.

     How many are afflicted now? None.

     How many are "at risk?"   Three.

     This disease is not in my family but I am writing for a
     /_/ Male   /_/ Female   Friend.

2.   Was the afflicted patient diagnosed in a doctor's office,
     in a hospital or in a nursing home?   Hospital.

     What problems had to be met? The emotional inability
     of my wife to accept her fate.

3.   After the diagnosis:

Did different living arrangements have to be made?

Yes. My wife was emotionally incapable of caring for our children, ages 3, 5 and 7. Every time I was able to obtain domestic help, she made the person's life so miserable that the help left after only a few weeks of service.

Were there any financial troubles?
None.

Was there an employment problem?

No.

How were your requests for assistance received or refused?

No requests made.

Was there difficulty with an insurance problem or disability payments?
No.

4. How has the presence (or threat) of Huntington's disease
    affected your social life?

    During the period of my wife's illness, she refused to
    participate in any social activities.

    Has there been extra stress placed on your children?

    Yes, the 13-year-old boy is a bit apprehensive. The girls
    do not yet realize the gravity of the situation.

    How many children do you have, and what are their ages?

    MALE   One, 13.   FEMALE   Two, 9 and 11.

    Do your children know they are "at risk?"

    Yes.

5. In the future, I would certainly appreciate and HOPE for:
    (check:)

    /X/ More and better research.

    /X/ Better public understanding of our problem.

    /X/ Better and less expensive nursing care for H.D.
         patients.

    /X/ RELIEF from financial burdens.

    OTHER:

New York, New York   September 22, 1976

MRS. MURIEL M. TOMPKINS
MOUNT VERNON, NEW YORK   SEPTEMBER 8, 1976

    Well, where do I start? We have H.D. in our family and
have had plenty of it. I am one of seven children--my mother
had it--her two brothers--my oldest sister and my kid brother.
I have two children of my own--so far I am okay, as far as I
know, but it is frightening and depressing to live each day
and wonder who in the family will be next.

    My sister has one son, an only son, who won't even go to
see his own mother because of this disease. I am the only one
in my family that goes to visit and I do not drive so I have
to ask a friend to take me. You see, I live in Mt. Vernon,
New York, and my sister is in East Orange, New Jersey, in a
nursing home (Park Avenue Nursing Home). She's only 58. When
I go to see her she does not walk or talk--she just keeps
moving uncontrollably. She sweats even in the winter. She
continues to lose weight because she can't swallow her food--
spits it up, gags on it. It's really heartbreaking.

    I have seen so much of this disease. I even volunteered
to go down to the Veteran's Hospital for the test they were
doing on H.D. relatives, but I told the doctor--if you find
any signs of H.D. in me, please don't tell me because I would
jump off the nearest roof.

    When I was a teenager, I needed my mom, but she was
already sick with it. I watched them take her away in a
straight jacket to Grasslands Hospital and then they put her
in Wingdale. She was not crazy, she was sick. She was there
about 5 years and died on Good Friday. Her brother had it
also and was in Wingdale also at the same time--he died a few
months later. I had to raise two brothers the best I could,
but they needed their mom. These two brothers remember my
mother twitching uncontrollably so they do not want to go to
see my sister.

    My brother, George, was in Montrose Veteran's Hospital
for 7 years with H.D., and I visited him also. He had been in
the U.S. Army Air Force for 18 years and had two years to go
to retire and they found George had H.D. He passed away at
the age of 46--very, very thin. Yes, I used to go see him by
train and bus in snow and rain; taking him some pudding and
trying to feed him. Brother George would stumble as he tried

to walk and gag when he tried to eat. Do you know what this
has done to my nerves? You know, I knew it was helpless and
that he would die and never get well, but it was my brother
and I was helping him. He, too, could not talk or walk anymore, but he was so young. He had a wife and a little boy he
left behind.

I really hope that one day there is a cure--some kind of
help--even a special hospital for H.D. victims. When I used
to visit, people would shake their heads and look at me hug-
ging my sister and my brother, and say--All you can do is
pray. Well, little do they know that's just what I'm doing--
praying that nobody else in our family gets H.D.

Yes, I would be willing to testify in person, but I do
not drive.

New York, New York   September 22, 1976

LUCY TRUGLIA
HUNTINGTON STATION, NEW YORK   SEPTEMBER 10, 1976

    We are one of many families afflicted with Huntington's
disease. It is very hard to see your loved ones taken so
quickly and feeling so helpless. The first member of our
family is our mother who was not diagnosed right away and she
died very young, age 48 years. We didn't know what she had
until she died. She also lost her three brothers at 40 years
and one 65 years.

    They were diagnosed a lot quicker than our mother, but it
was too late for them. Our dear mother was put into a mental
hospital with all the other very severe mental cases and never
returned home; she died there alone.

    This is one of the reasons why we need better hospitals
and more care for these Huntington's disease patients. They
should be by themselves so they can receive better care and
feel wanted.

    Our mother gave birth to eight children. So far we have
lost one dear brother at age 40. He was in the same mental
hospital our mother was in and he died alone. We have an
older brother 49 years who is in the more advanced stage of
the disease.

    Our sister is 47 years and in an advanced stage also and
in the same hospital with all the severe mental cases.

    We have three more brothers who are younger but as of
now do not show any signs of the disease. I am one of a set
of twin girls, our age is 37 years and show no signs of the
disease.

    We are all hoping and praying that there will be some-
thing done very soon, so we can all benefit from the help
that is needed so desperately.

New York, New York   September 22, 1976

JANET M. WENGERT
CHESTER, PENNSYLVANIA   June 2, 1977

RESPONSE TO QUESTIONNAIRE DISTRIBUTED BY CCHD, MICHIGAN CHAPTER

1.   About my family and relatives: How many have died with
     H.D.?   Two.

     How many are afflicted now? Two.

     How many are "at risk?" Six.

     This disease is not in my family but I am writing for a
     /_/ Male   /_/ Female   Friend. Husband.

2.   Was the afflicted patient diagnosed in a doctor's office,
     in a hospital or in a nursing home?   Hospital.

     What problems had to be met? Placed in nursing home.
     My husband is only 36--one child (son). His sister
     is 34 and has four children.

3.   After the diagnosis:

Did different living arrangements have to be made?

Yes. Placed in nursing home. Took him out; couldn't afford prices.

Were there any financial troubles?

Yes. When you own a home and have to meet a mortgage payment and repairs, $330 S.S. don't go very far. Oil price to heat your home, what's left for food? I (Mrs. Wengert) can't work because Mr. Wengert needs me 24 hours a day.

Was there an employment problem?

Yes. 100 percent disabled.

How were your requests for assistance received or refused?

Social Security -- no problems, but not enough money to handle coverage of bills and mortgage.

Was there difficulty with an insurance problem or disability payments?

Yes. No new insurance could be obtained.

4. How has the presence (or threat) of Huntington's disease affected your social life?

    People laugh and make uncalled-for remarks when I take my husband out. People stare at him.

    Has there been extra stress placed on your children?

    Yes.

    How many children do you have and what are their ages?

        MALE____1_____   FEMALE_____

    Do your children know they are "at risk?"

    Yes.

5. In the future, I would certainly appreciate and HOPE for: (check:)

    /X/ More and better research.

    /X/ Better public understanding of our problem.

    /X/ Better and less expensive nursing care for H.D. patients.

    /X/ RELIEF from financial burdens.

    OTHER:

New York, New York   September 22, 1976

E. WEXLER
NEW JERSEY   OCTOBER 7, 1976

     I've been advised that your organization may receive
federal funding to aid research needed to conquer Huntington's
disease. I am acquainted with the terrible effects this illness has on both the afflicted individuals and their families
and I want to add my voice to those who desperately wish to
see Huntington's disease vanquished. Thank you.

New York, New York   September 22, 1976

HENRY WEXLER, M.D.
NEW HAVEN, CT   SEPTEMBER 21, 1976

        This brief statement attests my deep concern with the
hereditary disorder known as Huntington's disease (H.D.), one
of many such disorders and one of the most tragic of them. I
have had personal and professional experiences with it. At
long last it appears that governmental forces are being brought
to bear on the care of those afflicted ones, and, equally important, is providing a funded organization for the vigorous
pursuit of research to further understanding and hopefully find
a cure for it. It is a heartening sign of the continuing development of civilization. I firmly believe that discovering a
genetic cure for H.D. will open the gateway to the cure of all
hereditary disease. I hope the current plans will provide for
a tripartite program to include: symptomatic medical care;
care on a long-term basis: medical, nursing in hospitals and
nursing homes; provision of half-way houses for the chronically
ill but ambulatory cases.

        Needless to say, it gladdens the heart of medical people
and of sufferers of the affliction, to say nothing of informed
citizens over the country to observe the continuing action of
their legislators on behalf of those many with the disease and
those at risk of getting it.

New York, New York   September 22, 1976

BEATRICE WHITE
WAYMART, PENNSYLVANIA   MAY 27, 1977

RESPONSE TO QUESTIONNAIRE DISTRIBUTED BY CCHD, MICHIGAN CHAPTER

1. About my family and relatives: How many have died with
    H.D.?   Three.

    How many are afflicted now?   One.

    How many are "at risk?"   Three - eleven.

    This disease is not in my family but I am writing for a
    /_/ Male   /_/ Female   Friend.

2. Was the afflicted patient diagnosed in a doctor's office,
    in a hospital or in a nursing home?   Hospital.

    What problems had to be met? First home care, then hos-
    pital. Money problems.

3.   After the diagnosis:

Did different living arrangements have to be made?
Yes.

Were there any financial troubles?

Yes.

Was there an employment problem?

Yes.

How were your requests for assistance received or
refused?

He entered a Veterans' hospital (son).

Was there difficulty with an insurance problem or
disability payments?

None.

4.   How has the presence (or threat) of Huntington's disease
      affected your social life?

      Change in jobs for him. None for me.

      Has there been extra stress placed on your children?

      No.

      How many children do you have, and what are their ages?

      MALE   One, 43 years, CCHD FEMALE   Two, 44 and 42 years.

      Do your children know they are "at risk?"

      Yes.

5.   In the future, I would certainly appreciate and HOPE for:
      (check:)

      /x/   More and better research.

      /x/   Better public understanding of our problem.

      /x/   Better and less expensive nursing care for H.D.
            patients.

      /x/   RELIEF from financial burdens.

      OTHER:

New York, New York   September 22, 1976

JOHN R. WHITTIER, M.D.
STONYBROOK, NEW YORK

    I am submitting the following statement for possible use
by the Federal Commission on Huntington's Disease and Its Consequences.

    Creedmoor Institute for Psychobiologic Studies became a
research unit in New York State's Department of Mental Hygiene
in 1950, located in Queens on Long Island.

    Prior to my taking responsibility for this unit in 1950
my training and experience in medical research was largely related to basal ganglia of the brain and their disorders,
including Huntington's disease (chorea). Observations on this
disease were continued as the unit evolved. It became increasingly apparent over the years that not only were there enormous
needs for research, education and services directed against the
disease, but that (1) these needs were unmet, and (2) the disease presented a unique opportunity to study methods for prevention of aging processes in human brain having heavy genetic
contribution.

    Interests of the staff in the laboratories of the unit
grew rapidly and so did the needs, in such a manner that during
the past decade staff and physical resources had been organized
into a program so comprehensive as to be apparently unique.

    The pressure of requests for services and education from
patients, families, medical and lay organizations exceeded
resources, and indeed threatened to subordinate research so as
to jeopardize the policy priority to develop means to control,
if not to prevent the disease.

    At the time of this writing, the unit was involved in the
essential cooperative relation required, in various ways and
degrees of intensity, with 144 families, having 272 direct line
relatives with H.D., in New York State alone, representing 2,000
individuals, 920 of those direct-line relatives who might carry
the gene.

As the program evolved, many principles emerged. We learned:

- That without prospective design, the genetic and natural characteristics of H.D. could not effectively be studied.

- That without reasonable stability of staff and resources, the continuity required for prospective design could not be achieved.

- That effort appropriate to the magnitude of the problems and opportunities presented by H.D. required a "center" concept.

- That the personal and time consuming nature of the genetic counseling function could not be minimized without weakening the prospective design; genetic associates (in training, from Sarah Lawrence College Human Genetics Program) were a very valuable supplement to our staff.

- That Laboratory studies not coordinated with comprehensive clinical aspects of family participants were by that much of lesser value.

- That diversion of resources from H.D. priorities beyond whatever necessary to keep perspective, inevitably diverted effort.

- That investigators outside the unit desiring access to cooperating family members were so numerous and dependent on provision of time and resources of the Creedmoor center as to require careful screening with regard to relevance of their interests, to ensure protection not only of participant family members, but budgeting of unit effort.

- That inviting studies of symptom-prevention, unless staff, budget, and facilities permit, continually threaten disease prevention, if the latter is a priority.

- That the disease presents ethical, moral and legal
  problems of the highest order. (Appendix,
  Creedmoor reprint, 1963).

- That there is justification for considering H.D.,
  even heuristically, as a "communicable" disease,
  and employing the epidemiological approach, and
  finally:

- That the natural history of H.D., with all its complexity and multiplicity of impacts on those affected
  and those involved, well merit the disorder high
  listing in a rank-order of disease by cost measured
  in misery and money.

Five reprints and one preprint of publications from Creedmoor Institute are appended and should be considered integral to
statement. The 1973 reprint is especially informative. Also
appended is a partial listing of operations in the Huntington's
Disease Program as it was structured in 1975.

From our experience we can recommend creation or recognition of at least one National Center for Neurogenetic Diseases,
with a specific Division or Section on H.D., and functions including but not limited to those listed for the Creedmoor Program.
Center activities should be adequately and continuously funded.

Regional Centers could be considered, the primary purposes
of which would be epidemiology and communications.

Collaborative arrangements with separately funded investigators would depend on local circumstances. Creedmoor Institute's
experience in becoming overwhelmed by the needs of the population
in New York State alone should be kept in mind. From rather
extensive studies, we believe serious consideration should be
given to feasibility or demonstration projects employing Neurogenetic Mobile Units. Properly managed, such units might be
very practical supplements to Regional Centers.

The report of the Federal Commission on Diabetes could well
serve as an example of a prior report, which in its recommendations,
could be directly applicable to H.D., allowances being made for
the great differences in prevalence between H.D. and diabetes,
and the already extensive and long existing clinical and laboratory facilities devoted to diabetes.

New York, New York   September 22, 1976

This report was prepared while Creedmoor Institute was undergoing reorganization, and relocation to Long Island Research Institute as Division VII - Psychobiology. In the new setting, the Huntington's disease program will be continued, and hopefully provided with new opportunities.

I wish to thank all the staff of Creedmoor Institute for their work on H.D. Special thanks is due Charles Korenyi, M.D., who is my associate in conduct of studies on Huntington's disease and who helped in preparation of this statement.

Opinions in this statement are personal and do not necessarily reflect those of the N.Y. State Department of Mental Hygiene.

New York, New York   September 22, 1976

JOSEPH ZURAWIECKI
JERSEY CITY, NEW JERSEY   OCTOBER 13, 1976

     First of all, I could not appear in person due to my
heart condition. My social functions are rather limited.
Never far from home or for a long period of time. In addition
to this, there is no one I could leave my wife with! But I
would be glad to answer any questions by mail or phone.

     And what more can I add to what I have already written?
Last year I took her to Bethesda, Md., where after a short
interview, they would not keep her for further observation.
Case too far advanced! So where is the help? This year I had
her committed to the Trenton Psychiatric Center thinking it
was for neurological tests. After ten days I signed her out,
against advice of physicians. I could not live with myself if
I left her there, being confined as a mental patient. She is
not that yet. So I'll do my best as long as I can.

     Help? In what way? I cannot get S.S. disability for her
because she lacks four quarters. No S.S. supplemental income,
no Medicare or Medicaid, because I'm collecting S.S. disability of $315 a month and this seems to put me in a millionaires
class! So where is the help to come from?

     There should be separate facilities for people with H.D.
and I don't mean psychiatric centers. N.J. just shut down a
facility at Mt. Kipp, Glen Gardner, N.J. This would be ideal
for patients and staff and neurologists, etc. But who is to
give it to us?

     Patient: Albina Zurawiecki

ANONYMOUS
NEW YORK, NEW YORK   SEPTEMBER, 1976

An H.D. family is a destroyed family.   It is an internal process that each member of the family endures in his own special way.

The disease member because:

1.   He had children before he knew he had the disease.

2.   He realizes a burden to his family.

3.   He is not sure from onset how long he can function.

4.   He feels mentally capable but is physically incapacitated for five-fifteen years.

5.   He knows there is no cure.

6.   He knows he is deteriorating when tied to his bed, can no longer eat or drink and tubes are placed in him to keep him alive.

7.   He feels life semi-consciously with no doctor truly knowing just how much he feels or senses.

AND HIS FAMILY WATCHES.   The children wonder:

1.   Will I get the disease (knowing the 50% odds)?

2.   What insurance company will give me coverage because of the family history even if I'm lucky and don't get the disease?

3.   Will my intended spouse want to suffer as my parents have?

4.   I know I must never have children because of the odds.

5.   Why do they allow an H.D. patient to live in the advanced stages of the disease?

AND HIS FAMILY WATCHES.

The other parent lives two lives...

1. He faces each moment with respect to the other members that look to him for hope and confidence.

2. He must be cheerful but aware in the presence of the patient.

3. He must be one step ahead mentally when confronted with questions by the offspring. Be honest but don't frighten--they still have several good years and you want them to function as teenagers and young adults.

4. He must make another life for himself to keep a sense of balance for himself and his children.

5. He must cry alone to relieve his frustrations.

THE NEED IS TO BE REALISTIC WITHOUT ALL THE BUREAUCRACY.

One agency--one coordinator--hundreds of branch research laboratories, with the ultimate goal--a cure.

Skilled, trained medical staff and hospital equipped to care for an H.D. patient.

Insurance available to pay for this long-term devastating illness.

The right to death at the onset of the final stage of being tied to bed, skeleton in form, incoherent and filled with tubes.

Signed--an insider knowing well the minutest details.

New York, New York   September 22, 1976

ANONYMOUS
NEW YORK, NEW YORK   SEPTEMBER 12, 1976

It is terribly difficult for me to write this letter.

I truly hope you will never know or experience the torment I am going through watching someone I love slowly die and feeling so helpless.

In June of 1975 my husband suffered from a severe reaction to the drug Prolixin (used to treat H.D.). He spent two horrible days at a hospital for Physical Disabilities where he was not helped at all. The neurologist on call was on vacation and the neurologist subbing for him never showed up. It seemed everyone was under the impression that H.D. affects the mind and that his problem was mental, not physical, which was not the case. He simply was suffering from the effects of medication which he could not tolerate.

I was told (after he was tied to his bed) that I must take him to the psychiatric section of the hospital where he would be helped. This I did. I was told by the admitting doctor that my husband would have to be "certified" by two doctors in order to be admitted. I was not told that "certification" was commitment. I might mention that I was in the room when the two doctors spoke to him. One was in a great hurry and nervously asked a few questions and left. The other doctor mentioned that he had seen a T.V. program where a doctor gets H.D. while operating on a patient. (His hands start to shake.)

After the two doctors spoke with my husband, two men came to take him to his room. I insisted on going with him to make sure that he would be settled comfortably. Thank God I did. They took him to a building where people were screaming and they locked the doors behind us everywhere we went. I said there was NO WAY I WOULD LEAVE MY HUSBAND THERE. I explained to the nurse on duty that he was aware of everything and just wanted to be helped because he was suffering from the effects of medication. I told her that he did not belong in a place like this. She said it wasn't so bad and that it would only be for a few days. I refused to leave and I told her that I was walking out with him and that they would stop me over my dead body. I told her I was going to the newspapers and to my congressman to expose the hospital. She then called the doctor who was to be assigned to my husband and we left that horrible building and were taken to a beautiful building on the grounds of the hospital, where I had expected him to be put in the first place.

We were very fortunate that the doctor in charge of his case was interested in him and really cared about him. (He was new to the staff and had been with the hospital about a week.) However, he knew nothing about H.D. and I gave him one of our pamphlets.

I might add, as an afterthought, that the doctor in charge of admissions also knew nothing about H.D. and had to look it up in one of his books.

My husband was released after two weeks in the hospital. Since then he has suffered from fears and anxieties. I still have nightmares about that building with the screaming people and the locked doors.

If my family physician had not been on vacation we would have gone to the local hospital and not lived through this horror. I was afraid to go to the local hospital because so few doctors and nurses are familiar with H.D. Instead I called the hospital of physical disabilities and they assured me that they were familiar with the disease and had a neurologist on call that would help him immediately. This, of course, was not the case.

I am telling our story because I hope no one ever has to go through what we went through because of ignorance about H.D.

New York, New York   September 22, 1976

ANONYMOUS
NEW YORK, NEW YORK   SEPTEMBER 10, 1976

SUMMARY

1. A woman of 52, who has been so much to so many people, is in a nursing home.....for the rest of her life..... with HD, not knowing what day it is, or even able to tell time anymore.

2. Nothing can be done for her: the facility is custodial, only.

3. Fear of the future devastated her.....and can do this for her husband, her children and others in her family, as well.

4. We need to do so much.....research in all aspects of this and other genetic disorders must be increased many-fold now, until these diseases are overcome.

My wife, who had her fifty-second birthday about a month ago, is confined to a nursing home, where she'll be for the rest of her life, because of Huntington's Disease.

New York, New York   September 22, 1976

　　　The disease was diagnosed in January of 1972 by Dr. Irving

Cooper of St. Barnabas Hospital in New York. Her deterioration

has been rapid: in about two years she changed from an extremely

intelligent, vivacious woman, most capable as a wife, a mother,

a gourmet cook, an artist, a pianist.....a person who could do

anything and was afraid of nothing.....to a fear-stricken

shadow. As of last January, her deterioration was such that I

had no recourse but to _sentence_ her to a nursing home.

　　　Fear of the future overtook her; she had seen what HD did

to her mother and to an uncle. Fear of the future often comes

close to overtaking me: I know what she is going through, I can

see what has happened to her in a short time, I worry about our

two grown children.....I'm sick with worry when I think of the

fact that my daughter has two young children who are "at risk".

　　　This has had a monstrous effect on our family. When my

wife and I were first married, we had never heard of HD. Later

her mother became ill.....but no one even had a name for the

problem for some time. We had our children....we then had

my wife's mother's diagnosis. Even then, when the doctors

talked of Huntington's Chorea, there was no dissemination of

intelligence pointing out that we were dealing with a genetic

disease, and that my wife and our children were at risk. We saw her mother waste away, racked with choreic movements! Her

primary medication consisted of tranquilizers, these did

nothing to control the poor woman's movements..... her constantly

moving feet would wear out pieces of carpeting put in front of

her chair in a matter of weeks. But, still we never were given

a reason to fear for ourselves.....on reflecting upon that period

and its lack of knowledge about HD, it seemed that we were going

through a Dark Age.

After my wife's diagnosis, the realization came that we are

still in a Dark Age. Medication - Haldol, Tofranil, Thorazine

and various tranquilizers - control choreic movements, but there

is nothing to slow down the awful deterioration.

When my daughter was married, she, of course, knew much

more about what could be ahead for her than my wife and I did

at that same stage. She chose to have children because she

didn't want to miss the happiness we had with her and her

brother. Fear is in the back of her mind, however -- she

is receiving psychiatric counseling in an effort to gain some

inner strength she may need some day.

Our son, with the same set of facts to evaluate, chose

to have a vasectomy when he was married recently.

When my wife developed her most severe symptoms, those of mental deterioration, I found it very difficult to do my job, which requires some traveling. I worried about her constantly, but realized I had to live, physically, emotionally and mentally, to take care of her and to give strength to our children.

It became obvious that I could not keep my wife at home, even with the nurses I had there when I was at work or traveling. So, she's in a "Chronic and Convalescent Hospital". She still has enough of her faculties to be horribly lonesome = with our children away, I am all she has. Her speech is deteriorating badly and the sparkling personality and the love of being with people that she had have been replaced by a total dependence on me.

As for myself, I never knew how a person could be so lonesome.....my home both stifles me and feels like the biggest, emptiest place in the world.

The nursing home does give me (and my wife) a sense of security; I can be at work or travel on business without worrying every minute. But, as kind as the staff is, they can only give prescribed medication and provide custodial care.

I _am_ bitter about this. Why "us" - why "her"? What is
our future? (I have nightmares (and know) that someday she won't
recognize me!)

My employer provides an excellent medical insurance program,
but expenses for the nursing home are not covered. Thus, well
upwards of one thousand dollars a month is spent there, and all
the living expenses normal for the two of us go on and on,.....
for how long can I do this?

What do we need? First, although it can no longer help my
family, we have to have a way to identify this genetic trait,
hopefully in the fetus. We need to learn how to overcome such
inherited disorders, and I well know how gigantic a task this
is. We need to have medical men who can recognize and treat HD;
I have spoken to otherwise capable physicians who know much less
about HD than I do! We need to be able to take care of people
who develop HD: private custodial facilities are not enough,
state institutions I have seen are snake pits that degrade and
dehumanize people. We must be able to give hope, both to those
afflicted and to those who love them.

New York, New York   September 22, 1976

ANONYMOUS
NEW YORK, NEW YORK   SEPTEMBER, 1976

At age 2, I couldn't realize the implications of my father's illness. At age thirty, it causes me nightmares.

It was with little regret that my family saw my father taken away one day, for, after all, we had all been subjected to such terrible beatings as to be relieved when we were free of his abuse. For he, like his entire family, was an alcoholic and "dangerous." He would beat my mother and two brothers unmercifully; make unreasonable demands under threat of harm; and generally rule the house with a demonic hand. The scars, under normal conditions would last a long time. The scars when accompanied by H.D. would last forever.

It was sixteen years later that my father died, having been hospitalized in a mental institution for all those years. During those years, he managed to escape several time--each time requiring the family to seek police protection. In his less violent times, he usually just sat mute, smoking, brooding, and VEGETATING. There were many bouts with pneumonia, and illnesses which I can't remember now. There was talk among the adults that the ward was so roach infested that the beds were raised on tin cans to keep the roaches out of the beds. Dream or reality, I can't say--even the reality seems like it must be a dream.

It was at his death that my brothers, sister, and I were told about my father's hereditary disease, and, of course, warned not to have children. The warning came years too late since my father had already been

*"blessed" with six grandchildren. There would be eight before the chain
would stop. The news was accepted with general disbelief and a feeling of
disassociation with "that man" who had been absent from our lives for so
long, and didn't know us when we visited him. It was at his funeral that
the reality of the news became more apparent, because it was there that his
relatives gathered to attest to its truth. The one brother who was not
institutionalized came a human wreck. Helped on either side by his wife
and daughter, he came to see his brother for the first time in years. He could
neither speak, nor understand, nor walk unattended, and like his brother he
was a skeleton of a man. The rest of the six siblings could not attend
because all but one, who had died many years before, were institutionalized
--all victims of Huntington's Disease. Unfortunately, our clan had live
up well to their Irish-Catholic heritage. Children abounded.*

*It was perhaps four years later that I realized the threat of
H.D. It was then that the younger of my two brothers (then in his late
20's) began to exhibit erratic behavior. What was once a bright, responsible,
sensitive young man was becoming "a chip off the old block." His marriage
was failing; his job was in jeopardy; and his drinking and violence were
becoming matter of fact. It wasn't long before he had no wife, no job,
no money, and no self-respect. As a teenager, I didn't realize the job
I took on when I promised him, myself, and God to see him through. Without
parents or other moral support, I took on the care and support of my brother.
It is only now, some eleven or twelve years later that I realize the toll
that care has taken. I left teenage years optimistic that the horror would
soon be over; I approach middle age convinced it never will be.*

There were so many obstacles to overcome. Problems with the Social Security office--is he eligible? is he ill? what is this strange disease? why can't it be diagnosed? It was the same with the Veterans Administration. At the Department of Rehabilitation, I was told point-blank "don't waste your time and don't waste our time. The man cannot be rehabilitated, do you know what I mean?" No, I didn't know what he meant, since "the man," at that point, had several working years left. So he went from an accountant to a floor sweeper, and then to no job at all. Throughout this time, there was misinformation--a male-oriented disease; brought on by rheumatic fever; etc.--and an arms-length approach to his treatment. It was as though the disease was not only hereditary, but contagious as well.

My brother's illness progressed insidiously throughout the years. There were hospital stays, and brain biopsies, muscle deterioration, and always another superhuman decision. Should I consent to a brain biopsy? Will it make matters worse? Is he ready for institutionalization? A nursing home? hospital? boarding house? How will I pay for the care? And so on, and so on. And almost without exception there was no one who could help. Go to this department of the Social Security Office; go to that department; ask Mr. So and So; ask Mrs. Such and Such. Always left on "hold."

And then the real bomb fell. My oldest brother was hospitalized for a "nervous breakdown." It wasn't long before we knew that his recent erratic behavior was attributable to his father's legacy. A sadder version of H.D. than his younger brother--quieter, moodier, and more resigned to his fate--he battled with the disease for about three years. Choking on his food, unable to find his way to and from work, frightening to his children, it was cancer that finally saved him from his brother's continuing degeneration.

He died in a V.A. Hospital of cancer. Throughout his illness, we were told

that the deterioration we were witnessing daily was due to H.D. It seemed

the very insinuation of H.D. made any further tests unnecessary. Although

far more experienced in H.D. than any of the staff, we were unable to convince

doctors and staff that the symptoms my brother was experiencing were not

common to H.D. and that further tests should be taken. By the time the

stymied staff began to suspect another culprit (some two months later), my

brother was too weak to be tested. He died a suffocating-kind of death,

full of cancer and devoid of hope.

It was a result of these sad experiences that I have come to view

H.D. as a horrifying enemy--senseless, demoralizing, never ending. In my

small efforts as part of an H.D. organization to try to raise money, collect

brain tissue, or disseminate information, I am more often discouraged than

not. The public is apathetic, hospitals and doctors unsympathetic, and

agencies too bogged down in bureaucratic red tape to be helpful. A recent

survey sent to nursing homes and shelter care facilities brought in negligible

responses by mail. Follow-up telephone inquiries as to whether or not H.D.

patients would be admitted into their facility brought responses such as

"our doctor told us to stay as far away from you people as possible." We're

unpopular to our families, friends, and to society in general. And the

problems go on.

Throughout all of the years contending with H.D., I often forgot

that young girls do things other than make awesome decisions and face

terrifying problems. Life has been too serious to be young at heart--personal *aspirations have been pushed aside. Although there's seldom time to wallow in self pity, it's often difficult not to fall into it when awakened by a ghoulish nightmare which turns out not to be a dream at all but just another day in the life of an H.D. family.*

New York, New York   September 22, 1976

ANONYMOUS
NEW YORK, NEW YORK   SEPTEMBER 10, 1976

After 10 yrs of marriage, I thought my husband had started to be come
an alcoholic, staggering down the street and becoming abusive, even
trying to choking me. In fact one time after taking a few glasses
of beer he took the car and could not drive very well(had taken the
test 9 times, when one inspector thought he was just nervous and
passed him) and left the children and I on the beach. I thought
he was having a nervous breakdown.

It was very hard to get him to a doctor and we didn't know what to
do or what was wrong. He thought it had to do with his feet and
bought space shoes. He kept falling at work since he was a salesman
and head of stock , he had to climb a ladder often. Finally he lost
his job. I was lucky my uncle gave him a small position with his
firm, and after a while I had to drive him to work every morning
before going to work myself but I still had to worry about him getting
home.

He finally went to the VA Hospital at Ft Hamilton because of a bleeding
ulcer--they would not do anything further to clear this other problem.
We finally thought all his trouble was due to a fractured skull he
got in the army, and told him he could get a pension. Again he went
to the VA--when he went through all the test, Dr Nostrand told us
it was Huntington's Disease (my brothers-in- law and I never heard
of this before) she told me it would affect his mind and the whole
nervous system. I asked when he should be hospitalized and her reply
was ---you will know!

When he had stopped working he would go out in the street for walks,
or to NY on the subway and just wander around--he never looked clean
even though I dressed him every morning in clean clothes, and bathed
him. One day he lost his pants in the street and my two daughters,
who were in school at the time, had to go to the police station and
bring him home.

When the time came to put him in the hospital I could get no help so
I had to phone the police and say he hit my daughter, who also has
Huntington's Disease, to get him in the hospital. They took him in,
then sent him home with a promise he would go to the VA the next
day. He signed himself in then they transferred him to Pilgrim State,
as they would not keep him there.

kept getting sick at business and being sent home, she was also very nasty and abusive. In the middle of the night she would pull me out of bed by the hair, light all the lights in the house and have fist fights with her sister. She went to numerous doctors, and once in the hospital for tests she started breaking bottles and everything in the place. They put her in a stright jacket. The doctor told me to bring her home, which I did. She was calm for a while--then one night when I came home she had broken all my nick nacks-knocked over a book case and had the gas on. I had to call the police again, as the doctor would not put her in the hospital. She was in Pilgrim State two weeks when her father passed away. She is now a patient there for the past 4 years.

New York, New York   September 22, 1976

ANONYMOUS
NEWARK, NEW JERSEY   AUGUST 30, 1976

        We are a family who is afflicted with H.D.   I say a family because
when H.D. strikes, it afflicts not only the victim but also the offspring,
their mates and their families.

        H.D. is a family disease--and once it strikes a family, all its
members spend the rest of their lives in fear and uncertainty.   The fear
is of the onset of the horrible symptoms; the uncertainty is for living and
planning.

        How does one who is at risk fall in love?   Marry?   Buy a house?
Raise a family???   He can choose to do none of these things and merely
exist instead of live.   OR he can make an attempt to live, but he does so
always with hesitation because he never knows if or when the disease will
strike.

        I married a man who is at risk with H.D.   He is 37.   He is the
oldest of three sons born to a woman who was diagnosed as having H.D.
in 1971--three years after we were married, one year after son number 2
was married and one year before son number 3 would be married.   The
diagnosis was made and fear and uncertainty set in.

        But uncertainty abounds with this affliction.   There is no one test
which tells doctors what a particular patient with peculiar symptoms has
H.D.   As a matter of fact, in Mom's case, she was diagnosed as having
Alzheimer's Disease in January, 1971; but in September, 1971, she was
diagnosed as having H.D.   Another hospital corroborated the findings in
1972.   The doctor in charge told us that there are three areas he looks
for to make a diagnosis for H.D.   (1) Heredity; (2) Spastic movements;
(3) Psychological change.   When we questioned that we could not trace
the heredity in Mom's case, he indicated that he believed that she is a
mutation.

        So here we are, five years later.   Mom's symptoms have progressed
to such a point where she is no longer the same woman we remember.   The
movements are not so great, but the mind is affected.   She is now 61
years old and seemingly very healthy otherwise.   She could live in this
state for another 10, 15 or 20 years!

Her neurologist, who admittedly knows very little about H.D.,
suggested that my father-in-law commit her to an institution. Since he
is the man without the funds to afford a nursing home, the doctor suggested a state mental hospital. After committing her to one of these
hospitals for 10 days, my father-in-law decided to keep her at home
as long as possible. People with H.D. have no options. It's either an
expensive nursing home or a mental hospital.

That is what happens when you are a victim. It is not so pleasant
to be at risk either. Son No. 1 and I have decided not to have our own
family. We hope that we will be able to adopt. Son No. 2, a doctor aged
31, and his wife think differently. They already have one son and plan
to have more children. As a doctor he does not really believe that his
mother has H.D. He feels the doctors made a clinical diagnosis. Son
No. 3 is 25. He is married and he told me just yesterday that he prefers
never to think about the fact that there is H.D. in the family.

Anyway, as far as I can see, the disease has splintered the family.
No one in the family likes to talk about the disease, and when they do it
is with a lack of understanding. It is too painful, but there is a definite
need here for some counseling.

My recommendations for the Commission are the following:

1. A cure--or at the very least--a control drug.

2. Federal aid for H.D. patients (particularly for women and
    non-veterans) for nursing home care.

3. Organized individual and family counseling.

Unfortunately, I am not able to sign this letter. It would not be
good for many reasons if it was known that my husband is at risk for
H.D.

New York, New York   September 22, 1976

ANONYMOUS
SPRINGFIELD, NEW JERSEY   SEPTEMBER 14, 1976

      My family is at risk because my mother-in-law died nine years
ago, after lingering for many years with this vile disease that few doctors knew anything about.

      While in the early stages (in her forties) various doctors mis-
diagnosed it as "nerves," alcoholism, (she rarely drank and then only
wine), Parkinson's disease, and finally when a neurologist was called
in, he labeled it Huntington's chorea. But giving it a name with little
information was no help while watching this once healthy woman waste
away physically to just skin and bones, incapable of doing anything.

      Eventually, she had to have constant care in a nursing home, but
when the financial burden became too great, she was committed to a
public institution. This became a horrendous experience for the family
with tremendous guilt feelings since OVERBROOK in Cedar Grove was
always known as the "nut house" where insane people were put. In addition, the fear that went hand-in-hand with the guilt is beyond comprehension.

      She had two married children and they had a total of seven chil-
dren (four are now of marriageable age) and all of these human beings
are at risk, wondering and waiting with various stages of emotions as to
which one will be next. This makes daily living HELL.

      I cannot understand why nothing has been done to help the H. D.
families. This disease has existed for more than 300 years in this
country, yet the medical profession is ignorant. Why isn't there government funding for research? Why isn't there a diagnostic clinic or an
evaluation center available? Why isn't there therapy available, not
just for the victim, but the family as well? Why aren't there social
services available to help the families without funds? Why are we being
ignored?

      Due to the social stigma and jobs being lost and insurance policies
cancelled, the H. D. families are not as public as the Cancer or Heart or
the many other "popular" diseases that get attention. However, due to
the 50-50 hereditary factor there are so many at risk and perpetuating

this risk with each generation, a genetic time bomb situation is created, destroying any possibility for normal living.

Does one marry and plan to have children? Or is this perfectly normal function denied? Is one married or not, while the beloved spouse is committed for years to a mental institution to waste away until release in final blessed death?

How do we cope with our childrens' attitudes when they refuse to work or continue school because they feel it is a waste of time if "the curse is upon them."

My family is now watching and waiting for the second H.D. victim to slowly die. A cousin in his sixties with a wife, three adult children, and eight grandchildren, all in various stages of anguish and panic, wondering when it will strike them.

HELP US PLEASE. DON'T DENY US A FUTURE. WE ARE ENTITLED TO MORE THAN BECOMING A LIVING VEGETABLE.

New York, New York   September 22, 1976

ANONYMOUS
PATERSON, NEW JERSEY   OCTOBER 12, 1976

        The heartbreak of Huntington's disease is devastating.
The agony the patient endures, plus the heartbreak of his
family watching this is indeed very painful.

        My husband was stricken several years ago, and I have
just about tried everything, but to no avail. He has gone
through all kinds of tests, the doctors experimenting with
tranquilizers which only made him so depressed and not at all
with it. He has had eleven acupuncture treatments, but
nothing happened. Now he is getting progressively worse; the
walking is so bad and his speech is affected. He goes to the
doctor every three weeks and gets a B-12 shot and the doctor
checks him over. He is at least trying to keep him in the
best possible health.

        When are they going to really do something about this
horrible disease? I do not understand how something like this
can go neglected for so many years.

        Millions can be spent putting a man on the moon, but when
it comes down to caring for our very own here on earth, we
seem to be forgotten.

        To think that someday my lovely children may have this,
is more than I can endure.

        Please, please I beg of you to please try to help us,
for God's sake.

        I do not wish to sign my name, but I will sign it "Heart-
broken." Thank you.

New York, New York   September 22, 1976

C.W.
NEW JERSEY   DECEMBER 16, 1976

My mother-in-law and my husband both are victims of H.D. My husband was diagnosed as having H.D. about 18 months ago when he visited the doctor complaining of falling and dizziness. On the basis of this and the fact his mother suffers from an undiagnosed neurological disorder (she's been in and out of mental hospitals for the past 15 years and is presently in a nursing home) it was felt we are an H.D. family.

Now that we know about H.D., I realize there were signs of the illness at least three years prior to the final diagnosis.

The doctor was very kind and gave us the address for CCHD. This organization has given my family strength and courage; their newsletters are uplifting. The Delaware Valley Chapter has been helpful in providing information and encouragement. Before I made contact with CCHD, I felt so alone, the disease so frightening. I still feel the disease is the most devastating for complete families of any disease; but I no longer feel all alone with my concerns. When I attend CCHD meetings and hear doctors speak of their research, I gain hope. I pray for help for H.D. families. I have two sons at risk.

The public must be educated about H.D. This is made difficult because of the stigma attached to H.D. Victims fear job loss and discrimination, so they hide the disease as long as possible. This is where CCHD has been so very beneficial to my family: with members we can be honest, express our fears, show how terribly vulnerable we are.

When I first learned my husband had H.D. I became very emotional. Our neurologist was very kind but also very honest. A very helpful thing he said to me was, "Just because I've given a name to some problems your husband is experiencing doesn't mean that he's a different man all at once. This did not happen overnight."

I feel that not only the public, but social services agencies need to be more aware of H.D. At the time H.D. was

New York, New York   September 22, 1976

diagnosed, my family was attending family counseling sessions
once a week trying to resolve family problems that were being
caused, in part, by the personality changes H.D. causes. No
one at the guidance center realized my husband had H.D. After
the neurologist visit and we discussed H.D. in our therapy
sessions, family life became easier for us all because the
therapy began to work for us. H.D. families need to know
what they are battling, and so do therapists in order to help!

New York, New York   September 22, 1976

ANONYMOUS
MATAWAN, NEW JERSEY   SEPTEMBER 12, 1976

    My first encounter with Huntington's disease began at age
seven, when my father was hospitalized in a State hospital
with a "nervous breakdown," and who was to remain there until
his death 16 years later. Before his hospitalization, he had
turned life into a nightmare with his drinking, which resulted
in fighting, unprovoked beatings for his wife and children,
irrational behavior, and a suspicious nature toward all.
Subsequently, all of his five sisters and one brother were to
be in and out of State hospitals for the next twenty years.

    My sister and I do not have symptoms of H.D. However, my
two older brothers both contracted H.D. within the last ten
years, and we have watched them change almost on a daily basis
from highly intelligent, motivated individuals to an awesome
deterioration of both mind and body. The older of the two,
who contracted H.D. within the last five years, was stricken
down one and one-half years ago to the point that he could
just about make it from chair to chair alone. The doctors
felt that it was not unusual in some cases, for the deterioration to progress at a rapid pace. When they hospitalized him,
he was in and out of extremely heavy sleeping, his mind was
completely in a fog, and he couldn't walk. Because of his H.D.
history, the doctors assumed his symptoms were relative to it.
It wasn't until three weeks or more had passed that they
started making tests for other causes of his daily worsening
condition. X-rays and a Bronchoscope showed something suspicious on the lung, but because of his condition they could not
operate on him. The suspicion turned out to be a cancerous
tumor, which proved fatal to him a month later. The frightening aspect is, if he did not have H.D., they would have tested
him for something serious at a much earlier time, before it
proved to be too late.

    We have two children, who do not know anything about the
H.D. factor in our family, nor the anguish we go through as to
when is the correct time to tell them. My prayer is that when
the time does come to inform them, there will be a cure.

New York, New York   September 22, 1976

ANONYMOUS
METUCHEN, NEW JERSEY   AUGUST 29, 1976

The National Huntington's Disease Association, New Jersey Chapter, has asked me to outline to you my own personal experience with Huntington's disease. As my husband is a victim of this cruel and heartbreaking disease, I feel I am very well qualified to relay my story to you.

My husband, age 56, who should be in the "peak of his life" is a living vegetable, unable to think clearly, unable to concentrate to read or watch television or to hold any kind of conversation. Why--because he was unfortunate enough, through no fault of his own, to inherit this defective gene which has deteriorated his nervous system and brain cells.

My husband was a good living man, devoted to his family, his church and his country and worked hard during his working years, which terminated at age 49. Now when he should be enjoying the fruits of his endeavors what is he--a living vegetable and as senile as a ninety-year-old man--living a life of just plain HELL. To me, his wife, and our three children it has also been a life of Hell.

His illness was first diagnosed in October of 1969 when he was unable to perform his duties at work as a telephone equipment installer. After complete neurological tests at St. Peter's Hospital in New Brunswick, N.J., it was diagnosed as Huntington's disease. In February of 1970 he attempted to take his life on the railroad tracks, but jumped off just in time. He was then admitted to Marlboro State Hospital where he remained for four months and then was released. He stayed at home from April of 1970 until 1971, when he was again readmitted to the State Hospital, due to the fact that he wandered from home and was missing for several hours at a time. On one occasion he walked from Metuchen to Newark, N.J., a distance of some twenty miles, and we, his family, had no idea where he was. The State Police and local police forces were alerted to his being missing, due to his mental condition. He remained at Marlboro State Hospital for thirteen months, coming home weekends after three months. The doctors there felt he was deteriorating so rapidly, they thought he would do better at home and he has been here at home for the past four and one-half years.

To enumerate the many things he does, due to his premature senility, would take pages of writing, but to watch a man of only 56 years put his pants on inside out, spill his food (which has to be cut up in small pieces as a child's), all over himself and the floor and is unable to perform everyday functions such as taking a bath, shaving himself, etc., would tear the heart out of even the coldest person.

We have three grown children, ages 28, 25 and 22 and to look at our three children (two married and one about to be, and our two-and-one half-year-old granddaughter) you cannot get it out of your mind that they have a 50% chance of ending up a "vegetable," like their father in their forties. This is a cross which is almost impossible to bear. The only thing that keeps me going is the hope and prayer that medical science will discover how to correct this defective gene so that my three children and the countless thousands others who have this "nightmare" in their families, will have peace of mind and will be able to live normal lives. The only way this can be done is for appropriating the necessary money for research on Huntington's disease and other diseases which bring nothing but heartache to the families involved.

Regarding my husband's family history--his Mother died at age 51 when Tom was only 12 years old. According to other relatives she at that time showed no signs of Huntington's, but no doubt, carried this defective gene. She did have a brother who was supposed to have some sort of seizures, which they thought were epileptic, but no doubt were symptoms of Huntington's. Then in the late 1950's one of his brothers, age 40, was diagnosed as having Huntington's disease in the Veterans' Hospital, Bronx, N.Y. He died in the early 1960's of drowning.

Another brother who was an engineer for Western Electric, has been having involuntary twitching and movements for the past ten years, which forced him to retire from his job. But this brother, so far, has not turned mental, the disease being evidenced so far by his twitching and involuntary movements. Just one year ago another brother, who was a Department Head at Western Electric, was forced to retire on disability, as he was unable to perform his duties due to his deteriorating mental and physical state. Out of his family of seven, four of the male members have inherited Huntington's disease, leaving one brother, age 53, so far seeming to have escaped it. But, needless to say, his mind is a hell to him, not knowing if he will show signs this year or the next or the next. The two female members of the family who are now ages 65 and

63, show no signs of this "nightmare." The offspring from my husband and his three brothers who have or had Huntington's number 13 and so far, about 20 grandchildren. From this you can see how this disease will snowball through the generations unless something is discovered to eradicate this defective gene.

My husband is now an outpatient of Marlboro State Hospital, going to the Rutgers Mental Health Clinic here in Metuchen once a month for medication. He is taking Valium and Thorazine, which are only tranquilizers. I might add that one of our sons has consulted a nutrition specialist and he recommended that he give his Dad Vitamin E, Calcium Magnesium and iron supplement and bone meal, which has seemed to have helped his involuntary movements, although he is failing more and more each day mentally. Whether the vitamin supplements have helped, or this is just another stage of the disease, I do not know.

To summarize, I have tried to give you a description of how Huntington's disease affects a person in the prime of his life and how if affects the family of the victim. To say it is a life of Hell for the victim and his family, is putting it mildly.

I know eventually my husband will have to be admitted to a nursing home but I intend to keep him at home as long as possible. I had to go back to work after nineteen years at home for financial reasons. He receives a small pension from Western Electric and does get Social Security Disability, but this sum is not nearly enough to run a home with today's inflation. So far my health has held up sufficiently to be able to work, although in three weeks time I have to go to the hospital to have a cataract removed from my left eye, which was due to radiation I had to have after having cancer of the breast in the spring of 1969, just before my husband was sent hom from work. I know now that he was not acting normal at that time, and in fact, two or three years before that was not his normal self. With the help of my 80-year-old Mother, who lives with us, and the three children, I hope things will be alright, as I will be unable to take care of him for a few weeks after the operation. I will have to depend on my sons to give him his bath, shave him, etc., and my daughter and daughter-in-law to help with the cooking. Luckily, our children live within a ten-mile radius of Metuchen.

So, please, I beg of you, to do all in your power to appropriate the necessary money for research to find the cause and cure of Huntington's disease.

New York, New York   September 22, 1976

ANONYMOUS
NEW JERSEY   SEPTEMBER 14, 1976

On February 1, 1976, my husband,   died in

Marlboro Hospital, after many years of hospitalization

due to Huntington's disease.

It started 27 years ago with a personality change --- a man

who was thoughtful, generous and a good hard-working man,

turned into a suspicious, arogent and very difficult man

to live with. As time went on, he also developed a leg

tremor and his goit became very apparently effected.

No one knew why --- until my husband's sister came down

with the same disease. A small town doctor in Pennsylvannia

diagnosed the case as Huntington's disease, only then the

family admitted that their father must of had it.

Twenty years ago, getting help was an impossibility. I

went to my family doctor who suggested I go to my spiritual

advisor. My spiritual advisor listened --- then turned me

back to my family doctor. I knocked on doors, for years,

until a social worker in New Brunswick took pity on me

and helped me with hospitalizing my husband.

In Marlboro he was diagnosed as a schizophrenic, paranoid in earlier

years.

Our family life was a torment. Living with a person that exploded

at any given moment was not easy on me, but, also, the children

were greatly effected --- they were frightened -- confused, and,

often beaten.

Not only did Huntington's disease create problems at home, but also at his place of employment. Due to his inability to control his temper, he became abusive to anyone who disagreed with him. His coordination became erratic and he could not perform on the machines. This did not escape his employer's attention and 13 years ago he was laid off --- they said there was no job for him.

Eight years ago he was committed to Marlboro after he became uncontrolable in St.Peter's hospital while he was there for some tests after a visit to a neurologist. I informed the neurologist that I felt he had Huntington's disease.

It was urgent that he be hospitalized as he had strong sexual desires for all the young neighborhood girls. He also made advances toward many of our female relatives and friends.

Enclosed please find copy of a letter from the Office of County Adjuster. Not only did we suffer during the victim's life, but, the disease has taken its toll, financially.

I also have a Mother's worry. The disease is hereditary and my children have a 50-50 chance of going thru life like their father.

This has been extremely difficult to write, to bare my life, and much as I would like to block out this segment of my life, I need to fight for help for myself and other families afflicted with Huntington's disease.

Thank you.

New York, New York   September 22, 1976

ANONYMOUS
McALISTERVILLE, PA   SEPTEMBER 9, 1976

    In your continued effort to combat Huntington's Disease I'm
sure you hear hundreds of personal experiences every day. Could
you use one more?

    My husband spoke to you recently because now he has become
personally affected by the consequences of H. D. Not physically,
but just another example of the lives it touches and the toll it
takes. Here we are two perfectly healthy people otherwise, but so
preoccupied with my daughter's welfare that a normal life and
marriage is impossible. Yes, I'm speaking as the mother of a 29 yr.
old daughter with H. D. (Johanna Bell). She was born in 1947 with
what seemed like a lot going for her, that is to healthy, well adjusted parents, etc. The one thing missing, however, was a Grandmother Bell, for her father's mother had died in 1941 at age 57.
I had not heard or asked very much of the circumstances surrounding
her death but it was quite evident that her illness had been lengthy
and very hard on the family. The family had become separated with
the six children being split up between relatives. Then, about
age 30, my husband & Johanna's father started having a lot of "nervous"
problems to the point of personality changes causing loss of job after
job. Hospitalization insurance ran out after lengthy psychiatric care,
electric shock treatments and you name it to treat this mental disorder.
Finally he was admitted to St. Elizabeth's Hospital in Washington, D. C.,
a federal institution for the mentally ill. This happened to be the
same hospital at which his mother had died. Yes, they really tried

but didn't know at all what the real trouble was. Then, quite by
accident it was discovered that another male patient by the same
last name was there in the hospital with very similar symptoms except
much worse. It turned out that they were brothers - the oldest and
the youngest children of the Bell family. I believe the doctors were
on the right course of diagnosing the older brother's case when they
began to compare notes and the final diagnosis of Huntington's Chorea
was made for both men. These brothers had not known each other since
the family had been separated many years earlier. The older brother
incidentally, had three grown children and my husband and I had the
one young child.

To get back to myself and daughter's case. By now we knew that
daddy would not get well and he was in the meantime sent to a V. A.
hospital for long term care which lasted eight more years. Actually,
memories of her father are only of a sick father. Life was certainly
not easy for either of us for while I worked two jobs to support us
she was kept by a sitter. She had to assume many responsibilities
around the house and much too early in life she became the "sitter"
for her father who was at that time still able to come home for visits.
While I would work weekends, she tended to feeding him and helping
with his personal hygiene. Then when he could no longer come home
life still revolved around him and she and I spent every Saturday or
Sunday making the long drive to visit him. I look back now and think
perhaps some things could have been different but the fact remains that
her early life was certainly much different than all her friends.

I feel that her anti-social behaviour must have been partly caused by this early background, however, it still occurs to me that there may be early signs which bear looking into in connection with research of Huntington's Disease. About the only blessing in that respect is that she did not choose to marry and have children for now she is the victim of H. D. herself. I might mention that her first cousin, daughter of the oldest brother whom I mentioned earlier, is now in the last stages of H. D. and confined to a nursing home in Northern Virginia. Psychologically, all this adds up to a great depression for it's all too clear that life now consists of a steady decline in health and eventual total incapacitation. These real miseries you have seen and heard over and over again. I keep saying there just has to be something done to stop it from happening to other people, yet I'm sure I'm most wrapped in my own personal problems. We need help! Johanna was a well trained secretary earning a good salary in Washington, D. C. and strictly independent. I had in the meantime remarried and moved to Pennsylvania to start a new life. At about the same time as my marriage she began to have symptoms- so slight and sneaky that it took two years to really register on us that H. D. had struck again. By that time she was in desparate need of help and we brought her to live in Penna., away from all familiar surroundings and to people who cannot cope with the situation. Her behaviour just about drives us to distraction. She has lost so much reasoning power and I am continuously making excuses to her step father for her actions. The result is constant friction and un-happiness for all of us. She has run away from home and recently took an overdose of sleeping pills. It is true she is still mobile and

probably capable of doing much on her own with the proper motivation.

This is not to be had at home, however, and neither can we seem to find

where it is available. We've been told that all inquiries must go

through the county Mental Health Center. She had a case worker- but we

cannot even get an appointment with the medical director, their

psychiatrist, to make an evaluation of the case as to whether or not

she can take care of herself, needs hospitalization or referral to

some other resource. It boils down to this- I love her as much as

ever, but also love my husband and do not fault him for not being

able to cope with the situation. Even if I traded in my marriage for

a life of taking care of my disabled daughter what would be the price?

Could I do it financially or physically? Don't I also have an obligation

to my husband? He certainly didn't bargain for taking on the heartaches
of a wife and a mature daughter with H. D.

      I realize we're just three unimportant people caught up in this
situation, peculiar to this immediate area because the average person
has never even heard of the disease. There must be hundreds of similar
situations and many other lives at stake. If something isn't done and
soon, the multitude can only grow. I don't understand why so much
government money can go to foreign aid , moon shots and the like while

we have here in the United States something so terrible and the Health

& Welfare bills still having so much trouble being passed.

      Thanks for listening, Marjorie, I'm just hoping that since you

have already made some break through to the people in control of the

taxpayer's money that you can continue on our behalf. *God Bless*
you for all your effort.

New York, New York   September 22, 1976

ANONYMOUS   AUGUST 28, 1976

       I am enclosing a copy of a letter sent to "Newsday" on
Long Island. This letter speaks for itself.

       Personally I feel that hospital staff, doctors, and
particularly, social workers should be enlightened regarding
Huntington's disease.

       It would take pages to go into my unhappy experience with
Brunswick Hospital of Physical Disabilities in Amityville,
Long Island, but I would be glad to discuss it with anyone,
any evening after 5:30 p.m. or weekends.

I am writing you in regard to my concern with Huntington's Disease and its many side effects. I am an at-risk
patient and my mother, who was afflicted, was one of twelve
children exposed to the risk of inheriting Huntington's
disease. Four of the children have died of the illness, one
is still afflicted, four died of other causes before the age
of forty and three survive (each around the age of 60).

A three-out-of-twelve survival rate is very dishearten-
ing, and worst of all is that the twelve children fostered
from my mother's generation all live in fear of the illness.
And the sixteen children in the subsequent generation will
also have to be warned of the implications. I dread the
thought of having to tell my children that before getting
married their respective partners must be advised of the
potential consequences. The thought that this situation will
continue for generation after generation is frightening.

Amongst my relatives I am the most knowledgeable about
the disease, having read many articles on genetics related to
Huntington's disease. Because of the nature of the illness
and its association with mental illness (insanity), very
little discussion about it takes place amongst us. And
yet various relatives have been told by personal physicians
of the "severe mental deterioration that takes place" (which
is not always true) and that the disease can skip generations
(also false). My efforts to set them straight proved futile
until they heard it correctly from one of the doctors at
Columbia Presbyterian Medical Center. To have such a concentration of sickness within one family presents a severe
strain to the normal family relationships.

As for my immediate family members, my wife is very
fearful of the consequences of the disease and we seldom
discuss it. I once attended a gathering of at-risk HD patients at a person's home for coffee and cake and conversation. All I sensed all night was the feeling of doom hanging
over each one of us in the room. I haven't been to one
since.

Various members of my family have as a group participated in research programs at Columbia Presbyterian Medical

New York, New York   September 22, 1976

Center. I myself attend a research program at Creedmoor
State Hospital (physical testing and genetic history). In
one of the recent tests given to family members for a potential detection method, we were informed that the test was a
kind of longshot and that the ultimate hope for a cure in the
near future was nil. It was explained that a number of dis-
persed, unrelated research programs were being performed without an appropriate exchange of information between the various
research groups. It would certainly seem that a coordinated
effort could be made on behalf of everyone involved to aim
for a common goal.

Perhaps the most frustrating aspect of the disease is
the "not knowing who will be afflicted and when." Having
lived on an "at-risk" basis for 40 years is such a mental
strain that even if one "escapes" the direct effects, he
suffers indirectly for the major part of his lifespan. Needless to say, the other members suffer as well.

It is my hope that a concerted effort 1) can be made to
inform physicians of the disease; 2) towards a detection
system which will be implemented to spare unnecessary grief
to many families; 3) is directed towards eliciting more researchers
for the fight against Huntington's disease.

It is only with this kind of an attack that this ugly illness can be prevented from spreading to more and more families
and from generation to generation.

P.S. It is requested that this letter be used anonymously--
      Thank you.

New York, New York   September 22, 1976

September 11, 1976

ANONYMOUS

When I was nineteen and planning to marry in the near
future my father decided to tell me about Huntington's
disease and my mother. I had always thought she was just
clumsy. I had no idea she was sick or that her sickness
might affect me. I became very caught up with it. Things
became very tense and emotional in our house. My mother
would not admit she was sick. No one dared mention it. My
parents had pretended it didn't exist for such a long time
that it was a forbidden subject. My mother had an emotional
breakdown. She became impossible to live with. She saw us
as her enemies out to condemn her to a life of sickness.
Nothing we said or did was right. The night before my
wedding she threw me out of our house. Soon after we began
seeing a psychiatrist (against her will). We would lie to her
to get her in the car and once we got her there she was
totally unreceptive and irrational. One time Dr. Greenberg
said "you know you have Huntington's disease." I was shocked. No one had ever said that word in front of her
before. I cried and she screamed. Soon after she was taken
to a psychiatric hospital. At first we weren't allowed to
visit. When we finally were I was frightened. Afraid of
how she would be and how I would react. There was no need
to be. She was totally submissive. She was heavily
drugged. She still hated her doctor.

It was here I think that she started to see her
neurologist, Dr. Fahn. When she got out we continued to
see Dr. Greenberg, with no noticeable progress. She was
still seeing Dr. Fahn also. He was giving her drugs to try
to temper the effects of Huntington's disease. They were
experimental. How well each one worked is hard to tell.
Her condition was steadily worsening. After a while we
stopped seeing Dr. Greenberg although my parents continued
to see Dr. Fahn. She lost her resentment for us (her 3
daughters) a lot sooner than for my father. That took quite
sometime, but once it did she began looking to him as a
father rather than a husband. She made no decisions no
matter how small.

A great deal of time has passed since then. The only
family problem we have had to deal with since then has been
getting her to give up driving and allow someone to take
care of her. It was difficult. We went to a psychologist
who specialized in Huntington's disease patients to talk it

over with us. She gave in reluctantly. What her problems
are is sometimes hard to say. She is quiet most of the
time. Life sort of goes on around her. Soon she will need
full time help to sleep in. We are very lucky that my
father can afford to take care of her.

I don't dwell on Huntington's disease very much
although I'm sure it has made many subtle changes in my
life. I tried joining the local chapter of CCHD, but found
it very boring. I lost interest quickly.

The only time I really dwelled on it was when my
husband and I had to decide whether to bear our own
children. It was a difficult decision. We finally ration-
alized our way into it, hoping that by the time they
are 35 - 40 there will be a cure.

New York, New York   September 22, 1976

ANONYMOUS
NEW YORK, NEW YORK   SEPTEMBER, 1976

    I've always had difficulty coping with life's problems.
When I learned several years ago that my husband's father had
died of HD I tried to escape that knowledge through alcohol.
By the time we discovered two years later that my husband had
early symptoms, and that our two daughters and our son might
also get the disease, I was a full-fledged alcoholic. I was
drunk most of the time and on those few occasions when I was
reasonably sober, the guilt caused by my drinking drove me to
more drinking and the point of suicide. A friend finally talked
me into attending a meeting of Alcoholics Anonymous. Through
AA, I have found sobriety and a measure of serenity and peace.
My husband still has HD and our children are still at-risk, but
I no longer need to drink alcohol or take pills in order to cope
with this. Because of AA, I am in a condition and a position to
at least try to help them and others who suffer from HD.

    My reason for writing this letter is this: I know of other
cases where either the HD patient, the spouse, or the offspring
have turned to alcohol making a tragic situation intolerable.
With this thought in mind, I am suggesting that one of our chapter meetings might be devoted to the subject of alcoholism.

New York, New York

September 22, 1976

ANONYMOUS
PHILADELPHIA, PENNSYLVANIA

JANUARY, 1977

It's pretty hard for me to write this autobiography of my life with or in relationship to Huntington's disease for a number of reasons. Most difficult is I'm not too good at writing, and secondly, I'm not sure what exactly you (whoever you are) are looking for. So please bear with me.

My father is the one in my family who has H.D., and he first told me he had it when I was about 15; I'm not exactly sure. But he told me while we were eating lunch alone. Ruined my whole fucking lunch too! I can't honestly say it was that much of a shock to me, even though he was supposedly in just the beginning stages of the illness. I noticed his slowness in doing things and his reluctance to perform any real kind of fatherly duties, except financial. I guess if I had to pick one thing that bugged me the most, it was his attitude that as long as he was "working" and we were eating, he was perform- ing his role as a father. That's total bullshit; I don't believe it. And I don't think I've had any kind of real father figure for the past five years. I know it has some kind of effect on me, but it's not something that I could easily put my finger on.

I guess my first reaction was one of rebellion. I'm not sure if that was because of the H.D. or whether it was just that stage of my life, or what. Right after he told me he had it was when I started smoking a lot of grass and drinking. My parents said I was what you might call a real asshole. I suppose it was my mother who was hurt the most by what I did. I think I was trying to force my father into some kind of dis- ciplinary action, which he never did, and that flung my mom right in the middle of the whole mess.

Well, I guess as I've been maturing and slowly coming or came to the realization that either my father couldn't or wouldn't lift his hand to stop me from doing whatever I damn well pleased; even now I can ask him for just about anything except anything emotional or physical from him and the odds are 100-0 that I'll get it. I guess in that sense I'll remem- ber him as secondly a great guy who didn't want to be a father to me because it would hurt his image, and primarily a soft touch.

That's basically the way I see it now.

At the moment, I'm 19; I live away from home 12 months of the year and I only go home for about 5-6 days at a time before my home life makes me want to scream. When I call home, I don't even want to talk to my father because it's the same old bullshit. He doesn't have the slightest idea what's going on in my life and I know just as much about his. The reason for that is if I went and asked him how he's getting along with H.D., he'd say, "Oh, the doc says I'm doing fine." I know. I've asked him. And he doesn't do anything else. I guess I could tell him what I'm doing with my life, but I think that's just another aggravation he could do without. He wouldn't understand.

My elder brother is an asshole plain and simple. It's really hard to talk to someone who knows everything. I talk to him because it makes my mother happy. I mean, I go to art school. I'm a pretty good photographer; I've been doing it long enough and I've seen enough of it to think I have a fairly good idea of what I'm talking about. So how come he's better than me and knows more than me in photography? I don't know.

He'll ask for my opinion and then tell me I'm wrong. Either he'll change or I'll have to learn to live with it.

My younger brother I really feel sorry for. My whole family (me too) have done a supreme number on the boy's mind. He's a paranoid, a hypochondriac, he has absolutely no friends, no social graces, and he's got the laziest mind of anyone I've ever met. He'll really have to get his act together soon. People are getting tired of the shit he's giving them.

My problems, I feel, are less serious than those of my brothers. Sure I'm paranoid; maybe I drink too much, and I'm definitely stuck up. But I think that's to cover up for my other problems. I'm creative, I know what I want to do, I'm self supportive, I'm delightfully insane, and not too hard to get along with.

My mother plain and simply has got the troubles of the world on her mind.

I've run out of gas! I hope this helps you! I hope you can help us! I trust you! Do something for my Dad!

New York, New York   September 22, 1976

ANONYMOUS
HARRISBURG, PENNSYLVANIA   SEPTEMBER 25, 1976

My testimony of H. D. as I have seen it from the time I was 13, and
my niece was a year old, is as follows. My niece who is now 36, and
has the disease, and has had it for several years now. She hasn't been
able to work since she was 29. Had a really nice job as a private secretary. Had to give it up when she was between 27 and 28. Got jobs as she
could after that. Couldn't support herself after 29. Became pregnant
and had a child when she was 30. Child has very dark skin. She doesn't
know who the father is or when she became pregnant. Her doctor in New
York told us she is vulnerable to rape, being murdered, getting hit by a
car because she can't walk without staggering. All this was when she
was 30. She was an A student in school and college. Her doctor told us
when she was 30, you would never have known it. She was more like a
retarded person. She was very beautiful and meticulous about her appearance. Now she looks as though she's on dope. Her hair is matted and
dirty. Her housecoats are dirty. She looks dirty. She smokes continuously. Doesn't eat much and only cares and loves her child. It is very
heartbreaking to have watched this beautiful person go down to this level.
Why is she like this? Because she has inherited the dreadful disease,
H. D. , from her father who died of it when he was 53. He too started
with the disease when he was in his early 30's. By the time he was in
his late 30's, early 40's, he couldn't walk a straight line. In fact, he
would walk two steps and stagger backwards three. He went from 188
pounds to under 100 pounds when he died. He died in the mental hospital where he lived seven years before he died. He didn't look like his
daughter looks because my sister kept him from looking the way she
does. She doesn't have anyone such as a husband to look after her.
She can only do the best she can. Her child was taken from her because
she can't look after herself, let alone a child. The thing that is so horrible is in the end they are usually put into a mental hospital. They
aren't always uncontrollable and it seems a shame they must be around
people who have mental disorders and must really be there. These
people suffer enough trying to fight the disease which in the end claims
their lives. They know it will. Some can't take it and end it before the
disease takes them. Research or rather more of it is needed so they
can be helped. Places should be had for them to be cared for, without
having them committed to the mental hospitals. My niece lives several

hundred miles away from her mother. She lives in fear of being committed. We never see or hear from her. What we send her is always returned.
She doesn't want us to see her the way she is. My sister was married
25 years. Five of these years were good years. Twenty of them were
hard ones for her and her two girls. Now she lives in fear for the younger
daughter. This daughter has three children. The younger generation
seem to think it can't happen to their children. Let us pray more is done
about it so they are right. Most everyone wants a family, but people with
H.D. really shouldn't have them. It may be the only way to stop the disease. It will be if more research isn't done in its field. In my brother-
in-law's family, there were ten children. Five got the disease, the other
five escaped it. Several of their children now have it. All of the five
died under 55. The hurt and destruction of families and lives is sad.
Seeing people you love being afflicted with the disease hurts because the
average layman isn't capable of coping with the people. We need to be
educated on the disease. The Committee needs all the help they can get.
We are hopeful they will get it.

New York, New York   September 22, 1976

ANONYMOUS
ST. MARYS, PENNSYLVANIA   MARCH 26, 1977

        It is my strong desire to express the feeling that one
of the main functions needing to be served by any group formed
is that of psychological counseling and support to all members
of the families of H.D. victims. Because of the horrid distor-
tion of personality early in the disease, the wife and mother
of the family with whom I am familiar is not even vaguely the
same human being they started with. Worry, hate, fatigue, and
resentment create a monster inside the members of the family so
that not just one victim is dying, but five. This disease is
distorting five personalities, not just one.

        Surely support systems can help prevent the waste of at
least four of these lives. The monster that lives in the body
of this victim has long since caused no request in our hearts
that this life be saved or extended to further suffer and cause
suffering.

        I'm sure prevention and early cure are strongly being
pursued. It is too late by far in our case, so my plea is to
help the minds of the families to cope with the overwhelming
disaster.

        I would not want my friends to know my name so please
withhold it.

New York, New York   September 22, 1976

ANONYMOUS
PENNSYLVANIA   MAY 16, 1977

RESPONSE TO QUESTIONNAIRE DISTRIBUTED BY CCHD, MICHIGAN CHAPTER

1. About my family and relatives: How many have died with
    H.D.? One.

    How many are afflicted now? One.

    How many are "at risk?" Two.

    This disease is not in my family but I am writing for a
    /_/ Male   /_/ Female   Friend.

2. Was the afflicted patient diagnosed in a doctor's office,
    in a hospital or in a nursing home? Doctor's office.

    What problems had to be met? Unemployment.

3.   After the diagnosis:

Did different living arrangements have to be made?
Yes.

Were there any financial troubles?

Yes.

Was there an employment problem?

Yes.

How were your requests for assistance received or
refused?

Satisfactory.

Was there difficulty with an insurance problem or
disability payments?
Six-month waiting period for Social Security disability.

4.   How has the presence (or threat) of Huntington's disease
      affected your social life?

      I think about it constantly. I try to push it out of my
      life in being optimistic I will not get it. However, the
      fact that my father has H.D., it is difficult to do this.

      Has there been extra stress placed on your children?

      N/A.

      Do your children know they are "at risk?"

5.   In the future, I would certainly appreciate and HOPE for:
      (check:)

      /X/ More and better research.

      /X/ Better public understanding of our problem.

      /X/ Better and less expensive nursing care for H.D.
           patients.

      /X/ RELIEF from financial burdens.

      OTHER:

New York, New York   September 22, 1976

ANONYMOUS
PENNSYLVANIA   MAY 16, 1977

RESPONSE TO QUESTIONNAIRE DISTRIBUTED BY CCHD, MICHIGAN CHAPTER

1.   About my family and relatives: How many have died with
      H.D.?   Don't know.

      How many are afflicted now? One.

      How many are "at risk?" Five

      This disease is not in my family but I am writing for a
      /_/ Male   /_/ Female   Friend.

2.   Was the afflicted patient diagnosed in a doctor's office,
      in a hospital or in a nursing home?   In a hospital.

      Any problems in getting a diagnosis?

3.   After the diagnosis:

Did different living arrangements have to be made?

Were there any financial troubles?

Was there an employment problem?

How were your requests for assistance received or
refused?

Was there difficulty with an insurance problem or
disability payments?

4. How has the presence (or threat) of Huntington's disease affected your social life?

    I'm scared that I might get it, because I live in a home for girls now. If I get it when I get older I don't want my children in a home. That is, if I have any.

    Has there been extra stress placed on your children?

    How many children do you have, and what are their ages?

    My mother has five children.
    MALE__Three-14, 15, 16____   FEMALE__Two-18, 19____

    Do your children know they are "at risk?"

    Some.

5. In the future, I would certainly appreciate and HOPE for: (check:)

    /__/ More and better research.

    /__/ Better public understanding of our problem.

    /__/ Better and less expensive nursing care for H.D. patients.

    /__/ RELIEF from financial burdens.

    OTHER:

New York, New York   September 22, 1976

ANONYMOUS
DELAWARE   MAY 20, 1977

RESPONSE TO QUESTIONNAIRE DISTRIBUTED BY CCHD, MICHIGAN CHAPTER

1.   About my family and relatives: How many have died with
      H.D.?   ?

      How many are afflicted now?   One.

      How many are "at risk?"   Seven.

      This disease is not in my family but I am writing for a
      /_/ Male   /_/ Female Friend.

2.   Was the afflicted patient diagnosed in a doctor's office,
      in a hospital or in a nursing home?   A Hospital.

      What problems had to be met? Had to prove he wasn't
      an alcoholic.

3.   After the diagnosis:

Did different living arrangements have to be made?
We had our attached garage made into a living room-
bedroom.

Were there any financial troubles?

Some; however, I had been willed some money and I worked.

Was there an employment problem?

How were your requests for assistance received or
refused?

It took several years just to get an aide to come twice
a week to wash and change him. Police answered calls of
violence very quickly.

Was there difficulty with an insurance problem or
disability payments?

No.

4. How has the presence (or threat) of Huntington's disease
    affected your social life?

    Only friends of long standing were allowed in. I attend
    nothing, not even church, in our town.

    Has there been extra stress placed on your children?

    I believe all five felt the greatest stress when in public
    high school, no one to turn to, in school or out.

    How many children do you have, and what are their ages?

    MALE _Three (19-24)_   FEMALE _Four (30-31)_   Grandchildren:
                                                        _(2-7)_

    Do your children know they are "at risk?"
    Yes.

5. In the future, I would certainly appreciate and HOPE for:
    (check:)

    /x/ More and better research.

    /x/ Better public understanding of our problem.

    /x/ Better and less expensive nursing care for H.D.
         patients.

    /x/ RELIEF from financial burdens. AND FAMILY COUNSELING.

    OTHER:

Seattle, Washington

April 14, 1977

TABLE OF CONTENTS

Chronological List of Witnesses
Seattle, Washington

April 14, 1976

Page

OMENN, Gilbert, M.D.
University of Washington   5-449

BIRD, Thomas, M.D.
University of Washington   5-455

ARKIN, Aaron
Social Security Administration   5-459

LESTER, Charles, M.D.
Seattle Visiting Nurses Association   5-463

THIESSEN, Harold
Seattle, Washington   5-466

WOLD, Hans
Everett, Washington   5-467

THULINE, Horace, Ph.D.
Department of Social and Health Services   5-470

SCHULTZ, Amelia, Ph.D.
University of Washington   5-472

HACKLER, Nan Frederick
Seattle, Washington   5-474

JOHNSTON, R. Sherwin, M.D.
Chehalis, Washington   5-478

THEVICK, Harold and Vivian
Seattle, Washington   5-483

THEVICK, Karen
Seattle, Washington   5-485

SMITH, Clifford, M.D.
United States Army   5-489

NIELSON, Fran
Woodinville, Washington   5-492

ATKINSON, Carol
Seattle, Washington   5-494

BERMAN, Wilma
Seattle, Washington   5-496

SWANSON, Phillip
University of Washington   5-499

CONRAD, Darlene, R.N.
Community Home Health Care   5-503

DENNEY, Merle
Everett, Washington   5-505

LIGHTBOURNE, Robert, M.D.
Western State Hospital   5-510

PLUMRIDGE, Diane
Portland, Oregon   5-510

RUNNELS, Stella
Kingston, Washington   5-512

KINGSTON, June
Ellensburg, Washington   5-519

HYATT, Donna
Mount Vernon, Washington   5-521

HUFFMAN, Lynn
Missoula, Montana   5-522

BERGESON, Kathy
Ellensburg, Washington   5-525

KARSTETTER, Randy
Seattle, Washington   5-527

Geographical Index

Alaska

McKinley Park

Pederson, Gretchen, 5-568

Idaho Boise

Klein, Milton G., 5-561

Montana

Missoula

Huffman, Lynn, 5-522

Oregon

Portland

Buckner, Mrs. Norman, 5-537

Plumridge, Diane, 5-510

Washington

Bothell

Dahl, Hjordis, 5-543

Taylor, Jennig, 5-543

Bremerton

Lewis, Marti, M.D., 5-564

Walker, Janice R., 5-587

Chehalis

Johnston, R. Sherwin, M.D., 5-478

Ellensburg

Kingston, June, 5-519

Everett

Denney, Merle, 5-505

Kreucher, Helen, 5-563

Palmer, Densley H., 5-567

Wold, Hans, 5-467

Kingston

Runnels, Stella, 5-512

Mount Vernon

Anonymous-1, 5-594

Hyatt, Donna, 5-521

Othello

Wilson, James G., 5-589

Renton

Gitchel, Deanna, 5-549

Ritzville

Sprenger, Ernest H., 5-576

Seattle

Arkin, Aaron, 5-459

Atkinson, Carol, 5-494

Bergeson, Kathy, 5-525

Berman, Wilma, 5-496

Bird, Thomas, M.D., 5-455

Bucher, Carolee J., 5-534

Conrad, Darlene, R.N., 5-503

Hackler, Nan Frederick, 5-474

Hackler, Nan Frederick, 5-551

Karstetter, Randy, 5-527

Lester, M.D., 5-463

Lightbourne, Robert, M.D., 5-510

Motulsky, Arno G., M.D., 5-565

Omenn, Gilbert, M.D., 5-449

Schultz, Amelia, M.D., 5-472

Smith, Clifford, M.D., 5-489

Solis, Mrs. Alex, 5-574

Strown, Arlene, 5-534

Swanson, Phillip, M.D., 5-499

Thevick, Karen, 5-485

Thevick, Vivian & Harold, 5-483

Thuline, H.C., M.D., 5-582

Thuline, Horace, M.D., 5-470

Snohomish

Thiessen, Harold, 5-466

Soap Lake

Jackson, Mary R., 5-560

Spokane
    Duncan, Eleanor, 5-545
Starbuck
    Cook, Shirley R., 5-538
Stratford
    Roach, Leona G., 5-572
    Team of Friends, 5-580

Vancouver
    Northup, Irma, 5-566
    Wilson, Mrs. Theodore, 5-590
Wenatchee
    Blumhagen, Marguerite, 5-532
Woodinville
    Nielson, Frances, 5-492
Yakima
    Kokenge, Roy F., M.D., 5-562

P R O C E E D I N G S

GUTHRIE: This is Dr. Aronson, who is a member of our Commission,
a personal friend, a dean of a medical school, and someone who has
been very concerned and interested in our problem. Over here is Dr.
Nancy Wexler, who is herself the Executive Administrator of our Commission, who's been going around the country organizing and helping us
to establish this opportunity to express our needs and to express your
needs in a very personal way. In a sense, if you can imagine, instead
of sitting here like we are in this formal setting, I wish you could
pretend that you had the opportunity to walk into a very small office
and sit down with your Congressman; and he said to you, "What's your
problem," and you could tell him one-to-one what your problem is in
terms of living with a disease like Huntington's. Then, if he asked
you, "What do you think I can do to help you," then, that would be,
again, your opportunity to tell him what you think. Saying it in that
kind of way will help us as members of this Commission to eventually,
through the data that we're going to collect, make recommendations that
we hope will help all people who are concerned with this problem. I
know that I personally feel a little bit nervous when I see this kind
of formal setting, and that's why I said what I did.

We're very fortunate that Dr. Gil Omenn is here today to bring us
a message from your Governor, which I've already heard, and I just
think it's so nice. I'm delighted to ask you to please come up and
let's put into the record the good words that we heard, Gil.

TESTIMONY OF
GILBERT OMENN, M.D.
DIVISION OF MEDICAL GENETICS
SCHOOL OF MEDICINE
UNIVERSITY OF WASHINGTON

OMENN: Welcoming statement by Governor Dixy Lee Ray:

As Governor of the State of Washington, I, Dixy Lee Ray, welcome
Mrs. Guthrie and the members and staff of the Commission for the Control
of Huntington's Disease and Its Consequences to this public hearing on
Huntington's disease. I am aware of the personal tragedy in Mrs.
Guthrie's family and in so many other families affected by Huntington's
disease. I am aware that many families in this state need and have
received genetic counseling and treatment from their own physicians and
from the special services at the University of Washington and at the
Western State Hospital. There can be no doubt that much more must be
learned about the normal and abnormal functions of the human brain, so
that effective treatment and prevention of Huntington's disease and other
degenerative neurological disorders can be devised. As in many other
diseases, we must be supportive of the family members who bear the financial and emotional burdens of caring for loved ones as this disease
strikes.

I hope that your deliberations here today and in other cities throughout the country will bring forth practical recommendations for improvements in health services and novel ideas for new research. You may be interested to know that one of my first acts as Governor was the appointment of a select panel of citizens to examine the social and health services of our State government and the department charged with these responsibilities. I am eager to receive a summary of this hearing, including any recommendations that are particularly applicable in this State and to the medical problems being addressed at this meeting.

GUTHRIE: Thank you, Dr. Omenn. Did you want to make any comments of your own?

OMENN: I'd like to say by word of welcome and by comment that the Medical Genetics Clinic at the University of Washington has been very much involved in the care of families and patients with Huntington's disease, and for the many of you who are here today, of course. The clinic, founded in 1956-1957 by Dr. Arnold Motulsky, is, of course, one of the leading centers in the country, and he is one of the major figures in human genetics and in genetic counseling. He, unfortunately, this year for the purpose of this hearing--quite unfortunately for him I'm sure--is doing some very interesting work in Palo Alto. He has sent to us actually a copy of a letter to Dr. Wexler, a brief note, urging that others of us who are under his charge here at the University partici- pate, of course, in the hearings. I would like to read this brief letter from him because it makes a few points that are quite important:

"Dear Dr. Wexler:

"Thank you for notifying me about the hearings of the Huntington's Disease Commission in Seattle. I have transmitted the material to several of my colleagues in Seattle who will respond, as requested by you. As you know, I am on sabbatical leave. I continue to be worried about the proliferation of efforts for specific diseases in HEW and NIH. Special campaigns against a named disease--for example, diabetes, Hunt- ington's disease, and now many others--are not necessarily accompanied by granting of new funds. Consequently, funds will be siphoned off from general research allotments with counterproductive results in the long run. Success in creating special status for some diseases, which is not synonymous with conquest of the diseases, will encourage other disease- oriented groups to establish more and more such fragmented efforts, a move which may have serious consequences for a productive biomedical research enterprise in the long run.

"I realize very well the impatience of those who are afflicted with Huntington's disease, and particularly those who are at risk, with our current inability to come up with answers. I spent many agonizing hours during and following interviews with Huntington's disease families in my

capacity as a genetic counselor. Yet, our efforts to do something for
this disease should be viewed against the totality of the biomedical
research enterprise and the historical presence of possible research
leads coming from unexpected quarters. My involvement with the Biomedical Research Policy Committee of the Institute of Medicine of the
National Academy of Sciences has made me particularly sensitive to this
issue.

"Arnold G. Motulsky, Professor of Medicine and Genetics."

Now, I'd like to add a few remarks. As I said, the clinic here at
the University of Washington has been going on for now 20 years. All
of the staff, including the many physicians trained under Dr. Motulsky,
and including myself and Dr. Bird, who are here today, and Dr. Amelia
Schultz, who has been the social worker for the clinic for quite a
number of years, and my other staff, have taken special interest in
Huntington's disease and in the broad array of genetic disorders that
produce chronic and progressive illness.

We have a genetics center, one of several around the country, which
is devoted to combining basic research and clinical investigation with
the care of patients. We are doing the best we can, we feel. We are
eager, of course, for the input from families whom we see. We are
sometimes dependent upon their cooperation for studies.

Of course, we depend upon Federal and other outside support for the
funding of this research. I have another document I would like to submit,
which I think is in the hands of the Commission already. It is a report
of a work group on genetics, immunology, and virology. The Commission
requested of several people active in research and in the care of patients
with Huntington's disease to prepare reports that would be discussion
papers and would be incorporated into the final report of the Commission.

One of these work groups was chaired by Dr. David Comings, who himself trained here with Dr. Motulsky in the '60's, and is now at City of
Hope Medical Center in California. The other members were Dr. Motulsky,
Dr. Joshua Lederberg, Dr. Carleton Gajdusek, who shared the Nobel Prize
this past year, Dr. Margery Shaw, and myself. The document need not be
reviewed in great detail here, but I would like to highlight a few
aspects of it.

The first is that many of the research issues that are identified
in Huntington's disease apply to a good many other genetic disorders.
Last night, Mrs. Guthrie dramatically illustrated this with a diagram
on the board in a style of lay presentation, which she has found very
effective with medical students as well as lay groups. The point is

that the issues of figuring out what it means to say a disease is
inherited from generation to generation--some one dominant disorder--
to figure out how to study a disorder of the brain when in either brain
tissue or hopefully other tissues that are more accessible but might
share some of the same biochemical questions of presymptomatic detec-
tion--these questions are general issues cutting across a great many
diseases. On the first part of this report, there is a long list of
other diseases that for other families would be extremely important,
but here are simply illustrative of the class of genetic medical conditions which you and they share and which, in the aggregate, probably
in the sense of reaching your Congressman, might have important impact
in deliberation and in support for both basic and clinical research.
Then there's a detailed review of current studies, mostly biochemical
studies of the central nervous system and of accessible tissues (that
means blood cells and skin biopsy cells) work that is actively being
pursued these days, most of which wasn't even on the drawing board 5
years ago.

I hope that you are encouraged by the tremendous amount of effort
that good researchers are making trying to identify effects of Huntington's disease and hopefully mechanisms of Huntington's disease so that
there might be more reliable confirmation of diagnosis and more rational
therapy, more effective therapy, and finally the means of presymptomatic detection.

There is also in this report some discussion about immunological
and virological approaches, and there's a substantial bibliography of
the current research. All of this is simply to say that there is a good
deal of work going on--some of it here in Seattle, incidentally, in which
I'm partly involved, Dr. Bird is involved--and a good deal in other
centers around the country.

Now, I'd like to say one other thing. It's been my practice in
interviewing families and trying to deal with the complicated emotional
issues and straightforward medical issues, that as Dr. Bird will emphasize, the most important first issue is to be certain of the diagnosis.
It has been sobering to me to see how differently different families
react to what seems to me to be the same information--that there's a
50-50 risk for each child to either get the gene or not get the gene;
therefore, eventually get the disease if they live long enough. Some
are really assured that it's not 100 percent; and some are appalled
that it's 50 percent. In a few cases, as you will hear, we have found
that what was supposed to be Huntington's was not. So the medical
criteria, the actual neurological examination, is essential to rational
and genetic counseling.

Secondly, I'm impressed that for many reasons having to do with the
psychological effects, even within the same family, and also the period
of time... It is my practice, as some of you know, to ask, "If we had a
test available for detection before you have symptoms, would you want to

have the test tried on you? Would you like to know the results?" Some
individuals have told us, "Yes, of course. First of all, we'd like to
help research regardless of whether you tell us the results or not because many people realize that until you do the research and determine
how valid the results are, it's impossible to interpret them." Others
say, "We are willing to cooperate in the research, but we really aren't
sure we want to know; as long as we seem to be healthy, leave it at
that." Some have told us that—they must not be here today unless they've
changed their minds—"We came in today because Brother, or Sister, or
Ma decided we had to come, but you won't see us again." Sometimes we
do see them again after they've thought about it. The point is that we
are extremely respectful of the individual's feelings and understanding
of the disease.

This applies to other diseases as well. We are not in the business
of telling people what to do. We are doing the best we can to try to
explain what the facts are, and where the promising leads in research
and in care seem to be heading. I hope that today's session will identify
some more of those areas.

As I say, of course, we at the University are eager to see the results of your Commission's hearings, and I think you should take quite
literally Governor Ray's request that at an early stage, long before the
final report, she would like to have feedback from today's session.
Thank you.

WEXLER: I would just like to say to Dr. Omenn, who is somewhat
modest about his own research experience in Huntington's, that Dr. Omenn
has been a long-time supporter of research in Huntington's, an excellent
investigator and an excellent... I have a few brief questions. Is Dr.
Ray's select panel of citizens, is that to plan policy or is it essentially to review programs? Is it to plan new programs or to explore
what exists?

OMENN: The intention is that this group of 14 citizens from around
the State in many, many different constituencies should identify the
needs as best we can under one health professional member of the panel
in the area of social and health services, and to examine how well those
are being served at present by the department and other agencies of the
State, and to make any recommendations with regard to priorities, and
potentially new services that we think are in the best interests of the
people.

GUTHRIE: I just wanted to comment that, are you aware that there
is one state, the State of Maryland, who has established a statewide
ongoing Commission for Hereditary Disorders?

OMENN: Yes, I'm aware of that. In fact, Dr. Motulsky just testified out in Olympia on an essentially similar bill in our own State
Legislature. I think there's quite a lot of progress than can be made
in that general form. We, of course, are concerned about piecemeal
efforts by the State to mandate screening for phenylketonuria, now for

hypothyroidism, and especially in situations where screening is mandated, but no funds or mechanisms are provided for followup confirmation of diagnosis or treatment. So there's work along those lines in this State also.

WEXLER: I would also like to say that the points that Dr. Motulsky and you raise have been discussed at length by the Commission, and that all the Commissioners are very well aware of the problems that he raises, and we'll address them in our final report.

The last question for you--you were talking about the difficulties of prediction, particularly when we don't have really adequate treatment at this time. Would you recommend that before we have a predictive measure which can tell which child has the HD gene before they show symptoms, that before we have such a test (which probably isn't that far away from what people say), that there be some kind of a group that might make recommendations about how to administer such a test; that there be some kind of a protocol developed for the use of such a test so that each clinician doesn't just give the test to whoever walks into his or her office; so that there is some kind of preparation before and after?

OMENN: I think some such guidelines would be an appropriate outcome of the Commission efforts. I'm sure you are having plenty of discussion on this matter. Some of the work group reports that you have generated deal with this matter, and we already have experience with the much-publicized test, this pharmacological challenge with L-dopa in which it was considered proven 5 years ago that you could bring out the movement disorder of Huntington's in those who were genetically predisposed to develop it some years later, by giving the subject a large dose of a particular drug which is a neurotransmitter precursor. That study was impossible to evaluate, of course, because there was no clue as to how many people develop twitches who would not develop the disease later, and how many did not develop any signs who did develop the disease later. Without long-term followup, you would not know. The most serious problem--as is recognized in this work group report that Dave Comings and the rest of us put together, and I'm sure you've heard from many other sources, and it is the reason, I believe, the test is not used anywhere to my knowledge--is that it provides the test subject with an opportunity to make his judgment, possibly fallacious judgment under great anxiety as to whether or not he or she has signs of the disease under challenge. There have been some unfortunate followup experiences in a few of those cases, to my understanding. In any case, I would support the notion that there should be a rational review and guidelines for such testing, and that there should be adequate numbers, and that it should be reviewed before it's recommended widely for application.

ARONSON: I would hope, Dr. Omenn, that amongst the many guidelines, that your group would be sensitive also to the legal implications of an individual who is, assuming the accuracy of the diagnostic procedure, identified as being biochemically ill--that the civil rights of such an individual be protected for as long as possible, in such areas as a driver's license, etc.

OMENN: I think this is terribly important. In fact, the matter of the rights of the individual, once there is a clinical diagnosis, needs a good deal of attention. As Mrs. Guthrie has commented so clearly, there are many patients who have been properly diagnosed in the early stage of the disease, who can compensate adequately, and should not be treated the same as someone who's in the end stage of the disease. By the same token, there may be some situations in which family or some supportive personnel may need to intervene for the protection of the individual and the family. I think you've raised an extremely important area.

GUTHRIE: If there are no other questions, thank you, Dr. Omenn. Next, we'd like to call on Dr. Bird, Division of Medical Genetics, School of Medicine, University of Washington.

TESTIMONY OF
THOMAS BIRD, M.D.
DIVISION OF MEDICAL GENETICS
SCHOOL OF MEDICINE
UNIVERSITY OF WASHINGTON

BIRD: Pardon me for reading this. I don't want to appear too formal. There are specific points that I would like to make, and I want to be sure not to forget to make them.

I am a neurologist with a special interest in hereditary disorders of the nervous system. I have dealt with Huntington's disease at several levels, including diagnosis, clinical management, and genetic counseling. I have also been involved in clinical and neurochemical research in Huntington's disease and related genetic disorders of the nervous system. I would like to make a few brief comments regarding special problems with Huntington's disease that I have experienced in three fields: clinical management, genetic counseling, and laboratory research.

In the area of clinical management the obvious overwhelming need in Huntington's disease is to have a mechanism to prevent the development or the progression of the mental changes. Unfortunately, there is presently no solution to this problem, although it is an area under active investigation. I should like to point out that it is not necessary to know the cause of Huntington's disease in order to find a useful treatment for it. The classic example of this situation is Parkinson's disease, where the cause remains unknown but where there are a number of useful therapeutic agents.

Lacking a good treatment for the mental deterioration in Hunting-ton's, the resulting problem is the care of individuals who are beginning to show mental and behavioral deterioration. First of all, this is a difficult predicament for those who are showing early dementia but are not yet so severely involved as to require full hospitalization. They are a source of considerable depression to themselves and a cause of anxiety and emotional and financial burdens for their family and friends. Persons in this situation truly fall through the cracks in our health care deli-very system. There is a real need for some sort of sheltered protective environment for such individuals short of permanent chronic hospitaliza-tion.

Secondly, there is the problem of the chronic care of those indivi-duals who are severely demented. As you know, the trend in the last 20 years has been to decrease the facilities and bed space in psychiatric hospitals as a result of the successful pharmacologic management of patients with schizophrenia. However, there remains a need for chronic care facilities for severely demented patients which include not only those with end-stage Huntington's disease, but also a number of other degenerative neurologic diseases which are more common, such as pre-senile and senile Alzheimer's dementia. I see a need for a chronic care facility for patients such as these, where they are cared for with dignity by highly motivated personnel who understand both their immediate nursing problems and also their long-term prognosis. Perhaps the establishment of a few regional, highly specialized, well-funded chronic care facilities for patients with dementia should be a proposal result-ing from the deliberations of your Commission.

I have experienced two major difficulties in the field of genetic counseling of families with Huntington's disease. The first is often a forgotten problem, and that is the issue of accurate diagnosis. I have seen both false negative and false positive diagnostic errors. Some patients with Huntington's disease are initially diagnosed as having some other disorder. Equally as serious, and less well recognized, is the patient with a different neurological disorder who is labeled as Huntington's disease. The incredible consequences of this diagnosis to both the patient and his family emphasize the critical issue involved in accurate diagnosis. Physicians should be particularly cognizant of the fact that we presently have no test that is specific for Huntington's disease. If a patient is an isolated case of dementia and chorea, it behooves the physician to consider other diagnostic possibilities before settling on Huntington's. Even if there is a family history of a similar disorder, this does not necessarily imply that the diagnosis is Huntington's, particularly if the neurologic disorder has only occured in a single generation. The importance of a positive family history in at least two generations and the extreme usefulness of the documentation of Huntington's disease by autopsy examination on other family members cannot be overemphasized. By carefully evaluating these kinds of diagnostic evidence, we have been able to remove the label of Huntington's disease from at least three families visiting our clinics.

I am generally in favor of the establishment of a national registry of Huntington's families. I believe this would primarily be of diagnostic importance, particularly because both physicians and family members may be totally ignorant of the diagnosis having been made in other branches of the family. I recognize that such a national registry may be impossible because of the problem of invasion of privacy and, also, because of the potentially dangerous situation of a family being erroneously categorized as Huntington's. Such a registry should be able to give an indication of the degree of probable accuracy of the diagnosis.

The other problem in genetic counseling is how to determine who should be told what. The physician must balance a patient's "right to know" versus the consequences of raising the issue of Huntington's disease to a given individual or to a distant branch of the family. I have seen divorce, loss of employment, inability to get life insurance and rejection from armed forces all revolve around the diagnosis of Huntington's disease in a family. Nevertheless, we generally take the attitude that patients and families should be told the diagnosis on the general principles that knowledge is preferable to ignorance, and that the presence of this disease may have significant bearing on a choice of occupation, plans for the future, and family planning.

In the field of research we know that the underlying mechanism of Huntington's disease remains undetermined. Nevertheless, a number of neurochemical clues have been uncovered in the last 4 years. Funding of high-quality research in this area is crucial and, I believe, it should include a broad approach to all degenerative disorders of the central nervous system, including diseases such as Alzheimer's dementia, spinocerebellar degenerations, and other hereditary neurological disorders as well as Huntington's. One cannot predict where additional clues to underlying mechanisms will be found. The key to solving the mystery of Huntington's disease will be at least partially related to understanding the mechanisms underlying other autosomal dominant disorders of which we are mostly ignorant. However, even in the field of autosomal dominant diseases, progress is being made. For example, the elucidation of enzyme mechanisms in the hereditary porphyrias and cellular membrane abnormalities in familial hypocholesterolemia demonstrate that the puzzle of autosomal dominant disease can be solved, and makes me optimistic that we will eventually successfully treat and prevent the now-relentless degeneration produced by Huntington's disease.

GUTHRIE: Thank you very much, Dr. Bird. I'll just ask you-- because of your experience with the families as a neurologist, what would you say is the major problem after you have seen a family over a period of time, you know that the diagnosis is clear, you have all the guidance in terms of your social services to help you--how do you feel yourself?

BIRD: How do I feel in dealing with the family?

GUTHRIE: Yes. How do you feel as a physician?

BIRD: I feel frustrated. I think that's the best term. It's very frustrating. It's frustrating because we don't have a good treatment. We really can't do much about the disease. The best thing that we can do pharmacologically is decrease the movements. The best thing that we can with that. But other than that, it's primarily a social, emotional and supportive kind of tack that we have to take; and in the short run, we can be quite successful. I think with a lot of support particularly with help from the families, a lot of useful things can be done.

I feel an important point is to be sure that the affected patient doesn't get the feeling that that's it, I've got to give up. As we all know, people can have signs of the disease, and continue on for many years with a very productive, useful and interesting life; and we have to be sure that the individuals and the families know that, and that there isn't just a rejection of that individual.

GUTHRIE: I wanted the families to know that you also suffer, and that you also have frustrations in dealing, and that what you said in terms of the families, that you share that. I think sometimes the families put down the doctors so often and forget that you too suffer from these kinds of problems that you feel you can't deal with as well as you would like to. Thank you.

VOICE: May I ask a question?

GUTHRIE: We don't usually take questions from the floor, but I think that if it's a short one, and you're there, Dr. Bird, let's take it. Let's be different.

VOICE: My first wife passed away from the disease, and I had her over at your clinic in the final stages. You told me then, at the time, that if you had known 5 years ago what you knew then, you could have helped her. I was wondering if it's done anything on that line since that time.

BIRD: The only advance as far as treatment of persons with Huntington's disease has been in the area of controlling the problems they have with the movement, with the chorea. There are a number of drugs that are now available that can decrease the amount of movement and the amount of handicap that the individuals have. As far as having a medication or a treatment that actually slows the progression of the disease or changes the mental and emotional problems they develop, there really isn't anything very effective available at the present time.

GUTHRIE: Thank you. I've decided to call on Aaron Arkin, who is the Vocational Consultant, Case Review Section for Disability Insurance, Social Security Administration.

TESTIMONY OF
AARON ARKIN
VOCATIONAL CONSULTANT
CASE REVIEW SECTION FOR DISABILITY INSURANCE
SOCIAL SECURITY ADMINISTRATION

ARKIN: I'll try to pretend I'm talking to one person. We're
primarly concerned with the evaluation of impairment rather than the
treatment or with research, so I'm going to talk a little bit about the
Social Security Disability programs, some of the basic definitions in
the programs, and general evaluation criteria; and more specifically,
evaluation criteria for neurological impairments and Huntington's chorea.
To begin with, we have two basic programs. We have the disability insurance program; it's Title II. This is the program you hear about in the
news because of its funding problems. People pay into this program,
matching contributions are given by the employers, and these people are
covered until age 65.

We also have the Supplemental Security Income program. This is
on a needs basis. Payment for this program comes out of the general fund,
and basically, the definition of disability in both these programs is the
same. The definition of disability is the inability to engage in substantial gainful activity by reason of a medically determinable impairment
which has lasted or can be expected to last for 1 year or result in death.
Within this definition, substantial gainful activity means the performance
of significant services over a reasonable period of time for profit.
Medically determinable in this definition means an impairment that can
be objectively determined by a physician through signs, symptoms and
laboratory findings. Impairment is defined as a significant departure
from a normal condition. It can either be anatomical, physiological, or
psychological. There are two ways in which a person can be found under
a disability in the Social Security Disability program.

One is on the basis of the medical impairment alone. This involves
usually a severe impairment. The second way is having a medical impairment which is not as severe, but which, nevertheless, in combination with
adverse vocational factors, can qualify someone to be found under a disability. In order to provide disability examiners who make these decisions in connection with doctors in the Social Security system--in order to
provide these people with guides for determining disability based on
medical conditions alone, the Social Security Administration publishes a
listing of impairments. These listings, which are divided by body systems,
contain a number of the most frequently seen impairments. Body systems
include such things as musculoskeletal, cardiovascular, neurological, and
mental. Within each of these body systems, there are a number of impairments listed which contain descriptive criteria which, along with the name
of the impairment, establish the severity and, where necessary, the duration of the impairment. The Social Security Administration also recognizes
that there are numerous conditions which cannot appear in the listings.

There are just too many possible conditions or combinations of conditions, so they do allow for finding of disability based on medical considerations alone if a person has an impairment which, while not one specifically listed, nevertheless can be considered equivalent in terms of severity to a listed impairment. Now each of these body systems in the listings is prefaced by a discussion of the key evaluation concepts necessary to establish disability.

For example, in cases like cardiac problems, certain types of EKG evidence is necessary along with symptoms and signs. Likewise, preliminary function is necessary in cases of chronic constructive pulmonary disease. When you get to neurological impairments, however, the basic evaluative criteria apply only to epilepsy, and it breaks down epilepsy only because, unlike most of the other neurological impairments, disability based on epilepsy is due to the frequency of the type of seizure and degree of control that can be achieved. So you might say that neurological body systems are a little bit behind the times in terms of having good evaluative criteria. Most of the other neurological impairments have descriptive criteria which include such things as motor weakness involving two or more major extremities, coordination, and gait problems.

Until 1968, Huntington's chorea did not appear in the listings. It appeared in 1968 along with Friedreich's ataxia and spinocerebellar degenerative diseases. Unlike most of the other listings, there are no descriptive criteria associated with this listing. What this means is that most examiners, once they have this diagnosis as having been established, will allow the claim. The type of thing they will look for is the family history and a neurological examination, which show the typical changes, if there are such things as typical changes associated with Huntington's disease. What this means is that when it comes to evaluating disability for Huntington's chorea, nobody's really concerned with the amount of functional loss associated with the disease. Now, these listings have been in effect since 1968, and they are due to be changed.

However, in my last contact with the central office, no one could promise me when they would be changed. I did obtain a few statistics that you might be interested in based on classification of diseases. According to our data processing section back in Baltimore, they indicate that diseases that have an international classification code of 331, which includes Huntington's chorea, are seen in .031 of the applicant population. That was in 1975, and that was only under one program. It's hard to get more up-to-date data.

The interesting thing, though was that the data we did have showed that under Title II and under Title XVI the allowance rate for cases in which 331 was a diagnostic category was approximately 90 percent, which is very high, and which indicates that many examiners are adjudicating these cases based on the family history and established diagnosis together with support by a neurological examination, regardless of the actual functional impact of the disease. I'd like to entertain any question you might have.

ARONSON: Mr. Arkin, would it be possible, from the records that SSA keeps in Baltimore, to give some estimate of the numbers of individuals identified as having Huntington's disease who are currently receiving some sort of Social Security compensation?

ARKIN: It would be possible to break it down by the international classification.

ARONSON: Yes, but Huntington's is only one of many in that category.

ARKIN: I realize that. Outside of a manual tabulation, which probably for all purposes would be impossible...

ARONSON: Could you give us an educated guess? An actual number of American citizens receiving...

ARKIN: No, I couldn't.

WEXLER: You said that the criteria for determining the amount of functional disability is due to be changed?

ARKIN: Well, in talking to some of the policy people back in the central office, they indicate that the intent of the listing, although it never actually appeared in the listing, was to have some descriptive criteria which involved functional loss, motor loss, coordination problems, built into the listings. However, it never got there, and it is possible that subsequent issuances of the listings may contain more descriptive criteria for the finding of disability based on medical conditions alone.

WEXLER: Would you encourage these criteria to be made with these differentiations?

ARKIN: Well, it would be consistent with the rest of the program to require objective evidence, which would be in terms of symptoms, signs, and, where applicable, laboratory findings. So, inconsistent with that, it would be preferable to have those criteria included because it would lend itself to the consistency of the program.

WEXLER: But it wouldn't necessarily be of any advantage to the patient's family?

ARKIN: Not necessarily.

ARONSON: Mr. Arkin, on the basis of your experience with individuals distressed with Huntington's disease and similar disorders, and knowing as well as you do the ramifications of the Social Security rules and regulations, do you have any recommendations as to how these regulations should be changed to assist those individuals who are currently afflicted?

ARKIN: The only thing that comes to mind immediately, and this is in light of discussion that has gone on so far, is that the pigeonholing of diseases by strict diagnostic classifications sometimes does work to the detriment of individuals; therefore, it might be better to get away from very specific diagnostic labels in judging these impairments.

ARONSON: ...might be of assistance in terms of providing true social security?

ARKIN: Well, this takes it a little bit out of my area of expertise; as I indicated, we're concerned primarily with the evaluation of impairment. I think, speaking as a private individual in light of the discussion that's already gone on here, it seems to me that education, bringing these things to the attention of people who can supply funds and other kinds of support for existing programs or programs that you would like to see come into existence, this would probably be the best way to go.

ARONSON: One last question. I asked you earlier whether you could make a guess as to the number of individuals who are receiving assistance. Let's put it in a negative sense. Would you guess that there are appreciable numbers of individuals with Huntington's disease eligible for assistance who are currently not getting it?

ARKIN: I think that the Social Security Administration generally organizes the programs to bring as many people into the district office as possible to apply for programs they might be qualified for; that a large number of people do not get exposed or do not come in; or for one reason or another do not take advantage of or have not taken advantage of the existing programs.

ARONSON: Does the Social Security Administration have any mechanisms for distributing information regarding such benefits to physicians' offices?

ARKIN: Yes, it does. One of the things I have is a booklet that I will be glad to leave with your secretary on the evaluation of impairments. These are sent out on a regular basis to every physician listed within a community. It's sent out by various components of the Social Security Administration.

ARONSON: To all practicing physicians in the United States?

ARKIN: Well, that was the intent. Now, whether it actually got to everybody... The reason for this is because we depend very heavily on the local physician population to provide information in regard to their patients who have applied for these programs. So it's very helpful to get this information to the physician so he can see the types of evidence that we consider probative.

GUTHRIE: I think what you're implying is that we all have to do some work. Thank you very much. We're going to call next on Dr. Lester, who is from the Seattle Visting Nurses Association.

TESTIMONY OF
CHARLES N. LESTER, M.D.
SEATTLE VISITING NURSES ASSOCIATION

LESTER: I've left a copy of this with your secretary. I am a retired physician who is currently acting as the Executive Director of this organization, pending its election of a permanent Director. Our Director recently resigned. This agency has been providing in-home nursing services in this community since 1929. We presently provide, as needed and as ordered by the physician, skilled nursing care, home health aides, homemakers, physical, occupational and speech therapists, and social work services to anyone in King County and (within the available financial resources) without regard to the ability of the individual to pay. In 1976, we provided one or more of these services to approximately 6,000 persons, more than three-quarters of whom were over 65 years of age. Parenthetically, approximately half our patients are eligible for Medicare services.

Until two days ago, we had only one patient with the diagnosis of Huntington's disease within our case load in the past year. Interestingly enough, we had a second case appear just the day before yesterday. The local registrar of vital statistics tells me that without a computer printout, she couldn't be absolutely positive, but she is reasonably certain that there has been no death in King County in the past year certified to this cause.

I cite these facts to indicate the disease must be quite rare in the community or at least that in-home health services are rarely requested. In contrast, we have cases of Parkinsonism, multiple sclerosis, amyotrophic lateral sclerosis, as well as strokes constantly in our case load. The care needs are highly individualized in all cases of acute or chronic disease, and we do not envision the needs and care of Huntington's disease to differ significantly as a class from other chronic neurological diseases. We are prepared to provide needed services in the categories that I have enumerated in any instance in which in-home care appears to the attending physician and to us to be preferable to institutional care.

ARONSON: I'm intrigued by the fact that the nursing service in
King County has not encountered more than one case identified as Huntington's disease within a span of the last few years. Yet, we heard
earlier that there are--no figures were quoted--but numbers of families
with Huntington's disease seeking genetic assistance through the clinics
of the University of Washington...

LESTER: Well, my second point was that if it's not rare, at least
they're not being referred for in-home services.

ARONSON: Yet, I can think of no disease which would need such service more than Huntington's disease.

LESTER: Well, we can only take care of the cases that are referred
to us.

ARONSON: I appreciate that.

GUTHRIE: I think that I would like to suggest that--is there some
way that there--there are people in this community because we had a meeting last night, and I saw many, many families with this problem in their
home. I'm wondering if they know and are aware of what services you
offer. How do you let people know?

LESTER: Well, we've been trying to let them know in various ways
for many years. We've also tried very hard to let physicians know.
This has been a constant problem. If you have any suggestions for making
people read literature or read newspaper articles or other things, I'd
be very happy to hear them.

GUTHRIE: I think most of our people feel that nobody really cares.
They're so used to it that perhaps they don't read it with a positive
attitude. Maybe we can help you.

LESTER: We still have problems with physicians not thinking about
home care for the conditions as well.

GUTHRIE: We believe in home care. We think that many patients
could stay home with help so much longer than they do, and perhaps do
a very fruitful...

LESTER: I'd like to say that there are several other organizations
in the community which render some of these services, and I did not check
with them to find out what their experience is.

WEXLER: How is your service financially supported?

LESTER: Approximately half of our revenue comes from Medicare, and
then a quarter from Medicaid; the rest from private insurance, contracts
of various kinds, such as with the Cancer Society, and we are a nonprofit

organization. If you know anything about Medicare, you know that we have to be on zero-line, and any deficits in our finances are made up from United Way funds.

GUTHRIE: Well, I think I know the answer to what I said before, then. You see the problem I think that our families have is that they don't want to go onto Medicaid because it means depriving them of so many other opportunities for work or care for the rest of the family. In order to get rid of everything you own, in order to get the Medicaid you'd rather keep what you have and do the best you can without your services. So I think maybe we ought to do some thinking about how to reorganize that.

LESTER: Well, we are able to provide a certain amount of free service or a part-paid service with the United Way funds. But the United Way contribution represents only about 10 percent of our total budget.

WEXLER: With private insurance, what we found in other states, at least, is that private insurance won't pay for anything under unskilled care. Is that not your experience?

LESTER: Well, that depends on the insurance carrier. There is considerable variation in that some are more liberal than others. Of course, I can't speak with the experience in Huntington's disease because we've had so few instances; I don't know who is supporting the care in these two instances.

ARONSON: I can't imagine why it would be any different than those other diseases that you mentioned. It doesn't seem that it would be any different than Parkinsonism.

LESTER: I doubt very much that it would, yes.

GUTHRIE: I suspect that we have some work to do to try--maybe, is there some way that you might suggest for us to try to get Medicaid to change some of its policy in terms of making families divest themselves of everything before they can get the help?

LESTER: I haven't any suggestion.

GUTHRIE: I think that's something we'll have to work on. Thank you.

WEXLER: Do you have any literature about your organization? Perhaps we could provide it to the local HD health voluntaries to publish in their newsletter.

LESTER: I don't have it with me, but I'll be glad to see that you get some if you'd let me know how to get it to you.

WEXLER: Okay, I'll give you the address. Thank you.

GUTHRIE: We're going to have a very special experience, all of
us. Mr. Thiessen is going to present something that he has been doing,
and he and his son are going to take over, and we've been asked to leave
the table and sit in the audience for this presentation.

DEMONSTRATION BY THIESSEN
(Applause.)

GUTHRIE: I'd like to say that Mr. Thiessen and I have been corre-
sponding for several years, and when the article first came about him
in the newspapers, it was so thrilling to us at the National Headquarters that I reproduced it and I still keep it on our table, and
somebody walks in and tells me about their problems about Huntington's,
I say, "Did you ever hear of somebody living with Huntington's who's
having a good time? Well, let me show you this," and I take out the
article about you, and it's so nice to be able to come here and have
you with us and show us what you've done with the time that you've had
to the best of your ability. I think that there are some of us who
might like to ask you some questions.

ARONSON: Well, the questions that I would have would be purely
technical. I was thinking, and I don't think that the audience would
perhaps share my enthusiasm except may I just for myself express my
very deep thanks for seeing this. I'm so impressed with what people
do with abilities rather than disabilities or in the face of disabilities.
This is an extraordinary degree of dexterity, artistry, and imagination
and creativity. I am profoundly impressed. Thank you for letting me
look at it.

WEXLER: When can we come and watch it?

THIESSEN: You're welcome any time.

GUTHRIE: I would like to because I think it's important for documenting for the purpose of this Commission--could you tell us, first,
how long has it been since you had Huntington's disease?

THIESSEN: It was 5 years ago with the doctor's diagnosis.

GUTHRIE: Do you remember before the 5 years now in retrospect
what signs there might have been that indicated that there was a problem?

THIESSEN: The first thing that--there were several. The cops
asked me to walk a straight line because I drove a car like a drunk
person. Of course, you know, your feet are affected. The feet were
the first thing that were affected. So, I lost my driver's license,
and it's awful for almost any man not to be able to drive a car anymore.

It's one of the real discouraging things. It was really a little while before I really got over that. I really enjoyed driving, but it compensated.

GUTHRIE: Can you tell us when you discussed your problem with your family?

THIESSEN: My mother had it, and, of course, at that time, there was that 50-percent chance. Twenty years ago, when we lived in the St. Louis area, then we went to the neurologist at the university there, and there was no sign. Since my mother had it, we had, my wife and I, gone back to college realizing that 50-50 chance, and she got her teacher's training. She finished up at the small college, where our daughter is going. They graduated at the same date at the college, my wife with a teaching degree and our daughter with something else. They were in college together.

GUTHRIE: You know, I told you last night and I'll repeat again today that for those people who are here today or who may see you, it means so much to them, and I was told this morning by a young man how much it meant to him to see a man living with Huntington's. Your presence here is very, very important to all of us, and we really do appreciate your being here. I want to thank you for all of us.

THIESSEN: I'm very thankful, and I certainly, I really feel that confidence has been a strength for me. My first 2 years I kind of let go and resigned and didn't do anything. When I saw Merle Denney's husband, and the plight of their family, it really shook me up. I just decided that I wasn't--in our family, it's coming much later than theirs--and I just decided that it wasn't going to be with me that long episode. All of our many good friends were there with great encouragement.

GUTHRIE: Thank you so much. Our next person to speak before us is going to be Hans Wold from Everett, Washington. I wonder if we could ask Doctor Horace Thuline also to come forward. He is from the Birth Defects Study and Counseling Program, Department of Social and Health Services. I think we're going to try to move along a little bit, and so perhaps combine several speakers.

TESTIMONY OF
HANS WOLD
CCHD
EVERETT, WASHINGTON

WOLD: I'm Hans Wold, and I work with the Huntington's Committee and Merle Denney in the Everett area. Also, I'm a teacher in Everett.

Seattle, Washington   April 14, 1977

        THULINE: I'm Horace Thuline. I'm supervisor of the Birth Defects
Study and Counseling Program, which is in the Department of Social and
Health Services.

        WOLD: I've prepared a statement, but I think I'll talk. I thought,
as I was sitting there, you know, my brother died of an incurable
disease. Our family lived in fear of that for a long time, and it
wasn't Huntington's; it was tuberculosis. I thought as I was hearing
what the doctors have to say that we have hope that Huntington's will
go the way of tuberculosis. I'm going to talk about fear, and I think
some frustration because I'm going to speak from my family's standpoint
because we have Huntington's in our family. We have probably in our
family I think 37 people that are at risk or have been diagnosed.

        Now, the frustration is that if you are attempting to help members
of your own family, you're going to be up against--it seems maybe from
the outside, but you're going to be up against some things that are the
result of fears. I'm just going to talk about two cases that we know
about personally. The first fear, I think, is the fear of rejection.
I'm going to talk about Ardell's case. Ardell is one of our older
sisters; and not long ago, my wife received a telephone call and it
was from Merle Denney, who was head of our Committee. She said that
the hospital had called her from Everett in the psychiatric ward, and
that her sister was there. Her older sister had not been diagnosed
as Huntington's earlier, but we hadn't seen her for some time. We
suspected that she was beginning to show some signs. She is married
but had no children. Now when they arrived there, no one knew that
she was there. Her condition was the result of, as we found out, de-
hydration and starvation really. Her husband's reaction was to be gone
7 days a week, 12 hours a day working, ostensibly to meet those bills.
He really, he told the hospital authorities that no one in the family
was concerned. Now, his reaction was out of a kind of fear of rejection, I think... His wife does not accept the idea that she has Huntington's and the first thing she said to us was "I've got a clean bill
of health, I don't have HD," when, in fact, she did have it. We were
able to take her home, and within a week she was rational again just
by that kind of--just by taking care of her physical needs.

        I think that the reason I'm bringing this up is that it points to
me that by going to her psychiatrist to arrive at visiting care, I
think that we need to have someone sort of outside of the family
circle be called in in connection with a case that the doctors come
across, and see what the needs are in that home. As a result of this,
she's gained 30 pounds and is being able to move around. But we would
never have known about this except for an accident which came to us
really through our own Committee. It was just an accidental connection. Literally, she may have died in that condition.

The second case that I want to talk about is a younger girl, 40 years old. This is my mother-in-law's youngest daughter, and this is her situation. Now the mother cared for her husband for probably 20 years, and he died at home. So, he was cared for in the home all these years. The daughter had had three children. Two of these children are 11 and 13. They're living at home. It's very difficult for anyone from the outside to tell them you will do so-and-so; we're going to help you now. We're going to tell you how to handle this. If you try that, you're going to run up against another kind of fear. I think this is--it manifests itself in a kind of family denial in the hostility. Why does this happen? There are other members of the family who really don't want to admit that they have this problem.

So, it's very difficult for this kind of people to get any really effective help. She has a husband who seldom comes home and doesn't support the family. They live on whatever the relatives provide, and the mother's Social Security. They have very little health care, the children particularly have very little health care. They have educational problems; that is, they don't get to school regularly. They are not properly clothed unless somebody watches them. What I'm suggesting, then, from these two cases, here are some of the needs that I think I see.

We need a kind of public advocate for these people, that the doctor can refer them to. This person will go out and see what the need is and contact the sources--the people who provide the nursing care--do some of the things that the family can't do. Sometimes, the closer you are, the less help is going to be accepted. The second, I think, is we need to do something for the children of these families. They need someone to be sure that they are really being adequately cared for in terms of their health, their education, and of their guidance. I agree, also, that we need now in this particular case...what is going to happen to this young woman when her mother, who is near the end of her life, is gone, when her husband has abandoned her, and she no longer has people to turn to? All right, her relatives will provide assistance, but what if she had no relatives? What are we going to do about terminal care for these people? Not putting them into an institution for someone who is deranged, but into a real care situation.

Also, I think that, indicative of this research or care center thing, there should be a public involvement, and I was interested in terms of your brain banks, your autopsy things, the things that we, as the public, can do and members of these families can do to provide help and input into these kinds of centers.

GUTHRIE: I'll just comment, if I may. Let me ask a question.

In other words, are you suggesting that this Commission should make every effort to look for the outside resources so that they are available to families like this?

WOLD: I think the resource has to come to the family. I think the families are not going to come to the resource for reason of over-riding fears that are simply immobilizing, and oftentimes make them reject help from their own families.

ARONSON: Earlier today, we heard what I think is a very legitimate concern expressed by Professor Motulsky of the University of Washington regarding the purpose of named commissions, and I share to some measure his feelings. But I think that the purpose of a commission goes beyond the designation of how funds should be used in biomedical research. It also performs what we have been listening to very carefully in the last half-hour, namely, the exploitation of certain social resources in the community, perhaps changes in legislative regulations so that these resources can be brought to the attention of those individuals afflicted with Huntington's disease. I think a Commission such as Dr. Wexler and Mrs. Guthrie are managing might very well be the catalyst to translate these things into reality.

I think your recommendation of a spokesperson or ombudsman for HD families is an excellent one, and one that, in fact, the Commission is considering; your testimony gives support to this recommendations.

TESTIMONY OF
HORACE THULINE, PH.D.
BIRTH DEFECTS STUDY AND COUNSELING PROGRAM
DEPARTMENT OF SOCIAL AND HEALTH SERVICES

THULINE: I, Mrs. Guthrie, presented written testimony to the Commission. I will not go over that. I would just like to highlight what I think comes from experiences of professional dealing through my professional years with handicapped individuals, primarily in the field of the retarded. That is that many times a professional is caught in the bind when he considers the dictum "Do no harm." I would like to comment on two instances that have occurred that brought this to mind.

Several years ago, Dr. Clark Frazier, who is a human geneticist for McGill, in an address to the American Society for Human Genetics pointed out his experience in dealing with a family, particularly a young woman, who had had a parent with Huntington's. Cautioning those who were involved in medicine and in genetic counseling from isolating the disease from the person and from the family, he was very much concerned that people get into the habit of dealing solely with the disease without considering other factors. He pointed out that in Huntington's in particular, this was a very important consideration. That, at that time, didn't make too much of an impression upon me, but later on, we had the situation in which a mother who had had a husband commit suicide because of a recent diagnosis of Huntington's and with four minor children state, when asked about counseling, that she was not going to tell her children, and she did not wish for us to do so either. She brought then to the floor the question of whether those who do not yet know that they are involved have the right not to know. I would ask that the Commission take into consideration this aspect. I think we proceed pretty much in the medical model that it is good to know, everybody should know, without taking into consideration that we may be creating for those people 20 to 30 years of problems for which really we have at this time no adequate answers.

Without dealing with the question of the right not to know, I think it would be hazardous for a strong effort to be made, particularly in the direction of a registry, and also as has been said by others, in terms of a test. I would like to bring up two other aspects to this.

One is the right of the child, the unborn child, to be born without this disease, which is nil. I do not know whether the Commission has intended to consider that aspect of the ethical problem or not. The other one is that we have already as a precedent for infectious diseases a social action to limit the spread of disease. In other words, we already, if you wish, are willing to override certain individual rights and freedoms if they are infectious to other people and infringe upon their rights. I would wonder if the Commission might not consider the analogy, if you wish, of infectious disease, in terms of legislation concerned with Huntington's disease.

ARONSON: I suspect that were we to explore the last issue that you raised, Dr. Thuline, I think the rest of the day and perhaps the rest of the week would be occupied. I don't quite know how you would go about enforcing a proscription upon procreation.

THULINE: I'm not saying that I should. I'm asking that it be considered.

GUTHRIE: I think that this is something that is going to be considered in some of the deliberations of the work groups, and we will no doubt hear a great deal about this problem. We discussed this recently at a meeting in Denver, and they talked about it for 3 days. So, I can't say that we've gotten much further. At least it is being discussed, and I'm sure the Commission will be interested in all points of view.

THULINE: Thank you.

GUTHRIE: Thank you. We have a treat, according to our managers.

We can all stretch our legs for a short break, calling it a coffee break.

TESTIMONY OF
AMELIA SCHULTZ, PH.D.
MEDICAL GENETICS AND CLINICAL RESEARCH CENTER
SCHOOL OF MEDICINE
UNIVERSITY OF WASHINGTON

SCHULTZ: I'm a social worker at the Medical Genetics Clinic at the University of Washington Hospital. In my experience there, I felt that a major problem with families is their despair in regard to finding long-term care for the patient with Huntington's disease. Nursing homes and state institutions arouse strong, often justified, fears. Will the father, mother, spouse be accepted in the first place? Will the care be compassionate and appropriate, and will the patient be kept when the care becomes heavy? Because of what they have experienced or heard about in these areas, a family will try to cope at home long after their physical, emotional and financial resources have been exhausted.

In my opinion, the solution will not be found while nursing homes are a private, profit-making business staffed at the lowest levels by untrained, overworked and underpaid aides. Often the big, beautiful places are the worst, while the few modest, small nursing homes have unpretentious publicity and programs but give good care. Another aspect of the problem, again something that concerns not only HD patients, but all of us, is the spread between those, who by some fortunate circumstance, a Veterans' Administration service connection for example, have all kinds of equipment and services available; and those who, by some unfortunate circumstance, such as not enough quarters of Social Security coverage to be eligible, cannot even qualify for Social Security Disability grants. Even a very modest income can disqualify a family for state--it's called Medicaid in this state--financial or medical aid so that we have had occasionally to advise a spouse to divorce the patient so that the spouse can manage to support the children.

A problem which is minor compared with some of the others that patients and families face, but still very perplexing, is how to handle the matter of a patient's driving a car when his judgment and coordination are no longer adequate, and his driving is hazardous. But either he doesn't see the danger, or his family hates to deprive him of his last freedom of movement; or if he happens to be an irritable person, they don't want to antagonize him.

In this state, we have a Driver Improvement Division in the Motor Vehicle Bureau, who will keep in confidence the name of anyone who

writes and suggests that a person's driving may need to be retested. A
license may be renewed with limitations. Nevertheless, physicians are
reluctant to report, for reasons of confidentiality, and families will
hold off for as long as possible. Several times, I have myself written
to the Driver Improvement Division, not in my capacity as a social
worker because I'm part of the medical group and I have to follow
the precedents, but either as a member of the Committee to Combat
Huntington's Disease or simply as a person who noticed the condition
of the patient, feared for the public and for the patient, and without
making any judgments myself I would ask that the possibility of retest
be considered. If, however, a retest is given, the patient may be
deprived of his license; but if he then continues to drive without a
license, there is no further way that I know of to help the situation.
It's possible that mandatory reporting by physicians when they feel
that that time has come might partially solve this particular dilemma.

GUTHRIE: I was thinking as you spoke of what Mr. Thiessen said
about losing the opportunity for mobility. Do you think that maybe,
Amelia, we could consider some kind of special program where people
can be helped to feel that although it is a deprivation, the educational and the harmful aspects of it maybe need to be emphasized more
in counseling? Maybe we haven't done enough in that area?

SCHULTZ: You mean to the patient?

GUTHRIE: Yes, to the patient.

SCHULTZ: If the patient still has very good judgment, there's no
need to explain. If he doesn't, it doesn't help. I've been wishing
that there might be something, and there may well be and I just don't
know about it, but some kind of technical way that the driving of a
car could be made safer? I just don't know if it's possible. I just
would appeal to anyone who was an engineer or anyone who's thought
about it to see if there's something that could be done so that a
patient could be done so that a patient could safely drive longer.

GUTHRIE: The other possibility, of course, is to provide somebody
else who will drive you where you have to go; and I know that there is
a program called "Volunteerism" where some people who have to go to see
a doctor or want to go some place for a vacation can call and get help.
Maybe that's something that might be a suggestion for this community.

SCHULTZ: There is a volunteer organization called FISH, and I
forget what the initials mean. I think they're less active than they
used to be, and they're more active in some localities than in others.

GUTHRIE: Now that you mention it, I just heard about FISH only
a month ago. A lady did come to our National Headquarters and brought
me the information. They do provide services of this kind. Maybe if
more of us knew about it, we could help in that way and provide transportation and help.

WEXLER: I was wondering if in your work there would be enough patients with different disorders who might need similar services. Many epileptics can't drive; also multiple sclerosis, Parkinson patients, and yet I think one of the worst things we've heard reported over and over is that a person is perfectly capable of doing things but can't get out of the house, and that the spouse is working to support the family, and the person with HD sits at home, watches television, feels depressed and miserable, as we all would. So I wonder if there might not be some program which might be, at least if it were headed by the medical or social work community, that would have access to patients with different disorders, organize these patients and families, and provide some kind of a transportation service or recreational service to take numbers of patients with a variety of different disorders. Do you think that might be a possibility?

SCHULTZ: I just haven't thought about it enough. If there are agencies already doing this, then multiplying them would not help.

WEXLER: I'm not so sure...FISH is the only that I've really heard about, and we haven't heard that it's--considering the number of disparaging remarks that we've heard over the course of the hearings--if those agencies are there, they're not very effective. My question would be that there might be some outside agency; but if the outside agency worked with someone in the medical community that was having more regular access to patients and families, that they might be able to be more efficient.

SCHULTZ: Certainly, it would be well worth a try.

TESTIMONY OF
NAN FREDERICK HACKLER
SEATTLE, WASHINGTON

HACKLER: I'd like to thank the Commission for being here, and for my being here, too. I did submit a rather long written report. I submitted a report with some letters from doctors which were not at all very helpful. I'd like to make just a brief personal statement beyond what I wrote. My name is Nancy Hackler. I live here in Seattle. I've only lived here about a year. My experiences with HD were mostly in South Bend, Indiana. I have a college education, and my husband is here doing graduate work. We have only been married for 6 months, and we have a very active, healthy life. We have been doing transcendental meditation for 2 years. I do yoga. We are vegetarians. We only eat foods that are good for us. We don't take any drugs or smoke or do any of these harmful things.

As far as we're concerned, we have a very good, healthful, happy life; but I am at risk for Huntington's disease, which is a really heavy thing to have to live with--to have that cloud always there.

It's not like knowing that cancer is caused by smoking, or that one out of every ten women is going to have a lump in her breast. There's a 50-50 chance that you live with. If you had to put money on a horse with those kinds of odds, how much money would you put? If you had a 50-50 chance of crossing a highway and getting across alive, would you cross it?

Would you marry someone with Huntington's disease knowingly? My husband knew it before we were married. We would like very much to have children. This is something we'll really have to decide after he is out of graduate school, and this decision largely will depend on what comes out of this Commission. I think I could live with the knowledge of Huntington's disease for myself, but to live with the guilt of knowing that I passed it on to my children without knowing that everything possible is being done--I don't think I could live with that. I think when we decide to have children, it will depend on what is going on, what research is happening, what is known. If it looks like there is going to be a breakthrough, it will be a whole different story.

We learned about Huntington's disease in about 1970. My aunt was diagnosed, and at that time, my mother, who had always been emotionally unstable, she just absolutely fell apart and was put in the hospital. We went to the doctors. We said HD has been diagnosed in our family, does Mother have it? This was in South Bend, Indiana, which is a big city. We had M.D.s; we had psychiatrists; we had a neurologist. They all said, no, this woman doesn't have HD; she's just crazy.

So, we have an aunt who was on medication for HD who was doing fine; and she's cheerful. My mother was having shock therapy; they put her on some tranquilizers and sent her home. For 5 years, she went to psychiatrists at $35 a whack for 40 minutes, who told her you don't have it. Any symptoms that you have, any movements that you have are just because your sister has it; you're just relating to that. She went into this psycho ward two more times with what they just termed "nervous breakdowns." About 2 years ago, she went to England on a visit, and her behavior just became so uncontrollable that my stepfather took her to a doctor there who was just horrified at the treatment she had had, or the lack of treatment; it was obvious that she had Huntington's. So she came back here; unfortunately, she didn't stay there and get some further treatment. She came back to our local small town doctor, who hadn't been much help before. We tried to find another neurologist beyond the one who had seen her before. The local doctor just wasn't any help at all. I found the name of a doctor through the National Committee, who referred me to a local committee, who referred me to a doctor and offered to provide transportation whenever it was needed.

I think this lack of doctors being able to recognize it is what is so desperate. We need a test so that people know that it's there.

They just say, well, we can only trace it through family history; if it's in your family and you have symptoms, well, then it's easier for doctors to make a diagnosis. Well, it was in our family, but all they remembered was a great aunt who had the shakes, and my mother's father had died young before it had been diagnosed. It was in the family, but it just wasn't known. There must be so many, many people like that; so many people who are at risk but don't know it because of parents who died young, or not even knowing who their parents are, maybe.

I've never admitted to anybody beyond the family that I am at risk because of the lack of knowledge that people have. What you read about it is just so terrible and basically so untrue you feel like the first day someone sees you drop a cup, well, in 5 years, she's going to be an idiot. That's about what you read about it. There just isn't any knowledge for the layman--through what I've found out through doctors, very little knowledge. Most doctors I've come in contact with, I knew more about it than they did even on the second visit when they'd had time to research it, which is very discouraging.

I would like to see more done with just basically getting knowledge out to people, having it become a better known disease so that people who have it know who to turn to; so that doctors way back in South Bend, Indiana, know what's going on in Seattle, know where the resource centers are so they can refer people to them, what is available.

I'd also like to see just for my own personal lifestyle, I guess, having a healthy body, having a healthy mind before you develop it, what this can do. The sounder you are to start with must cause the disease to develop more slowly. How healthy you are in spirit emotionally, the less impact it's going to have on you. There is such a thing in TM as cosmic consciousness, too, which is--TM has been pretty much documented--it's in the brain waves and all this. What does cosmic consciousness send in Huntington's disease? How do they go together? These are my thoughts. Thank you.

ARONSON: Thank you.

WEXLER: You give our Commission, I think, quite a large responsibility. I think that there's a tremendous amount of research that's going on right now in the basic causes of the disease, and I think that it's quite possible and probable that in the not-too-distant future, that research is going to lead to a predictive measure. I think that there's going to be much less going on after this Commission is over. We have only 1 year to make certain recommendations. We want to make sure that the work keeps going on after we're through.

I think that the decision that you make about children, though, is a very wise one--that you want to wait and see because I think that there are so many things that are happening so rapidly that you can give yourself time to make a more informed choice, and I think that's a very intelligent way to approach the problem. Of course, I'm biased because that's what I've decided for myself also; I agree with you. But, I hope that we're given more time to prove ourselves than September when our Commission report is done.

GUTHRIE: Nan, I just wanted to ask in thinking back about your family, do you remember what you might recall as a child the first memories of what you saw in your mother that you now can say were the early signs of Huntington's?

HACKLER: Definitely. Even when she was a child, her parents had died young, and my mother said that she was told as a child that her nervousness all her life was due to the fact that she was premature, and her nerves hadn't developed right.

GUTHRIE: That's what she was told?

HACKLER: Yes.

GUTHRIE: What do you remember, if anything, that you saw?

HACKLER: I think we just always saw Mother and our aunt as being just nervous.

GUTHRIE: Can you describe what you mean by nervous? What did you see?

HACKLER: Movements.

GUTHRIE: You did see involuntary movements?

HACKLER: Yes. In our aunt, there were definitely movements. There were little humming noises that she made when she talked. Especially in driving, we noticed that the car was just always--even when we were little--it would go fast, slow down, go fast, slow down.

GUTHRIE: I was looking for early signs--if we had any keys that people remember --so it's important to try to think. Psychologically as a youngster growing up with your aunt and your mother, do you remember about thinking about what you thought might happen to you as a child thinking about it? When did you start thinking about it? About yourself?

HACKLER: Worrying about myself as far as... Well, even after my aunt had been diagnosed and the doctors said no, your mother doesn't have it, we knew there was something wrong with Mother. We were relieved. We didn't pursue the diagnosis, I'm sure, because I'm sure we were happier to accept the fact that it wasn't hereditary. We had no reason not to trust what the doctor said. I think growing up as a child, knowing that it wasn't a hereditary thing--I mean we didn't even know about HD. There was no question of anything. It was just growing up with a mother who was maybe not as capable as other mothers.

GUTHRIE: Thank you. Dr. Johnston, another dear friend from a long time ago.

TESTIMONY OF
R. SHERWIN JOHNSTON, M.D.
COURTHOUSE ANNEX
CHEHALIS, WASHINGTON

JOHNSTON: I'm Dr. R. Sherwin Johnston, Health Officer for the last 20 years in Lewis County. I had a small health department in Colorado before that; but I come not to you as an M.D. or an expert in this field at all, but as the husband of an HD case.

I finally reached the end of the rope. I have been able to sustain my own wife by my above-average income, true faith in the Lord, belief in the sanctity of marriage, good sense of humor, and 4 years of varsity wrestling. But all of those finally collapsed. While I lie down on my back taking massive doses of cortizone to try to keep from...I dreamed up a report. Fortunately, I will not read it to you because I am the only nonreader that ever got through the University of Colorado Medical School. I ought to condense 30 years. Actually, my Dorothy has only shown symptoms for 20, but 10 years before that, we had--I found out for the first time--the true diagnosis of my father-in-law. He had been reported as heart disease. We had to decide how to tell two boys that they shouldn't have been born, and certainly they shouldn't duplicate this error we made by having another child. I never did get the answer. They worked it out themselves. So, since I can't condense 30 years in 10 minutes, let me give you just two things--one a slogan and one a story.

The slogan that I've found is that when you inherit Huntington's disease, then you inherit nothing else. My wife's father was a wealthy real estate man, owning farms all the way from Iowa through North Dakota clear up into this country up here into British Columbia. I did not ever know my father-in-law. His wife worked for 20 years, supported herself, then I and the rest of the family supported her for another 20. At the time of death, there was nothing left. Then in my case, I take another look at what this disease has cost. As you know, the M.D.s today are all very wealthy, and through this courtesy, we have gotten in on the great handouts from the higher-ups. Unfortunately, I didn't. I've been a health officer, and I didn't get in on Medicare. One of the reasons I took that was because I could be free to take care of my own. So I have done a great deal of the care of my wife myself, and this can't be measured. But in costs that can be measured, this 20 years has cost about $75,000. Now, I again remind you of my medical degree. That's with professional courtesies and no medical charges because I found no M.D.s that knew any more than I did until I met these gentlemen here today; apologies to them. They have passed me, and I'm tremendously pleased that they have. $75,000 without medical costs, without specialized nursing care; out of this, there was a very small amount that I could actually deduct from income tax. There was very little help I got from that. The last 4 years have cost me about $20,000 because I could no longer carry her myself and had to put her in professional care, and at the same time I was granted an opportunity to pay $13,000 to the Federal government, who has offered no help. Except that I discovered last night that that's not quite accurate. Through this clinic and this young lady right here, I have had some help, and I appreciate it very much. You can see how I've had a better than average opportunity to know of the disease, and certainly a better than average income which has been just smashed by this devastating disease. In some ways, cancer is kinder--it kills.

The other thing I wanted to tell you was a story. I hope maybe you'll ask questions. My two boys, ages 3 and 4, that's about how old they were when I first discovered the disease, and they wanted a pony very badly. Christmas morning they came tearing down under the Christmas tree. There was nothing there but a great big pile of manure. Ralph said, "Oh, shoot." I think that's what he said. As I was beginning to start to turn away, Spencer came down and said, "Ralph, quick, come get a shovel. With all this manure, there must be a pony somewhere." That son now has a Ph.D. in genetics, and he's still digging. [Applause.] That pony they wanted, obviously, I didn't really do this, but that pony they wanted was just the right that every average citizen had to live in this wonderful country of ours, and in this respect, to live out a full natural life. Spencer is still digging. Ralph and I have gotten tired. We will welcome anybody with any size shovel to come and help us.

Another thing that kind of ties into this story is that we three know that there are other people who have lost their pony, and in the course of this meeting, if we can find some other people's ponies, that would help us, too. We would be happy to do that. Now, I am retiring from public health and starting my third life. My first was getting trained; my second was working as an M.D.; my third life I would like to devote to helping others so that I'm not available to you just 10 minutes, I'm available to you and the Commission and the United States, the Governor, any individual, for as long as my breath holds out--recognizing that it's been temporarily somewhat limited, and my economic state is at a very low level.

If I may, I've got to mention this, too. Dr. Lester, a friend of mine, spoke about how few cases have used the home health service. That was part of my job at one time. I was the Director of Home Health Services. I couldn't think of a thing that they could help me with

in the whole 20 years. It wasn't skilled nursing I needed. I
needed somebody to clean the house, some little things that I needed;
and there were some times that I desperately needed somebody that would
be like a paid neighbor, but not skilled nursing services. I'm not
surprised that the number is small.

I think somebody else mentioned the fact that vital statistics
had a very poor count. As I said, my father-in-law was listed as
having died of cardiac. His brother was electrocuted. Can you imagine
the motions on the high-tension line? He didn't last very long. The
one brother suicided. Another one, because his driver's license was
taken away, he got a motor scooter, and he stepped off the motor scooter
in front of a truck. He didn't die of Huntington's disease. His was
an accidental death. Choking is very frequent, and one sister died in
a hospital in Colorado. Starvation was what she died of, but they were
trying to take care of her and just didn't know how.

One final comment, I have found Social Security to be the worst
investment the world has ever known. I've paid maximum all this time,
and when the hospital twice sent me down to get help, I never got past
the front clerk. I'm busted now, and I'm counting on them helping me
next year.

Would you try questions, and if you think of questions later, I
told you I'm available as long as I have breath.

GUTHRIE: Well, first of all, we're not going to let you get away
with just doing nothing. You know that. Merle Denney and some of the
people in this local community are going to see to it that you are occupied 100 percent of your free time, and obviously you're a very good
person to be occupied with. I just want you to know that you have
announced publicly that you are going to be at our service, and you
can't get away with it now; you can't pull back.

In terms of questions, I just want to ask you--you mentioned the
money in your personal situation--you've lived all these years this way.
If we had better medication, if we had had it for your wife and you had
started to use the medication way way back--you did keep your wife at
home all these years--do you envision that what you did would be good
for other people, or are you aware as a physician that not everybody
can keep a patient at home? I just wondered how you feel about that.

JOHNSTON: Let me try to answer in this fashion. My son, the
geneticist, told me 2 or 3 years ago that there's no problem in
eliminating Huntington's, you just don't have any children. Three
months later he called up and said, "Guess what, Dad, we're awful
happy, but my teaching sure got shot down." He said, "What should we
do?" I couldn't tell him. I knew that it would have killed his wife
if they had to kill that baby that was started. I told him that even

with what limited knowledge I have, I can guarantee you 10 more years
of function, and I was able to deliver for your mother. Our time bomb
seems to go off at about 40, and he's in his thirties; he has 10
years that probably he'll function fine, then if he loses his 50-50
bet, I think I can give him another 10 years. Then, I told him, you'll
be 50; you're going to get old anyway.

GUTHRIE: You didn't get my question, or maybe I didn't say it
right. I think that some people might admire what you did, and I
happen to be one of them; but there might be others, that's why I'm
playing devil's advocate, who say, "I cannot live with this patient in my
home; I just can't take it; I don't want to be faced with it every
day. This is my wife, and I can't look at her this way. I'd rather
have her hospitalized." I think that there are people who might want
to listen to how you feel. Do you understand the other side of the
coin?

JOHNSTON: There's enough in the family that we've got almost
all the ranges. My sister-in-law was married to an airline pilot, and
he just said, "I can't fly an airplane and take care of her." So he got
a divorce, and she's the one that starved to death in the very good
care of a hospital. She only lived to be 53. I've already got my
wife 10 years over that. So, TLC can do it.

I've been in an exceptional situation, as I said, through even the
4 years of varsity wrestling, it made it possible. If she had been the
one who had to take care and I had been the person that was ill, she
couldn't have done it. I'd have been hospitalized until I starved to
death. It's because it's a failure of the system, and you're either
starved to death or you fail to swallow well, and you're very liable
to choking. I've given both nursing homes where my wife's been written
notice that I expect them to use all possible quick things, but I will
not hold them liable for choking death. I recognize this. It's very
possible.

GUTHRIE: I just want to say I also agree with you that maybe if
we could provide better homemaker services, that would be of a great
help to you. I know that in Australia we had a very nice communication
that eight patients with Huntington's disease were taken on a vacation
for the first time in years by some wonderful volunteers, and the purpose of it was to give them an opportunity to have a little vacation.
Well, of course, what happened was not only did the patients have a
vacation, but the families of the patients had a vacation, and it
was mutually beneficial. So I think that your suggestion that we
seek or address ourselves to possibly getting some services of that
kind might be very helpful.

JOHNSTON: I fortunately could do this, but all I ever asked was
give me a break so I can take care of my own. I am pleased now, for a

homemaker, I could deduct that. At the time that I paid a homemaker,
I couldn't. They would only allow it to be deducted if it had been a
nurse. I couldn't afford a nurse and didn't need a nurse. What I
needed was somebody to keep the house together, and another glimpse
of the economics of this thing is in the last year, my wife's care
cost was only 2/5 of my income, but it came out 3/4 of my take-home
pay. That's to pay this high Social Security. Anything that could
be done, I'm an advocate for somebody who has some income, and anything
that could be done to keep them from being crushed because it's so
devastating.

     I do like your idea. One of the other things I was thinking of,
I was happy to keep my wife at home, and I don't want the hospitals
way off, but if we had had even a regional center it would be helpful
in research and at the same time be some place where she could have
gone for a month out of this 20 years, I might be functioning better
today. I'm exhausted.

     ARONSON: A very intensely personal remark, if I may; as a physician,
I'm deeply honored that you're in our profession. A question also.
Given the Social Security regulations as they presently exist, what
changes would you recommend?

     JOHNSTON: I think consideration for these long-term chronic
diseases is going to have to come in somewhere. I suppose what I'm
asking for is not quite so cruel. I was turned down all these times
just because I walked in the door, and they said I was an M.D., I was
making too much money. Out you go again. A year ago, because I was
already having some physical problems, I thought of retirement, and
then I discovered I couldn't support her under retirement pay without--
I would have had $200 a month left afterwards under my retirement, if
I retired a year ago, and I suppose that's... Well, I know some people
on welfare better off than that. So, I drove myself another year to
keep on employment and not retire. There's something wrong with that
system that forces me to stay employed. This year I'm being just plain
carried. I've been on sick leave 2 months, and I'm going to take a
vacation in 2. I don't think I quite answered your question, but I
believe the answer is in more consideration on when you can cash in
on your Social Security because I have paid 35 years under Social
Security, and when I was exhausted, I was still paying in high
numbers.

     ARONSON: You would agree, though, that these regulations
should be re-evaluated?

     JOHNSTON: Definitely yes. They're cruel, and they work all right
in short-term illnesses; in long-term illnesses, they're not.

     WEXLER: If we wanted to get more specific documentation of some
of your problems, can we give you a call later?

JOHNSTON: I'm available to you any time.

WEXLER: I guess the other is just a comment, which is I suppose working day in and day out on this Commission on the HD problem and working with Federal programs that I feel like I've been mucking around all year, but there are beginning to be a few rewards there...

JOHNSTON: I've done all that I can for my Dorothy. I've fulfilled the one and only promise that I made her--that she would never end up in Western State; and that sounds vicious as hell, but in the course of this family, I represent the University of Iowa's Hospital, the University of Colorado's Hospital, Arizona's State Hospital, and Western State here. I'm not picking on a single one of them, but none of them are satis-factory, and I promised her, because she was so fearful of it, she would never go to Western State. She's too ill, now; she'll never make it to go to Western State.

So, the rest of my life's devoted to see what I can do to undo the horrible pile of manure I dumped on those other two, and incidentally I have a younger daughter, too. We had a very careful examination, all the testing that was known, and when we were both 39, we got surprised again. Another careful evaluation said that she was not going to have Huntington's, so that that's the third error. We've enjoyed that error very much, but I can't feel anything but profound guilt for putting her in the position you are in, lady.

GUTHRIE: But you see that Nan's there and is doing pretty well.

HACKLER: I'm very happy to be here.

GUTHRIE: Thank you, all of you. We are now going to ask Harold, Vivian and Karen Thevick.

                          TESTIMONY OF
                    HAROLD AND VIVIAN THEVICK
                      SEATTLE, WASHINGTON

V. THEVICK: I'm Vivian Thevick, and this is my husband, Harold, and my daughter, Karen, and we have one son, Larry, who is age 29. Our daughter is 27. We have known for the past 11 years that my husband has Huntington's disease, but I agree with the young lady who was just speaking... Now we found out that in 1957 they had made a study on Huntington's disease, and they tried to locate all the Thevicks' relatives. They knew that there was one in Washington, but they didn't try that hard to find us. If they had, maybe things would have been a lot different. But, when he heard that he had Huntington's, he was really distressed, of course, and it didn't hit him until after he got home, and then he had more or less a breakdown and ended up in the hospital and had quite a series of shock treatments. He was in the hospital about 2 months before he was able to come back home. Then he went back to work. He was a CPA in Renton, a very good businessman, and worked at that over 20 years so he had a good income, and I worked along with him quite a bit. When he first knew about the Huntington's, he said to my son after he had been out to the University of Washington Genetics Clinic, he said to my son, "I'm sorry," that he had this. He said, "Don't worry, Dad. I'm just glad to be alive." But after that one breakdown there, then he was able to work for a few years again. But then he'd have these emotional upsets, and finally he just couldn't do the accounting business. It was too confusing. He couldn't concentrate well enough so the doctors advised him to then sell out his business.

So he started looking for someone to sell to. So he did sell the business and bought a fishing boat and tried operating it, but he was unable to do that, and he had to hire a couple of skippers, and then our son, after graduating from college, he went down and ran the fishing boat, and has been doing that ever since.

But I think if the public, too, were more aware--to think such an insidious disease and hard to diagnose --if they knew more about it, maybe some of these things wouldn't happen. My husband attempted to take his life at one time, too, because of the depression. For about 2 years, he mainly stayed in bed. I had trouble getting him up. I'd bring him breakfast, lunch and dinner in bed. Then he'd be up a couple hours a day.

Then, he served for a time at the Veterans' Hospital and they put him on different medication. I think he's been better ever since then. That was about 3 years ago. During the time when we were going from doctor to doctor, we spent a lot of money, of course, and we didn't have that much hospital insurance. Now he is on Social Security Disability. He has been on that now about 3 years.

I think it is hard to live with a patient having Huntington's, but I think I have a more easygoing-type temperament. There are many times I've wondered if I could cope with it, but I try to be as patient and understanding as possible. He's been very good, but at times he explodes. My daughter says she remembers him breaking peanut butter jars on the counter or something--that type of thing. Maybe my husband would like to say a few words.

H. THEVICK: Only that I have a real good nurse here. (Applause.)

V. THEVICK: One thing I want to add, though--I think it is quite a stigma on the family when the children are growing up if they do have the parents in a mental hospital. His sister made that statement, that she always remembered kids teasing her and all. Of course, they know more now than at that time, but she was placed in the State Hospital, and they knew she had a nervous disorder. When we were first going

together, my husband said he thought it was due to the menopause.
That's all he knew about it.

Now my son's married, and his wife is diabetic, and because of
the two problems, they have decided not to have children. I don't know
if they would ever adopt, but none of their own anyway.

GUTHRIE: I just wanted to ask about--you mentioned about your
son conducting the business. Does your husband have an interest or
any role to play, even now in that business?

V. THEVICK: Up until about 3 years ago, he did work with my son
some and had an interest. But then he wasn't able to do much at all.
So my son bought out his interest in the fishing boat, so he does not
have any interest in it anymore. There are times, though, that--my
husband is still pretty mentally alert--he comes up with answers for me
many times. Tax questions, he'll answer for me. There are times he
might be a little confused, and then he'll remember a little later,
oh, I gave you the wrong answer. When he gets something on his mind
that he has to figure out, he doesn't let it drop until he figures it
out.

GUTHRIE: That's what I was interested in. Although his speech
is somewhat impaired, he is still functioning, and he knows when he
sees a good nurse--he's got one.

V. THEVICK: Oh, yes, and we have some property below our house,
and he's been handling that deal with the real estate man. It seems
whenever there is something like that, he seems to get a little better
and picks up more. I try to get him to be interested in some activity
or hobby, and he just doesn't have the interest. He gets tired easy.
Maybe if I'm there to do things with him, he'll do a little. On his
own, he doesn't seem to have the initiative.

GUTHRIE: Maybe now that he saw what Mr. Thiessen's doing, maybe
he could find a nice hobby. I see you're smiling.

H. THEVICK: Yes.

V. THEVICK: He still has a good sense of humor. Sometimes he
comes up with something pretty funny.

TESTIMONY OF
KAREN THEVICK
SEATTLE, WASHINGTON

K. THEVICK: It's hard to say what I feel, but so far in my life
(I'm 27), I've decided not to have children, which would be like my

contribution to life maybe in <u>not</u> recreating life, so that I could
change a little bit of suffering in the world. But I have a really
wonderful boyfriend, and I feel sorry for him that he wouldn't be
able to have children if he decides to marry me.

I have often felt within myself that I may be getting Huntington's
because I feel at times that I am uncontrollably just really mad. My
friend has talked to me. He said that you're of Norwegian descent, and
they used to be people that were called the "berserkers" that went
through Europe and stormed England, and they couldn't control them or
understand them because they had such a wild ability to fight, I guess.

So I think that it would be very interesting to try to trace the
disease back to its original beginnings, and I think the most important
thing would be to try to find a test that could test the children of
the parents so that they could plan ahead.

My life has often been one of feeling that everything is going to
terminate at any moment. That makes it so you don't really plan for a
future, and that makes it (I guess maybe that is my own fault), it makes
it not as full of life as it could be. I guess that's all I'd like to
say. But with my father, he's a marvelous person, and I do think that
because he has had this nervousness, and in order to combat that, he
sort of put a cap on himself, which--in a way, that's how he has attempted
to overcome this disease. I think that is really beautiful.

WEXLER: I would just like to say that having a legacy like Huntington's is enough to make anybody angry, whether you have the gene or you
don't have the gene. I think that those of us who are at risk can really
get to the point where you're questioning every move, every time you drop
a cup, every time you're furious with somebody, which increases the
tension and increases your anger. I think that since there is no predictive test at this moment, I think that you need to live in many respects as if there is a future, and you'll find out when there isn't
one. But if you stop it of your own will now, it's much harder to pick
it up later on if you find out that you don't have the disease.

K. THEVICK: That's true. Although I never did feel that I would
get it, I always felt very optimistic and I didn't--the temporariness, I
guess, was with my father's possible death. I always felt that even
driving down the streets, I would memorize streets and buildings because of
some overview of everything being temporary, but I, myself, I never felt
that I would get it. It never became an overshadow on my life.

WEXLER: Did your family ever have genetic counseling or just
counseling so you could talk with anybody?

K. THEVICK: We went to the University of Washington. They had
counseling, and each one of us, my brother and I, we had a little test

like to stick your tongue out and put your hands together, and they did say that I had certain signs with my tongue, but they said that it was probably personality, and that it didn't have anything to do with the disease at that time.

V. THEVICK: It wasn't really counseling. It was just something that one time.

WEXLER: That doesn't sound like counseling. Do you think that would be helpful to just have somebody to just go and talk to, somebody outside of the family?

K. THEVICK: Yes, I think that would be very good.

WEXLER: I think that there are people right here, people in this very room that could give you a place and a person.

K. THEVICK: I think that would be good.

V. THEVICK: I don't know if I made this statement, but I think we need, as Dr. Johnston said, some care where they would have unskilled or lay people to take, like say myself, take care of some Huntington's patients in a person's home where they wouldn't have to pay such high wages to a person and would have the understanding. Because I certainly don't think the mental hospital is the place for Huntington's patients and probably for a lot of other patients with neurological-type diseases.

ARONSON: I keep harking back to something. I agree with you that a mental hospital is not the place for a patient with Huntington's disease who requires hospitalization. But knowing some of the mental hospitals, I don't think, either, they're the place for mental patients. I think that one should not discriminate against any variety of human distress, whether it be psychosocial or organically originated, whatever; this is humanity and should be dealt with compassionately. So, I hope that your concerns are for all individuals who have a somewhat sheltered existence.

K. THEVICK: I worked at a nursing home. I'm an LPR and from there I noticed as much as you try to motivate people to get outside or do anything besides smoke cigarettes and watch TV, a lot of it has to do with how they feel themselves. Unless you have a facility which would have--I don't know what it would have to be--it would have to be acres in the woods with the sea and all kinds of inspiring things in order to really make people want to get outside and do things, I would think.

GUTHRIE: I don't think it's just that, and I don't want to ask for the impossible. But I do think that what we're stressing, we're

saying that humane treatment and permitting people to be who they are
to the best of their capacity for as long as they can--and sometimes
that doesn't necessarily mean it has to have the trees and the sky--
it does mean good relationships with good people who care about you.

K. THEVICK: I see.

GUTHRIE: So, I think that the Commission is very interested in
trying to establish, if we can, what we'd consider good care facilities,
as we say, for all kinds of patients, and we're going to be working on
that.

WEXLER: Do you remember the name of the drug that seemed to be
helpful for your husband?

V. THEVICK: Well, when he went up to Veterans' Hospital, they
gave him lithium carbonate and Thorazine as tranquilizers. He takes,
well, they had recommended five capsules of the 300 milligram lithium
carbonate a day. But it seems that his movements are less than they
used to be. He never had as many movements as some of the patients
I've seen. Now he's had a twitch in the face, and at night he does
move his, mainly when he's laying down in bed, he's continually moving
his feet or legs.

WEXLER: What does he take now?

V. THEVICK: He takes the lithium carbonate and Thorazine. He
takes the Thorazine two tablets in the morning and two at night. I'm
not sure if this is 50 milligrams each. He's had this pain along with
the Huntington's, and I understand Huntington's does not give a person
pain. He's had that pain all along, and that's what he's complained
about more than anything, and I do believe that a lot of the doctors
thought maybe that it was psychosomatic; but I think that the fact that
he had two operations, he had two of these neurotomies, has not helped
the situation, and maybe it's even made that feeling worse. I'm trying
to think of the scar tissue that you get.

ARONSON: They're called traumatic neuromas at the point of operation.

V. THEVICK: That bothered him quite a bit, and along with the
Huntington's, now someone said maybe he's using that pain as an excuse
not to admit that he has Huntington's. That was a few years ago. One
of the doctors made that statement. He's been out to the University of
Washington Pain Clinic in the last three weeks, and they're trying a
new thing for his pain. It's a nerve stimulator. It's called a [neurmon],
where you have electrodes in the back. He isn't wearing it right now,
but I think that's helping his pain. So maybe that will help him get
around a little more, although his legs have gotten weaker the last

few months. But, just recently, he's been getting on his bicycle exerciser, which he hasn't done in a long time. He's been getting on that about 5 minutes a day. So that's encouraging.

GUTHRIE: I do believe that the more you can motivate a person, whether he's got Huntington's or not, to do exercise and really build the body is very important. I think it would be very encouraging if you could get him to do more and more each day.

V. THEVICK: He does go out for walks around our home. He does not like to dress, however. I try to get him to dress. I work, so I'm gone and I come home at lunchtime. He'll stay in his bathrobe and go out and walk around the neighborhood. He'll do that a couple times a day. Of course, all the neighbors know him and speak with him.

ARONSON: I hope you exercise, too.

V. THEVICK: Well, I do get one day, and go golfing in the morning. I finally started doing that.

GUTHRIE: We're going to take a break now for lunch. Thank you. Because we're running a little bit behind schedule, let's all hurry a bit and try to get back within 40 minutes or so.

GUTHRIE: We're going to resume our afternoon session. Dr. Aronson hasn't come back, but we're going to hope that he'll be back shortly. He had some calls to make. Dr. Clifford Smith and Fran Nielson, would you please come forward? Dr. Smith, if you will first give us your name, address and affiliation.

TESTIMONY OF
CLIFFORD SMITH, M.D.
UNITED STATES ARMY
VERMONT

SMITH: My name is Clifford Smith. I'm a resident of the State of Vermont. I am presently employed by the United States Army. Members of the Commission, I gladly accept this opportunity to submit this testimony to the Commission for the Control of Huntington's Disease and Its Consequences as a reflection of my personal experience in dealing with the disease.

My father was a merchant seaman, a strong and vigorous man. Unfortunately, he was also the carrier of the Huntington's gene in our family. As his condition worsened in his late forties, he was forced to retire without any pension, which he lost because he accepted a position lower than captain on his last voyage due to disability.

Taking my father off the sea was very difficult for him to accept; his periods of depression manifested themselves by hostility and anger to
the point of beating his wife and children. His condition worsened
rapidly and he died 4 years later after his physical deterioration.

My mother had chosen not to tell us of my father's disease. Re-
trospectively, I don't question that judgment. The problem it's created,
though, is that of our feeling that our father was either crazy, or
worse, that he didn't love us. My mother had to work exceptionally
long, hard hours to keep the family afloat, all the time knowing that
in all likelihood she would see one or more of his children develop
this same disease that robbed her of her husband.

I didn't uncover the cause of my father's death until I was in
medical school, and I'll never be able to accurately describe the
impact it had on myself and my wife, both personally and professionally. I didn't know whether or not to finish medical school or to go
into a career that didn't require such an extended period of training.
We didn't know whether or not to have children, but our thinking was
that if we were going to have them, it should have been right away, so
I would have been older if and when I developed the disease.

We, and I underscore we, decided that I should finish medical
school. God decided that we should have a child. My wife became
pregnant very unexpectedly. We, I should say I, considered inter-
rupting the pregnancy, but thank God we didn't, for we both love and
cherish our daughter very much. The news of my wife's pregnancy should
have been received with joy, but instead it represented an agonizing
decision and the beginning of many more such agonizing decisions.

Depression, severe and episodic, is one facet of this disease that
I have the most difficulty dealing with. My wife senses this, and frequently tells me that I think about it too much—absolutely correct.
There isn't a day that goes by that it doesn't enter my mind, always
casting a great cloud over my existence. I think about it every day
because there is an infinite number of long-term preparations that
need to be made.

It took me 6 months to get life insurance that wasn't rated 100
percent. Still with no disability clause. I have yet to find disability income insurance. Just getting an administrative leave day
to come here represented a hurdle. What should I tell my associates
when they ask out of professional curiosity, "What's the meeting about,
Cliff?" Because of the extreme sensitiveness about the situation, I
have elected only to tell a few individuals about my predicaments.

This brings up another aspect of the disease that I think is
extremely difficult to cope with, and that is isolation. I have
found it virtually impossible to discuss this with other people,
especially other older physicians whose guidance I was desirous of
seeking out in reference to my career. I even find it a difficult

subject to discuss with my close friends. In a sense, your frustration and despair are locked inside. To a certain degree, this even happened within your own family structure.

Eventually, I'll have to decide whether or not it's advantageous for me to stay in the Army. It represents a decision that I'll have to make with absolutely no reliable, steadfast information. By that, I mean the following: I could elect to stay in the Army for 15 years, or thereabout, and then develop the disease and be retired with a very, very small pension. Against that, I have to weigh the possibility of being stricken with the disease early in life as a civilian without having had time to have built up any equity in my practice. It might offend some of the audience because of the financial advantages afforded physicians, and I accept this as a valid criticism.

The fear and concern are the same, though: that of leaving a wife and child without any financial resource, like my father had the misfortune of doing. I had thought of finishing this little piece of testimony by posing this question to the Commission, what would you suggest I tell my daughter? I soon realized, though, that the Commission wouldn't have any answers. More importantly, though, I realized that the question stemmed from the same uncertainty, frustration, and despair that I've tried to characterize briefly for you.

GUTHRIE: Doctor, just let me inform you that I happen to know a physician with Huntington's disease who is still practicing in Massachusetts, and his wife happens to belong to the Committee to Combat Huntington's Disease and serves on our board. She was in New York just lask week at one of the Executive Committee meetings. She's remarkable in her own understanding of the course of the disease with her husband. He is still practicing, and just this week when I asked her how he is doing, she said fine.

SMITH: That is certainly very heartening information to hear. Especially of my own where I've had relatively little exposure to others who have developed Huntington's disease and, therefore, only have my father's poor unfortunate instance to think about. In all likelihood, his course of the disease is probably much more complex and severe than I think need be the case today if people are more educated, both the families and the communities, in how to cope with the problem. I think that possibly represents one of the interests of the Commission.

GUTHRIE: I would hope so. I really sincerely do, and I think that our people should know that the members of the Commission, by listening to our families, are learning this from our own families. Where there is tender loving care, we see a different kind of disease developing, not that it doesn't go on, but it isn't quite what it used to be. I'm very happy that you are here so that I can tell you about this physician.

WEXLER: It would probably be too lengthy to go into here, but if we had additional information about the difficulty you had getting life insurance, that would be very helpful to us because we are making recommendations about the problems that people at risk have in getting these kinds of insurance.

SMITH: That's a very complex question, and some of it came up last night in the small meeting. I haven't really spoken to anybody who has experienced this same kind of problem, but I can tell you it was unbelievable the amount of red tape. I had a very dogged insurance agent, and that's the only time that I've ever thanked God I had a dogged insurance agent; and he, I think from a newly organized insurance company, who wanted to sell lots of insurance, we managed to stake out a relatively large sum of life insurance, and I just praise God that we had the opportunity to do that. I'm not sure that you will be able to coerce the major insurance companies into insuring people at risk because you'll be asking for an accepted status in that instance because they do exactly the same thing for people with severe pulmonary disease, people with severe cardiovascular disease, they rate their insurance. They're money-making operations.

GUTHRIE: Well, there's another answer, you know. That we all have to fight for together, and that is catastrophic illness. It is on the books as a possibility, and after it does happen or doesn't happen, the next step may be some kind of a national health insurance. Our problem is one of many people who have similar problems. What we have to be is a strong constituency that can fight for what we need for our people as well as the others, because if you have enough people, then you have a stronger possibility of getting what the people need. It's not as hopeless as it looked 2 or 3 years ago, frankly, but it will take a lot of work on all of our parts, and that's why it's so important for all of us to be aware of what's coming and what you can do to help make it come sooner.

I'm sure Nancy would like probably some more information, Doctor, from you if she may as our Executive Director, perhaps be in touch with you and get more details. Is that right, Nancy?

WEXLER: Yes.

GUTHRIE: All right, may we hear from Fran Nielson?

                    TESTIMONY OF
                    FRAN NIELSON
               WOODINVILLE, WASHINGTON

NIELSON: My name is Frances Burhart Nielson, 18211 N.E. 189th, Woodinville, Washington.

My former husband's, Darrol D. Burhart, first sanity hearing was
held at Harborview Hospital in Seattle on June 10, 1971. The disease
of Huntington's chorea had been diagnosed just 1 year earlier but he
could not accept that and live in a family situation. He was sent home
from that hearing, but Darrol did agree to take prescribed drugs which
helped him control his temperament considerably. Darrol lived at home
until October 1974, when he was admitted to the Seattle Veterans' Hospital against his will. To that point, there were many problems that we
worked out as we went along, such as Darrol's driving, getting him to see
a doctor, his trying to hold a job when he was already sick, the treatment our two sons had to live with from their father, financial hardships, and buying a home. There were many hardships and sadnesses that
we went through and I know other HD families share many of the same experiences. All of these we were able to face within our family circle
and go on.

But in January of 1975, the Veterans' Hospital decided that Darrol
(he is a veteran) could not be retained in the Seattle Hospital and
should be sent to the American Lake facility. They did not tell me or
explain in any detail what that meant. Darrol was subjected to four
sanity trials in the ensuing months. American Lake would not take him
and he was sent to Western State Hospital for 3 months, which had always
been a dread to Darrol because his mother died there. Finally, in mid-
1975, American Lake Hospital did admit Darrol until February of 1976, at
which time they discharged him without my permission or knowledge and
sent him to a nursing home in Seattle. He was in this nursing home
under Veterans' care for 6 months. I was contacted by a Veterans'
social worker that Darrol would have to be moved since the nursing home
would not keep any new public assistance patients and the Veterans'
Administration was relinquishing all claim for Darrol.

In August 1976, I went door to door of nursing homes in the north
Seattle area trying to find some place that would take a young man with
HD, partly on public assistance and Social Security. The search was very
frustrating and frightening. I did find a new, large home in Edmonds,
and Darrol is still there; but I received a call last week that they will
not be able to keep him because of his fighting over the TV, if something isn't done to control him. And there is the fear again, where
would he go from there? I haven't any idea. Western State Hospital,
I suppose, would have to take him, but that place makes me sick. Besides
the fact that it would be an hour and a half drive for me one way to
visit him and he would be left there just by himself, this is a terrible
feeling, not knowing of anywhere that will be willing to take care of him
and see that he gets good care and someone really caring about him.

We have two sons growing up, ages 10 and 14. Since I have remarried and the boys are no longer living in and with HD, HD is not an
open subject.

It is very hard for me to bring it up at all, yet I know the boys
need to know what could very well be a part of their futures. This is

very hard and heartbreaking for me, and I do not know how to face this at this time.

GUTHRIE: I don't think I have any special question because the things that you have said I know only too well because they're true. I think that this testimony along with so many of the others is going to be very important in terms of this Commission documenting the fact that we don't know what to do because the patients are being turned out. Thank you very much for this opportunity.

WEXLER: I would just like to say that I wrote a note to myself to send your testimony to the VA because we will be talking to them about their VA programs, and I will send it verbatim to the Head of Neurology in the VA next week.

GUTHRIE: You might be interested to know that we've just finished a survey of the VA, and we found 500 inpatients with Huntington's disease in VA hospitals, and another 500 who have been discharged either to a home or a nursing home or who are outpatients. So, with those figures we are ready to go back to the VA, and your documentation will be very helpful. Thank you very much.

Carol Atkinson and Mrs. Wilma Berman. May we have your names and affiliation?

TESTIMONY OF
CAROL ATKINSON
SEATTLE, WASHINGTON

ATKINSON: My name is Carol Atkinson, and my natural father has Huntington's chorea, and this is my mother, Mrs. Berman. I'm not prepared really too much, but I do want to say a few things.

My older sister who is 29 has Huntington's disease; I think, I don't really know, that she's accepted it all that well, and the one thing I wanted to say is that I feel she needs someone she can talk to because when she gets depressed, she calls my mother, and it's hard for her to know what to say to her.

I don't know what to say to my sister because I knew it for a long time before she knew it, and I didn't know what to say to her then. I couldn't bring myself to tell her I thought she had it, nor could I to any other family member if I thought they had it. That's a big problem. I feel that there is no place really you can go to talk to outside of Amelia Schultz has been a lot of help. When I was worried about my older sister, and I wanted my mom to know that I thought she had it, and a lot of doctors, I thought, did her a lot of injustice.

I don't know that my mother agrees because she has bad allergies, but the disease was blamed on these allergies for a long time, which I felt kept her from getting the help she needed then, and with my sister, the biggest thing I noticed in her which gave me an indication of it was that she hated people really easily or she loved them real easily. They were the two extremes in her life.

I feel that, and I mentioned to Dr. Schultz, when I had my daughter 9 years ago, I was pregnant before I knew anything about the disease, so I couldn't have prevented that; and when I had my daughter, I had her through the University, and they sent out visiting nurses then, which I felt was not needed; I personally feel that if they could take that money that they can spend on visiting nurses for women who have children and sent those people or people who would be paid to do the same thing out to visit people like my sister, I think I would really like to see that happen.

I wish I had more time to spend with her, but I don't, and I don't know that I'd be that helpful anyway because I don't know really what to do or to say. I would like to also say something about whether or not I think that people should be told, children should be told. I don't necessarily feel, I think if they're going to be--I can't say that if I had known, I wouldn't have had a child anyway, because I really believe I would have.

I don't look at the disease as a threat to me because I live each day at a time, and that's what is best for me in my life. But for other people who can't do that, I would think that maybe not to have children would be a good idea because I feel that if they did have children, they should tell the children at a time when they think they can handle or when they think it is necessary. But I think just to bring it up is really not all that necessary.

I know in my own family I think it wasn't talked about. I'm not sure really why, but I know one of the reasons is because our natural father--my mother was divorced, all four of us were adopted. I have two sisters and a brother. So that was one particular thing. We never really brought up our natural father because of our adopted father, and at least my personal feeling is that it would bring some pain to my father and to my mother. Even after we were told about the disease, I didn't talk about it too much because of the fact that it was my natural father. I didn't want to talk about it. But I felt it was necessary when my older brother, who is 28, went through a lot of bad times, I think because his girlfriend at the time read an article in the Ladies' Home Journal that said something to the effect that at the age of 13 a boy--and they sort of indicated in that article that it was male dominant, and that females had no chance--and I really felt that was really wrong. What that article did to my brother, I felt, still really hasn't been undone. Also, I think one of the things should be to see to it maybe if people could--magazines or newspapers--if they are going to print articles, make sure you get accurate information. It's a little better now but just because of that article, that's when I decided to find out what it was really all about, and that was in about '72. Before that, I was just guessing and finding out what I could, wherever I could. Dr. Schultz and my mother told me everything I wanted to know about it.

I think probably another big thing that could be done is that more doctors should know about it because I've been to a lot of doctors myself, for I was having a lot of problems in my life. Well, I had a lot of problems with my marriage, which pretty much took my time, and with that I got into drugs and I felt I used Huntington's chorea as a crutch then; but looking back now, I can say those doctors didn't know enough. So I could use what I wanted to use. I took information to doctors, and it kind of made me feel uneasy because I didn't really trust anything they would have to say about it--other than the University of Washington, which I feel is a fantastic place.

I don't feel--I'll be 25 next week--and I don't feel that I am going to get it, that's just the way I feel. If I do, I won't be prepared for it because I don't want to be, but I do hope that there will be more help for my sister or for anybody else in my family and that's really about all I can add.

GUTHRIE: What that person didn't know was that if that doctor looked in a textbook up until a certain year, there was nothing in a textbook to find out. But now we have the information, and that's what's important. Mother, what are you going to say?

TESTIMONY OF
WILMA BERMAN
SEATTLE, WASHINGTON

BERMAN: I also wrote a letter to the Ladies' Home Journal and read the correction on it or the retraction. There are two things that I probably could add.

One is I found out about the condition of my ex-husband accidentally. We had been divorced for quite a few years when his case was diagnosed, and I found it very, very difficult to get information. I only had hear-say. It took a great deal of letter-writing and working through a psychiatrist. They would not give me direct information about my ex-husband's condition, which I felt I needed to know for the benefit of my children. Eventually, over a period of about 6 months, I was able to obtain the confirmation I desired.

The second thing that's been brought up before is about when to tell children or what to tell children or if you should tell children.

Well, in our particular case, we went out to the University of Washington Genetics Clinic, and we were advised to tell them. The unfortunate part in our case was the youngest was about 13 and the oldest was about 19. They were 19, 18, 17 and 13. I think that the younger the child is when they learn about it, the better chance they have to correlate it into their lives to cope with it, to grow into it gradually, as you said on TV when I saw you; I concur with that. I think the worst time for children to learn about it is in their late teens: 17, 18.

We ended up with my middle daughter, as she said, has turned to drugs, and since has been rehabilitated. We're very, very proud of her on that score. The boy became an alcoholic, and he's conquered that and has gone back to college. He's 28. And, of course, the oldest one is diagnosed. I think that if the timing of telling the children can be controlled, it's better that they know at an earlier age.

GUTHRIE: Again, I have to--as a comment as a parent--I don't think there are rules. I think that we all have to work this out with our families. What might be good for me might not be good for someone else. I don't want to say that because I felt that it was important, everybody should do what I do. I think it depends on who is talking to whom at what time, but I would make a very interesting observation that people don't realize, and I learned in my own family, which was that when I thought that my children knew everything that I thought they should know, I discovered that one of my children knew more about genetics than I thought he knew. When he came and questioned me in a special way, it turned out that he didn't think that his mother, who had been a dancer, knew anything about science. He had just studied heredity and genetics in school. His feeling was that if his mother didn't quite understand that he had a 50-50 chance, he was not going to tell me to protect me. So we don't know always what our children do know.

BERMAN: Have a long talk with your children. You'll learn a great deal.

WEXLER: I'd just like to ask a question of clarification. Did your ex-husband's doctors know that he had Huntington's disease?

BERMAN: Yes, they did. So did the Veterans' Administration, and they would not give out any information. I worked through a psychiatrist. I wrote the letters, and they sent the information to the psychiatrist. Actually, for definite confirmation, we traced it back a second generation to my first husband's father, who had the disease, which is one reason I didn't believe it when I first heard, is because I knew he died in prison at the age of 70, and that's a long life. So I assumed that it was untrue. But I did write to the prison where he died, and they did confirm that he did die of Huntington's chorea.

GUTHRIE: In prison? That sounds like it used to be.

WEXLER: What reason did they give you for not giving you the information?

BERMAN: They said it was confidential and they could not give it without the patient's permission.

WEXLER: Your ex-husband was living at the time?

BERMAN: Yes, but I didn't know his whereabouts. I knew the general area, but I didn't feel that I really wanted to go to him and get his permission.

WEXLER: Okay. No one made any contact. The first that you knew there was something wrong was when your daughter began to have symptoms?

BERMAN: No, I got the information through the friend of a friend who happened to know my ex-husband, just by hearsay.

WEXLER: Otherwise, if your daughter began to have symptoms, it would have been totally out of the blue.

BERMAN: Totally out of the blue.

WEXLER: Also, would it have been helpful to you and to your family-- do you think maybe this happened, I don't know the sequence of events-- but when you were telling your children about their risk, if you could have worked with a counselor who could have seen each of you individually or as a family or had some more extensive period of talking through coupled with that information, would that have been helpful to you?

BERMAN: Well, we actually did have that because we were working with the Genetics Clinic at the University of Washington. Again, I have the highest praise for our local facilities. They are tremendous; we just don't know what we would do without them. They've been so wonderful.

WEXLER: Maybe I should rephrase. What I'm really asking is if you could think of any recommendation that might have minimized the trauma to you, to your brother, and to your sister? Is there anything in addition that you would like to recommend that would have been helpful?

ATKINSON: I feel that what you just said about a counselor, a drop-in clinic or even a call-in clinic would be helpful. Like I said,

as far as any other members of the family, like just one particular
member of the family noticing one other particular member of the family
and not wanting to bring it to anybody else. If there was some place
where you could just call where someone knew something about the
disease, and could maybe get the family more together in talking,
I think it would have been helpful.

BERMAN: At the time the children were told, we did make them
aware of the fact that Dr. Schultz was always available for counseling
and for consultation at the clinic any time they wanted it. So I don't
really think that there was a lack of facilities. I think that when they
learned, it was such a shock to them that they really didn't want at
that time to know any more. But this always was available, and they all
had cards for the University of Washington, so it was available to them;
but a shock like this, I think that it has to be perhaps assimilated
over a period of time.

I know that I didn't want to accept it for a long time, and I really
didn't want to tell the children; yet my oldest daughter was about to
be married, and I didn't feel it was fair to her respective husband to
marry her. This is the one who has the disease now. Without having
full knowledge of the possibility of what might happen, and in retrospect, I'm very happy that I did tell her so that she could tell him
before they were married because he has been just marvelous. He said
that for as much time as she has, he is going to make her life as good
as possible. He takes her out on his fishing trips on weekends; they
do things together. So it's really been good in that respect.

GUTHRIE: Thank you very much. We next would like to hear from
Professor Swanson, Merle Denney and Darlene Conrad.

TESTIMONY OF
PHILLIP SWANSON, M.D.
DEPARTMENT OF NEUROLOGY
SCHOOL OF MEDICINE
UNIVERSITY OF WASHINGTON

SWANSON: My name is Phillip Swanson. I am head of the Division
of Neurology at the University, and I'm a neurologist and am responsible
for the teaching of medical students and for the training of physicians
who are going to practice in neurology, which is the specialty medicine
that I think deals more with Huntington's and other neurological disorders. I have also done some research into the neurochemistry of
Huntington's disease. I'm not really sure what I should say today
because I am coming as a clinician and as a researcher; I find myself
rather frustrated much of the time in not knowing exactly where I'm
going or what it is I should be doing.

As a clinician, I see a certain number of people who have Huntington's disease. I see mainly outpatients, rather few people who come

into the hospital; and I follow some of these people, seeing them at
intervals, 6 months or a year. I think in analyzing what I do it's
really talking and listening and answering questions rather than anything that one might consider medicine. I basically don't feel that
the medications that are available really do very much. They may help
to a certain extent to control the movements in people who are really
severely affected, but they certainly don't change the course of the
disease, and I think they're very limited in what they do do.

As far as research is concerned, it may have already been mentioned
that financial support for neurological research these days is, I think,
at an all-time low. It may not look that way when one looks at the
dollar figures, of what is spent, but there are people in our group who
are on some of the study sections at the National Institutes of Health;
and in one of the last evaluation sessions where they evaluate the grants
submitted for approval, they funded three or four out of well over a
hundred that they approved and thought were worthy of support. This has
never been as bad as this as far as neurological support. Some other
researchers, I guess, are not doing so poorly. I think this is a very
frustrating thing for many investigators, neuroscientists, who are
trying to do research into the disease. However, I do feel that money
doesn't solve everything, and unfortunately, it's my view that most of
the research into the chemical things that have been found to go on in
Huntington's disease are really looking at the phenomena.

They're not really looking at the cause of the disease. There are
a number of biochemical things that have been found. I kind of think
they're effects rather than causes of the condition. This doesn't mean
that they're not important, because probably the same thing is true in
Parkinson's disease where the biochemical changes that have been found
have led to fairly useful treatment for people with Parkinson's disease.
I think the kind of research that's done is useful, but I don't think it
really gets to the heart of things, which is why genetic dominant
diseases cause the changes that they do in the nervous system. I'm
afraid that until we get to a point where genetic research really
understands what happens in other dominant diseases, that we're going
to be doing what I call "fishing expeditions" much of the time. I'm
afraid that I don't have any really good answers as to how to go beyond
that at the present time.

GUTHRIE: I'd like to just add my thoughts to yours. You know that
many of our people who are here today are not aware of the fact that you
just mentioned that neurology, the Institute for Neurology, has been one
of the least-funded of the National Institutes of Health, and that when
we get a firm coalition of constituents there's going to be an opportunity to increase that budget. But as long as there's not a strong constituency, it isn't going to happen.

This is one of the things that part of our education has been, to tell people that you are dealing with a neurological disorder, and that there are many similar disorders. When all of these people get together as a group, we're going to have a strong chance of getting better funding for the research. I believe your figure may not be quite accurate, but I believe I was told by Dr. Tower that 20 percent of the proposals were getting support this year; but I know at NIGMS, which is general medical science, at least 50 percent are getting their funding.

SWANSON: I gather that there are arguments that 20 percent or 15 percent or 7 percent or 4 percent, but that may be overall; but when it comes right down to it, the people in the study section can't understand--if it's 20 percent, why is it that only 4 of the grants that they approved were funded? They can't figure it out. They're unhappy about it.

ARONSON: The figure, Dr. Swanson, that I heard was 14 or 15 percent. I think 20 percent is an optimistic hope rather than a reality. Dr. Swanson, I'd like to ask, however, when Huntington's disease pops up in the undergraduate curriculum at the university?

SWANSON: Well, that opens a whole area of discussion. Certainly, every medical student that goes through the University of Washington has had at least one lecture in which the disease was discussed in relation to the anatomy and physiology of the nervous system, and they all have seen at least one patient on either videotape or film so they do, they have had that exposure at the very first part of their curriculum. However, there have been a number of curriculum changes at this medical school, and many are for the better, and there is some argument as to whether every change is for the better. But what has happened to the education of medical students in part has resulted in students finishing medical school who have an exposure to one thing, and other students not having an exposure to that thing.

There's much more in the way of elective choices. It used to be 10 years ago that every medical student essentially took all of the same courses, with maybe a little extra. Now one can elect, for example, to take a month in neurology or not elect to take that month. I think about 2/3 of the students do, but that means that 1/3 does not. So that third that has not had that exposure could probably have forgotten what was learned in the first year simply because there was no further exposure.

Also, I think that physicians who go on into further training, their training also has changed, so that some doctors who go into family practice, for example, will have had very little neurology because this isn't required during their training period. Most interns will, at least in this place, but in another medical school it may be different. So, I think it's understandable that many doctors don't know everything, and there may be some who are much less and some who are quite sophisticated about the nervous system.

WEXLER: When you see a Huntington's family, do you do your own genetic counseling, or do you usually refer to the Genetics Clinic?

SWANSON: Well, Dr. Bird, who I think was here this morning, is our neurology unit; and I think that we usually leave the detailed genetic counseling to Dr. Bird and the people in the Genetics Clinic, and I usually and others in the Neurology Clinic usually follow individual patients with maybe their spouse.

WEXLER: Are there any other referrals that you repeatedly make to Huntington's families--a psychology service or any other programs?

SWANSON: I don't do anything really routinely. I think it really depends on the problem at the particular time. I think that if there seems to be a vocational problem, then I would refer the patient to a vocational counselor, or there are just so many different problems that it's hard to be routine about anything. Certainly, I would refer a patient to anywhere where I thought the problem could be helped. I am never quite sure what to tell a patient if I think a patient has the disease, I'm pretty sure about it, but I'm not so sure the patient really wants to know, because I had one man who jumped into Green River Gorge when he was told that he had Huntington's disease. So I think that is a problem. It's difficult for a doctor to know whether it is right to be completely open or not, and I often let the patient sort of guide me on it.

WEXLER: Is there a period of time, just as a Commission, where you have certain suspicions but you can't be definitive? Does that extend for certain portions of the disease?

SWANSON: Well, that could extend for, I think, quite a while. That often is the way that I will actually approach it. If I see a person who's having restless movements, and I kind of think, I'm pretty sure in my own mind really, I might say that I notice that you seem somewhat restless, and I think it's possible that you have it without actually saying that I'm sure, which I may not be. I have a man who I see who really hasn't changed that much over several years. He's just a little bit fidgety and restless, and he's really been doing pretty well as far as I can tell.

I've also been influenced by a medical school physician. There is a professor of medicine where I went to medical school that has Huntington's disease; and I was very impressed that he was very productive. He was 60, I think, by the time I left, and although he certainly had involuntary movements that were evident to someone who knew he had the disease, he functioned quite well in the job that he had. So, again, that's made me somewhat less confident as to how strong the genetic counseling should be as far as having children is concerned. Certain people can be very productive and still have it.

GUTHRIE: All right. Darlene, I think you're next.

TESTIMONY OF
DARLENE CONRAD, R.N.
NURSING COORDINATOR
COMMUNITY HOME HEALTH CARE
SEATTLE, WASHINGTON

CONRAD: My name is Darlene Conrad, and I'm a nursing supervisor
with the Community Home Health Care that's here in Seattle, Washington.
Our agency is a Medicare-certified home care agency, and we provide
social and health services to a multidisciplinary team approach to patient
care in their own homes. The majority of our patients are the older
patients (disabled) whose services are reimbursed by Medicare. We also
receive some payments from Medicaid and some private insurance agencies.

Community Home Health Care is acutely aware of the limited services
available to the homebound patient suffering from a chronic, progressive
disease. Although our experiences have been limited with Huntington's
disease, we have had much experiences similar to this category, which
include amyotrophic lateral sclerosis, muscular dystrophy, multiple
sclerosis, Parkinson's disease, and rheumatoid arthritis. These patients
can have very heavy care needs, and they often receive only short-term
care in the hospital. The burden of their care, therefore, falls upon
their family.

Our home care agency can be of assistance in these situations. A
registered nurse is often needed to instruct the patient and family in
the nursing care need. This can include skin care and management of
bladder and bowels. A dietician can assist the family with nutritional
problems. A physical therapist or occupational therapist can instruct
regarding home safety in transit and in exercises that are needed for
joint mobility. A social worker can assist the family with financial
problems in making referrals to community resources. More importantly,
the social worker can provide support to these families by assisting them
in handling the emotional stress of these devastating conditions.

What these patients often need most in order to be maintained in
their homes as long as possible is the assistance of a homemaker home
health aide. These paraprofessionals work under the direction of a
registered nurse or physical therapist. They provide assistance with
the personal care needs of the patient and much-needed relief for the
family. Home care agencies have many limitations in providing this
type of service on an ongoing basis because of inadequate funding
resources.

Medicare covers for a limited period following an acute exacerba-
tion of the disease. The goal of our agency then is to assist the
patient to their maximum level of functioning, to instruct the patient

and family in care, and to set up a home management program for long-term care. Medicare does not pay for ongoing maintenance care of the chronically ill person. An exception is in those cases requiring inter-mittent visits to carry out specialized treatment, such as changing catheter every month.

Medicaid does pay for maintenance care, including home health aides, but the family must be very low income to be eligible for this coverage. Home care agencies lose money in providing services under Medicaid because the full cost is not reimbursed. Medicaid does not cover home visits by social workers, and this is often a primary need.

Private insurance often doesn't pay for any home care at all, and if they do, it is usually limited to the registered nurse or physical therapist. A social worker or homemaker home health aide is usually not covered. Families are, therefore, forced to provide all the care needs themselves, or if they have financial resources, they can hire private help or place the patient in nursing homes. We have even had cases where the couple has become divorced in order to become eligible for Medicaid assistance.

I appreciate the opportunity to share some of our frustrations in establishing ongoing home management programs to provide continuity of support and prevention of complications. This is something we consider an essential component of the delivery of quality patient care to these patients and their families.

ARONSON: Miss Conrad, earlier today, the representative of the Seattle's Visiting Nurses Association indicated that his association had seen one, perhaps two, patients with Huntington's disease within the last few years, which seemed to have been a discrepancy between that and the number of cases within the community.

In your association, would you recall offhand how many patients with HD have been seen?

CONRAD: Our agency is fairly new, but we have seen one.

ARONSON: Out of perhaps a few hundred patients altogether?

CONRAD: Yes. Again, I would guess that these people are often not in hospital situations. They're not discharged from hospitals so no one is thinking of discharge planning, and often the coverage is very inadequate because our cover under Medicare is very short termed, and often they're the only ones that provide coverage at all.

GUTHRIE: I have no other comment to make except that you are re-emphasizing, of course, one of the strongest needs for trying to get really catastrophic illness insurance or trying to get some kind of insurance that would help to get the right people to the people who need the help. Merle.

TESTIMONY OF
MERLE DENNEY
EVERETT, WASHINGTON

DENNEY: My name is Merle Denney. I work with the Committee to
Combat Huntington's Disease in the Seattle area. As President for this
chapter, I work with the Genetic Research Center at the University. I
was motivated to do this. My husband, Wayne, died of Huntington's
disease in 1974. He had been an invalid in a wheelchair and bedridden
for almost 15 years. He was one of the more severe cases.

At the time Wayne and I were married, or we were to be married,
Wayne told me that his mother had died of some nervous condition which
had no name, and that his grandfather had died of a nervous condition.
Wayne was aware of the fact that there were possibilities that he could
have it, but, of course, it meant nothing to me because I had not seen
his mother. She had passed away before we were married. Wayne was
22, apparently a healty, very handsome young man, so we were married. About 12 years after we were married, Wayne began to show
symptoms of Huntington's disease. As I look back now, I can see that
from the time we were married, these signs were present, some of these
signs, symptoms.

As the time progressed, I wondered if this was perhaps what his
mother had died of. And, of course, you live in a state sometimes and
you don't want to admit perhaps these things are happening; it was a
gradual thing so that in the meantime, we had three children, and so Wayne
was a military career man, an electronic technician. He did very intri-
cate work with his hands.

During that 12-year period of time, I did watch him progressively become worse, and eventually he was put into a military hospital,
U.S. Naval Hospital in Philadelphia, Pennsylvania. We had lived in
Colorado, and planned to retire there, and had a TV sales service store.
I realized in my own mind that there was something very seriously wrong
with Wayne. In the meantime, he had one year left of his service
before retiring, so he was transferred to Goose Bay Laboratory. As I
watched him, the night I took him to the plane, and everyone in the
airport was watching because he was carrying his bags; and the three children
and I were watching as he went down the ramp into the airplane, and he
was stumbling so badly that everyone in the airport thought he was very
drunk. My heart was aching because I knew there was something very
much wrong, and Wayne and I would not admit it to each other or talk
about the fact that there was something very wrong with him.

So 1 month after he was sent to Goose Bay Laboratory, I had to come
back to Everett because I had relatives here and I knew that something
was wrong with Wayne. So, during this month, he was put into the hospital, where they did not know of the family history; and whether or not

Wayne mentioned his mother's nervous condition, I don't know at this
point; but there was never the mention of Huntington's disease in the
family. For some reason, at the time, they removed all his teeth and
he was very frightened and scared, so when he was transferred finally
about 3 or 4 months later to Philadelphia, Pennsylvania, I left my
children in Everett and went to the hospital in Philadelphia.
He was diagnosed after 10 days of my being there; he was diagnosed
as having Huntington's disease.

When I went into the hospital, and I was unexpected, they had him
come down the hallway; they had me wait in a waiting room, and I saw
him stumbling down the hallway, a grotesque figure, with his teeth
removed. My first impulse was to turn and run. I was so frightened
and so confused that I didn't know what to do, but because of Wayne
and the compassion I had for him, I knew that I had to stay. So
this was my first reaction. So then after a few days the doctor
did tell me that Wayne had Huntington's disease.

The only thing I was told was that it was a hereditary, fatal
disease, which would last about 15 years. Then he would become
completely disabled, and mentally affected. This is all I knew about
it. So I left Wayne at the hospital without having talked to him
because they didn't want him to know yet. So I went back home to
my children with the determination that--the doctor did some counseling
with me about how to prepare myself in meeting Wayne again--whatever
happened, I would carry on.

So he was told and called me on the phone and sobbingly told me
that he had Huntington's disease. It was assumed that this was what
his mother had. I assured him that we would manage and not to worry
about it. To my knowledge, he was quite content. He was very placid.
He accepted things very graciously, which I'll admit that sometimes I
did not because I didn't understand.

The point I would like to bring out is that now we do have some
help, more knowledge than during the period about 7 or 8 years after
Wayne was diagnosed; and he was a very severe case. In fact, he got in
a wheelchair shortly after he was diagnosed, and there had been a great
deal of time before he passed away. But we did keep him at home most
of the time. He was in a VA hospital at one time. He was in a nursing
home where the VA put him.

I was turned down by the many nursing homes. Again, I am reiterating
that which has already been said, the nursing homes were not familiar
with the disease; they did not know how to cope or communicate with these
people, and I lived in an anxiety and a fear for those years not knowing

there was another soul in the world with Huntington's disease. I had
never heard of it.

Then Woody Guthrie died of it in 1967, and it was in the paper.
I didn't know who to go to or how to find out, but I at that time wanted
to know more about the disease, which none of the physicians I had been
to knew anything except a small paragraph which was in the medical books.

I finally contacted the University of Washington Genetic Research
Center; and after contacting Dr. Amelia Schultz in 1971, I began to
organize the chapter in this area for the Committee to Combat Huntington's Disease, realizing the need for sharing the need that other people
have to know that there is someone else who does have this disease, that
they're not alone in the world with it.

I work directly with the families. I have been confronted with
these families with all of the problems which have been mentioned here
today. Not knowing where to turn, not knowing who to turn to, nursing
homes not taking the patients, not being able to find financial aid:
Our welfare system certainly does need a reform. This is one of the
things I was going to recommend because I feel that the public assistance
money should be spent where it is most needed, and not on people who are
able to work if they wish to.

I can give you one good example of where a woman called me, and she
was very exhausted because she had taken care of her husband for 9 years,
and she had no relief from this; and I took her down to the welfare
office, and she was hesitant to go, she didn't want to go because of
the stigmas attached to it. So, we finally did. They took her husband
and placed him in a nursing home, where my husband was placed. They
left her with barely enough money to exist on. This is just one example.
She stayed married to him. They did pay the nursing home. She was left
with $186, as a matter of fact, and she had a $90 house payment and uti-
lities and other expenses. She could not go out and work because if she
worked, and made $500 a month, she was required to give $250 of that to
the welfare office, plus they would take away her $186 a month. Then
she had a small apartment in her basement which she rented out to the
college students. It was for $60 a month. She was no longer allowed.
She could rent the apartment out, but they would take it out of the
amount they allowed her so everything was futile for this woman except
to live from this. So, divorces are brought about for this reason. It
has been brought out earlier today.

Some of the legal aspects: I have been in court with many people
because a patient becomes incompetent (or perhaps incompetent is not
the word, but unable to manage their affairs or their monetary affairs
and so forth), and this happens sometimes before the family is aware
of which steps, legal steps they should prepare for.

Since I have been through a lot of the hurdles myself when there was no one to turn to--there were no committees, there were no doctors who understood or social workers who understood and so forth--I feel that I am able sometimes to see ahead what the next step is going to be in a family so that I can advise and help them in these ways.

I work with families in crisis situations. One thing I would like to point out is that the police departments in the city should be educated, the crisis clinics should be educated. I had a call from a lady who was absolutely frantic. I had been in touch with her for about 2 years, and her husband became very violent because he wanted the car keys, and she would not let him have them. So he absolutely destroyed the house. It was just a total wreck when I arrived.

She had called the police, but they would not come out because they thought it was a husband-and-wife dispute. They did not realize what Huntington's disease was. So, the crisis clinic was called, but they would not come out because they did not know what Huntington's disease was. So I went out, and when I arrived at her home her stepfather was there with her. My brother went with me because we didn't know what to expect, and so we did call the crisis clinic. I explained to them who I was and who I represented so they did come out after we spent 7 hours at the Harborview Hospital. They examined the man. By that time, he had calmed down, and he appeared to be normal. So, he had also threatened to burn the house down, and he had broken his little boy's finger previously. So how was this woman to cope with these things? Where was she to turn, because there was no one who would come out when she called? There was no one to turn to. So, we spent 7 hours convincing the psychiatrists that this man needed some professional help and this woman could not cope with it. They kept him for 2 weeks because he would not voluntarily stay. In any event, they kept him for 2 weeks. They then released him. Again, at home it was the same situation. So they had private psychiatrists, group therapies, and numerous things in order to try to help this man. This is one case I'm just citing to show that the police in our city, the crisis clinic, and professional people certainly should be educated as to what Huntington's disease is.

Finally, this particular person was uncontrollable at home, which some of them do become; he was placed in Western State Hospital, and that's where he is at this time. I really don't know what else to add except the great need for long-term care. At one time, I did a research survey over the state to find out where and what was available for long-term care for patients.

I found that the VA homes in this state were a disgrace to our country. What we call the "old folk homes." Channel 7, some of you may have seen it, did a story and kept in constant contact with the stuff that was going on because I found that in order to qualify, our veterans

had to be able to dress themselves, feed themselves, and go to the
dining room, and more or less take care of themselves, in order to
qualify to get into these VA homes. There are two in the state of
Washington. There is no other place for them. In the VA hospital at
American Lake they have to be considered psychotic or they will not
keep them. Therefore, the only other place for them is a nursing
home, and I was lucky enough, after being turned down about 10 times,
to get Wayne into a nursing home where Doris and I have become good
friends, and she's worked with our Committee. She learned about
Huntington's disease from Wayne and I, and she has taken other
patients and found that they can be successfully cared for in the
nursing homes.

Another thing I try to help with, and there is a great need for,
is to relieve the families of some of the guilt which I went through
in placing my husband in a nursing home in times when I truly had to--
when I was ill, when there were problems with my children, and I could
not take care of him at home. It is not easy to find someone to come
into your home, even if you can afford it; it's not that easy to find
someone to come into your home.

We have had some patients, my husband was one of them, who required
24 hours-a-day care. He was one of the more severe cases.   He
could not be left alone because he would harm himself or he smoked, he
would set fire to the house, which he did at one time. But I had a
guilt complex, which I carried through until after his death, in placing
him into a nursing home.

I can help some of these families through having been through this
myself, helping them realize that when a patient has reached a point
of disability, then the person really should be placed into a nursing
home and without any guilt feelings. There are numerous ways with which
I have been able to help, because of the hurdles I went over when there
was no one to turn to. That's why I feel that help to the family is
just as important as the research. I can't think of anything else at
this time.

GUTHRIE: Thank you. We're running short. I'm not going to make
any comments or questions, and I just want to ask in the audience
because we're questioning about the next few people, is Mary Jo Bixby
June Kingston, or Mathew Griffin here? Would you just see Mr. Booth
for a minute because he wants to reschedule you, and I'll thank you.
We're next calling Robert Lightbourne, Diane Plumridge, and Stella
Runnels. I just want to ask, is Lynn Huffman here yet? Lynn, this
is your lunch brought here by your aunt. Please take it off the table
before I eat it. I have been nibbling half of it already.

TESTIMONY OF
ROBERT LIGHTBOURNE, M.D.
NEUROLOGIST
WESTERN STATE HOSPITAL

LIGHTBOURNE: I do most of my work in Western State Hospital in
the Department of Neurology. In following patients with chorea, there
are three hospitals: Northern State, Eastern State and Western State.
We have just now confined Northern State, which is closed. Most of
them are in Western right now. I've been interested in this problem
of Huntington's disease since--for the last 19 years. I follow quite
a number of families.

I teach all the nursing students that come into training in
psychiatry; I have a film representative of the patients, a teaching
film of the Huntington's disease. That's about it. We have right
now just a total of 13 patients in the hospital. We've had as high
as 20. We're down to 13 now.

GUTHRIE: Can I just ask then what kind of therapy, if any, you
use for these patients?

LIGHTBOURNE: Our main therapy is[robofare], the drug that...
And in recent months I'm using the drug with the use for epilepsy.

GUTHRIE: All right. I just wanted to know what you gave as a
way of therapy for the people. I think we're going to move along.
Thank you. We'll go to Diane Plumridge.

TESTIMONY OF
DIANE PLUMRIDGE
SOCIAL WORKER
PORTLAND, OREGON

PLUMRIDGE: I'm Diane Plumridge, and I'm a social worker with the
Genetics Clinic, which is one of the programs of the Crippled Children's
Division at the University of Oregon Health Sciences Center in Portland.
I think I'm the only Oregon representative here today, although I had
five or six calls earlier this week asking, "Are you going?" and I said,
"Yes, I am." Several people were hoping they would be here, but I said
I would be here anyway to bring a report back, and I will be glad to do
that.

Oregon has about 65 families known to have Huntington's disease.
In the past 10 years, our center, which is somewhat similar to the
center here at the University of Washington, has seen 35 affected
patients with Huntington's, 94 "children" who are at risk (these are
adults) and 51 children (grandchildren) who are primarly at this age
still in the teen-age range.

We see about 36 spouses, and I have done most of my work in counseling with the spouses of those who are affected and those who are at risk.

I didn't have a prepared statement, but after listening today and listening to the many problems that sound similar, we hear again and again, I was really beginning to share in the frustration even more than I do at home. I was trying to think of maybe one or two helpful questions I might ask to deal with, since we can't deal with all the problems— maybe one we could start with.

The 2 things I'm most familiar with, of course, are the financial problems and the ineffective community and social support systems, particularly in the early stages of the disease. The tender loving care, the community support, everybody should be available to make life as meaningful and the quality of life should be maintained as long as possible.

There are two groups of people who have received a great deal of publicity the past few years and have had a great deal of political clout and now have quite a bit of financing. One is the area of aging, and the other is the area of mental retardation. Now, I started asking myself the question, "What do we learn from these successful programs, what could be adapted from them which is appropriate for adults—not only adults with Huntington's disease, but any adult with a neurological disorder—that could be used to help maintain this quality of life as long as possible?" I thought Huntington's might be a model as a pilot program to work with.

I know that not only is home health care terribly expensive, it's not always appropriate; much of it means skilled nursing care, which is not the question that's being asked at the time. It's been more of a home aid, and yet, even if you have the finances, it's very hard to find the appropriate people to help. I'm wondering if you have any thought of a day care program or a care program that could be worked through one of the local structures that already exists, say it's through the Aging department or through the local university, if you have an Aging program here at the University of Washington. It could be coupled with there being supervision during the day while a spouse is working; there would be appropriate nutrition, medical management; at the same time, there should be occupational therapy, recreational therapy, sheltered workshop for a different job, if this is still available. Many people certainly can work for many years at a different job. It could also be a center for counseling, either one to one, or families could drop in; there should certainly be a social work component. I'd really like to ask the Commission if they've given any thought to this, and most important, any thought to the financing of something like this, which I feel would be economically more appropriate for many people.

GUTHRIE: We've had some testimony in other cities similar to this, and I'm sure that we are going to consider this as one of the important recommendations, the idea of a day care center for the chronically ill or disadvantaged. I think it is a very good suggestion. I don't think we've found out how yet to finance it or just how to do it, but we think it's a very important proposal.

PLUMRIDGE: You say Huntington's as possibly being a pilot program, or are you thinking of starting a very large program to start with?

GUTHRIE: I don't think we've decided yet. I think this is still being discussed.

ARONSON: In the State of Rhode Island, there is a pilot program using the elderly, who formerly required nursing homes. A day care center has been established with the very characteristics that you've described: counseling, recreational therapy, occupational therapy, efforts in the direction of education. Many of the so-called encour-ageable symptoms assignable to the [synesis], some have diminished in these individuals, but they're able to go back to their homes in the evening (typically their children's homes), and there's a much greater degree of compatability. So, we're hoping in Rhode Island and hopefully in the other 49 states that such a program can be extended to other areas, such as Huntington's disease.

PLUMRIDGE: Who funds this in Rhode Island? Is it a state-funded program?

ARONSON: It's some private funding and the Blue Cross-Blue Shield.

GUTHRIE: Thank you, Diane, and now we will listen to Stella Runnels.

TESTIMONY OF
STELLA RUNNELS
KINGSTON, WASHINGTON

My name is Stella Runnels. I'm "at risk." My father, John W. Connolly, died of Huntington's disease (actually of cerebral hemorrhage) complicated by pneumonia. I'm 27 years old and have one living sister who is 30.

The first incidence I can really remember is when I was 7 years old. My father was hitting my mother with a fry-ing pan. My sister and I came out of our bedroom and jumped on Dad's back. He stopped hitting her and turned on us. That was the first time we "almost" left him. My father was 37 years old at that time. Those incidences of violence became more and more frequent as time went on. We related them to Dad having a drinking problem to just being a mean son-of-a-bitch.

We lived on an island in the Aleutians, Adak. There wasn't an awful lot of medical care available up there, but there were doctors. Dad had also been dehydrated so badly during the war that he almost didn't live through it. He had two-thirds of his stomach removed about 1962.

My mother, sister and myself finally left Adak without Dad in 1963. We came down to the Bremerton area, stayed 2 weeks, and then went back up there. There were a lot of promises which were not kept: the same physical abuse and Dad saying, "I don't remember what I did to you guys."

My sister left and got married in 1964, an escape marriage, and was in the States. She had always been affected more nervously than I had been, because I feel that everyone always said she was the spitting image of her father. Dad lost a promotion, and then experienced what they have called a breakdown in 1965. I don't know what actually happened to him, as my mother tends to forget the bad things, and won't tell us, or even acts like they didn't happen. He was sent to Elemendorf Air Force Hospital, then to Oak Knoll Navy Hospital, and kept there until May of that year. We left Alaska in June and moved to the Poulsbo area. Mom went down to Oak Knoll Navy Hospital and picked Dad up and brought him home.

He was given outpatient care at Bremerton Naval Hospital which consisted of Thorazine and other medications. Every 6 months he went back for "check-ups" which amounted to a quick talk with a psychiatrist and small physical exam, and then home again. He deteriorated rapidly in the first year and then seemed to slow down for about a year.

I married at 17, another escape marriage, and went to Texas. My marriage lasted just over a year and then I came home.

By this time, my mother had quit working and was an accomplished alcoholic. I lived at home off and on, and the violence was picking up again, as if the medicine wasn't strong enough, although they had increased the dosage as time went on.

In 1968 my father had to be taken from the house by my brother-in-law, and taken to the Naval Hospital. Mom could not handle him in her state of drinking and could not stop the drinking. He was committed that year to Western Washington State Hospital until there was a vacancy at American Lake Veterans'

Hospital. At Western Washington he was kept on a locked ward
with no thought of treatment or any study to diagnose the disease either. He became completely dehydrated due to what I
feel was lack of proper care and was kept in a ward until he
was able to get into the VA Hospital.

He was on several wards at the VA Hospital, most of them
locked wards with signs such as, "Keep door closed until
patient Connolly is restrained." Every once in a while we
would get there to see him and he would be on an open ward
with ground privileges and we would visit out by the lake
which he seemed to enjoy. He was brought home several times,
always to a similar routine of him deteriorating more and Mom
also.

I remarried in 1970 and in 1971 was going to Germany with
my husband, who was in the service. We went to see Dad for
my last visit before I went and he was allowed out of the
ward. The doctors were talking to Mom about taking Dad home
again and Mom couldn't really handle it with her drinking and
inability to cope with the reality of the situation. I told
them they couldn't legally or morally make her bring him home
again. Dad came out to the car with us after we had asked
them to keep him in until we had left, because he had started
getting mean and hard to handle. I ended up locking Mom in
the car and my last words to my father while he was alive were,
"I hate you."

That was September of 1971; Dad died in 1972 in July.
Apparently they had told Mom shortly before he had died that
they wanted to start studying Dad to see if they could find
out just what he had. We had been told Parkinson's, Pick's,
and just manic-depressant, to name a few up to that point.
My mother, sister, and I all remember different conversations
with different diseases. Well, their studies were not conclusive as far as Mom told us.

My sister had left her husband at the time of the funeral
and stayed in the States without her two children. She
remarried about a year later.

Mom was still at home drinking. I came home from Europe
in September of 1972 and Mom was so sick that she was admitted
into the hospital right after I came home with cirrhosis of
the liver. My marriage never really got off the ground, but
I left and lived in Lake Tahoe, Nevada with my husband and
got a tubal ligation there, which I had tried to do since 1970.
I had had an abortion in Germany. We came back to Washington
in October of 1973, and Mom had to go back into the hospital
again; this time it turned out she was diabetic.

My sister and her new husband decided that they wanted to have a child. I contacted the University of Washington's Genetic Clinic, and found out if they could try to diagnose Dad's illness properly. We went over there after they researched the autopsy findings, etc. and were told that Dad definitely died of Huntington's disease.

What are the special problems and recommendations associated with being "at risk" for HD?

Being at risk is never knowing. Even though I'm statistically young, when I get nervous about anything, or uptight, the tendency to think that it is HD is awfully strong. I've had therapy off and on for the last 6 years, but have never found anyone that could deal with me on the level of being at risk. It was good therapy as far as helping me get enough guts to face the future to the degree that I'm going to school now to become a medical assistant instead of just having the attitude that I'm going to get HD in a few years, so why even bother. But it hasn't helped me face HD any better, except my old standby, just ignore it until I get upset and then freak out.

I don't think I could ever emphasize the importance of some form of therapy to be made available to cover these particular areas.

What are the problems and needs associated with the period after onset of symptoms prior to diagnosis?

Since we lived on the Aleutian Island of Adak, there wasn't a lot of medical care available. The basic point to help other people with, is if someone in their family experiences extreme emotional changes, don't be afraid to find out what it is that is causing it, but to seek help. I'm sure that a lot of the reason why Dad did not seek out help was because of the fear of mental disease and the lack of emotional help from my mother and us kids also.

What are the problems and needs associated with the period during and after diagnosis?

Better treatment and emotional support is needed after a person is diagnosed, if they are properly diagnosed, and treatment besides medication is needed.

What are the problems and needs associated with the period after which the patient can remain at home but needs increasing support?

Families need to be given extensive therapy during the home care to better understand the phases of HD and not to resent the symptoms. I've since met people who knew their patient had HD quite early in the disease. Their whole outlook about the disease and life in general is so totally different than mine has been for so long, with the misdiagnosis and the nondiagnosis for such a period. Early detection of the disease seems like it can make all the difference in the world.

To experience your family and friends turning away, seeing your father deteriorate without an understanding of why, or even with an understanding, but no aid to help you cope is a very hard thing.

Very few people seemed to visit their family in Western Washington or American Lake. Getting adequate care is a problem that is closer to me now that time is going on. If you are service connected, it is easier to get into places, but it doesn't affect the care you receive. We just would visit Dad and then go home and "not think of him until we saw him next" type of attitude, or at least attempted to do that. I was gone when he died but was glad when he did.

We received medical care for Dad from the service, as he was retired Navy. It never was the best, but it kept the bills down for my mother. We never received a diagnosis until after he was dead 2 years, and then only because the University of Washington's Genetics Clinic was available to us. After we contacted the University, we were given accurate information on the disease and inheritance pattern. We were told that we could contact them, Amelia Schultz, and receive answers to any questions that we might have and also get our neurological examinations there. I wish to utilize this help more often, but have put it off as that is the way that I tend to deal with the problem: ignore it.

Dad was covered under military coverage that paid for the care. But his life insurance policies were changed after he became ill.

I have had an impossible time up to this point in getting health insurance. I had a blood disease as a child that is held against me also, and have not worked in the kinds of places where policies have been available, even if they were affordable to me.

There was so much that I wanted to state, but my mind is in a jumble getting this out. Since receiving the information that there was going to be a Commission, I have tried to sit down and get my thoughts together on all of this, with little success. It always seems that to ask for some kind of emotional support when so many other families are still with their affected person, and we are not, is selfish. But I want help to understand and to cope without messing up my life any more than it is. Someone to be able to reassure me that it's okay to get hazy-headed occasionally and to forget what you went to the cupboard for, without thinking HD.

GUTHRIE: I always feel, and you're bringing out a very important point, sometimes the unknown is so much worse to deal with than the known, no matter how bad it may seem. I felt that way, too. I really did.

ARONSON: I'm not sure if I heard you correctly. Were you suggesting that at one point a physician or a representative of the hospital withheld diagnostic information from the family?

RUNNELS: I made the statement that they started to view my dad about 2 months before he died, study him, to try to diagnose him, and then while--apparently, it wasn't conclusive, what the findings--he died 2 months later, and they weren't sure. But in the autopsy report, the University of Washington could tell what it was. I don't know whether my mother knew and didn't tell us; I don't know because she hasn't handled it very well.

ARONSON: There was a suggestion earlier today where an individual signified that her husband, from whom she had been divorced, had likely had Huntington's disease; but she had great difficulty obtaining the information because, as she stated, the physician was obviously reluctant to share with her because of the principle of patient confidentiality.

I would respectfully point out that that is only one of many principles of medical canon, and there are much more abiding principles; namely, that if another individual is at risk, you indeed do share that information. If you knew a person had tuberculosis, you have a moral responsibility to make sure that all the contacts are warned about this likelihood. Similarly, with genetically transmitted diseases, a registered physician has a responsibility to convey that information either to the person, assuming they're responsible to hear the information, or the surrogate of such individual. But somebody should be informed.

RUNNELS: Well, my mother told me last night something I wasn't aware of. She said that the hospital had told her it was Pick's disease, they thought. But, she told me that last night, so I don't know.

ARONSON: Well, I mean I'm not going to dispute what may be a very legitimate difference in diagnostic preception. I mean both the diseases that you mentioned involve changes in mentation, etc., so it's a possibility.

GUTHRIE: Thank you. We're next going to ask June Kingston, Donna Hyatt, and Lynn Huffman.

TESTIMONY OF
JUNE KINGSTON
ELLENSBURG, WASHINGTON

KINGSTON: I'm June Kingston. I'm from Ellensburg, Washington,
and I am at risk. My family has a considerable percentage of Huntington's, my mother's side of the family. She is still living in a rest
home here in the Kirkland area. She's been there since 1958. She's
the only one left in her family that still is alive. The rest have lived
to be 55, 65, but not her age; she is now 76.

I was just thinking, in the testimony that was given here about the
different services for senior citizens, maybe one of the tragedies of
Huntington's is no one gets to a Medicare age with this disease, or not
very many. They don't fit the criteria of anything, and I was reliving
the first experience of my family.

Living with this Huntington's disease is like the proverbial skeleton in the closet; everybody really slams the door in a hurry, and is
intimidated by the fact that they have this peculiarity in the family
that no one wants to talk about or to share or see.   I went to see my
grandmother, the first time I had seen her in years, and she was in the
Nebraska State Insane Asylum in 1939 or 1940. I was very young, and
it made a devastating impression on me although I couldn't understand
what in the world I thought. I thought I understood insanity, and yet
when I left, the last thing the psychiatrist said to us was, "But she is
not insane." I stood inside with my insides screaming," For God's sake,
why is she locked up in this place if she's not insane,"because she was
so happy to see us. The family seemed to mean so much to her, and there
was such an inadequate feeling when you left--if she wasn't insane, she
shouldn't be there, if she wasn't a criminal, but we weren't about to
take her home with us because she was a threat to us when she had her
temper tantrums.

So I don't think times have changed an awful lot, except that
people are not hiding it as much from the younger generation. Because
in our family it comes in the later years, around 45 or 50,
and by that time, the grandchildren are already there, the generation
is moving into a new life and moving away from each other, and we don't
see this disease as it progresses in the rest of the family.

In my instance, I was intimidated by this Huntington's to put up
with a bad marriage for quite a few years. I had all of the symptoms.
I was depressed; I was furious; I was violent, I suppose, because I was
having tantrums. I was falling; I was dropping things and cutting
myself and burning myself. I had all the symptoms except one--I felt
like all right, if this is it, I want to die. If I can't diagnose it,
if I don't know I really have Huntington's, what's going to happen now?

I want to know. I still couldn't get any answers, which is really
frustrating when you think maybe you have it. People say, "You're just
like your mother. You make the same gestures; you are just as ornery
as your mother was." With these kinds of things, you begin to believe it
yourself and wonder if you really are affected.

If there's anything else that I have as a message for everyone, it's
to make sure of what's frustrating you, make sure of what is intimidating
you before you determine that your life is ended, because I finally made one
decision that was right. I did decide to leave a bad marriage, and I
went over to the other side of the mountains. I found out I needed
glasses. I quit burning myself, and I quit falling, and I wasn't nearly
as frustrated. I made a few decisions right, and I felt like a new
person. I haven't been all that bad off, but if I had stayed in that
circumstance, I would have committed suicide, or I would have given up
and wasted the next 10 years. I hope I have 10 years yet. I'm still
not sure whether I have it. I wiggle my toes when I knit, and I play
with my dentures, and I do a lot of other peculiar gestures, but I'm not
sure. I think I have accomplished an awful lot in the last 2 years, and
if the next 2 years are as profitable, I will not have wasted any time
waiting for the Huntington's to get me.

I may be a fatalist in some respects, but I feel like the day when
my family sees me getting to the point where I can't handle it, there
are some of them who are willing to step forward and lovingly say, "This
is something that we'll help you with", not say, "You're just like your
mother, and we're going to go lock you up." I believe those were the
primary things.

I was hoping for funds for the study of the diagnosis because I do
feel this is very important.

Amelia has been a lifeline for me, and she has been a good friend
besides assisting me through some of the Huntington problems to sort out
what things really were Huntington's, and what were my problems.

Dr. Bird also was very helpful and very good to me. In thinking of
the testimony here, whether you should tell your children, whether you
should tell the patient, all these things are very individual, and I
feel like if I had known a few years before, I may not have handled it
as well because I hadn't been driven to the point of going to somebody
else and saying, "Look, I have this skeleton in my closet, and I don't
know how to live with it."

GUTHRIE: Thank you. Another very moving story for me because I am
meeting people all over the country, and you remind me again of the
people who think they have it, and then don't have it, and take on the
symptoms who don't really have the disease. Apparently, there is a
population among us that takes on the mannerisms without really a diagnosis. It's important to have this documentation from you. Thank you.
Donna.

TESTIMONY OF
DONNA HYATT
MOUNT VERNON, WASHINGTON

HYATT: My name is Donna Hyatt. I'm from Mount Vernon. My little
girl has Huntington's. She's 9 now. She was diagnosed 2 years ago.
Her problems first appeared when she was about 6, but the doctors assumed
it was something else. She was premature. They thought maybe she had
some brain damage. I was living on the other side of the state when she
first had a little bit of trouble. Coordination was the first thing.
It was a year and a half before we got the diagnosis here at Children's
Orthopedic, but meanwhile her father and I were divorced.

She's 9 now. It's been 2 years. There's been quite a little bit
of change. She attends public schools. She has speech problems primarily. She has a great difficulty communicating verbally. What I would
like to see more than anything else is information for her teachers
because they have never, never dealt with a Huntington's child before,
and they don't know how to deal with her. They don't know what to ask
of her; they don't know what her capabilities are; and they're almost
a little afraid of her because she's emotionally unstable. She seems
probably more about 7 years than 9. She's very capable of learning,
but her teachers don't know how much they should try to teach her.

I've asked her doctors to help them, and the only help they've been
able to give me so far is to ask the school to give her aptitude and
intelligence tests. That's really not enough, I don't think. She's
had those before. It tells them at what point she is at the present,
but the teachers don't know how far to push her. I don't know what to
tell them. I think that if they could get some information from other
teachers who have dealt with Huntington's, it would maybe more than
anything else reassure them.

GUTHRIE: I can only say that this is something that we are going
to have to talk about and work on. I don't think we have the information. I think this is something that in a sense we don't really have,
and education to teachers would be vital.

I did visit the school for special children here in the Washington
University med school and saw children with other disorders, handicaps
of various kinds, and people are just beginning to understand those
handicaps, let alone something like Huntington's. I would say that's
brand new. We know of children now, but we don't know very much about
what we can do for them. I think that your testimony today again is
going to remind us that this is something we must start looking into
and perhaps begin to find some answers for you. I don't think we have
them. Lynn.

TESTIMONY OF
LYNN HUFFMAN
MISSOULA, MONTANA

HUFFMAN: My name is Lynn Huffman. I'm from Missoula, Montana. I drove all night to get here. As I drove, I tried to think of what I was going to say when I got here. The overwhelming feeling that I had then and that I have now is that I don't know what I'm going to say because there is so much that I don't know.

Montana is a very big state. There aren't very many people who live in Montana, and Huntington's is extremely rare. You heard Mrs. Guthrie tease me about my lunch over there, and it was brought here today by a lady who is my aunt, that I haven't seen for 20 years. That's symptomatic of my family. They to this day treat one another as lepers, a very disarming situation for the younger people in the family who don't understand what's going on. I couldn't understand why things as simple as greetings in my family seemed to be very difficult.

I guess I'm what's called an at-risk patient like many of you people are. My mother has Huntington's. She lives in Billings, Montana. Her mother was 41 years when she died of Huntington's. They didn't know what it was 40 years ago in a small farming town in Idaho, and they put her in an asylum and gave her shock treatments. My mother feels that those shock treatments are probably what killed her, and not the Huntington's. My grandmother, as I just said, died before I was ever born. She claimed that she never knew her father, and my mother received some very old letters in the mail which indicated that not only did she know her father very well, but that he committed suicide as did several of my grandmother's brothers and sisters. You see, she claimed to not have known her father to her children so that she didn't have to discuss it with them. She knew that she had the same affliction when it probably as near as I can tell, she probably had Huntington's, she got it when she was about 35. She lived for another 5 or 6 years after they put her in the asylum.

It's astounding to me to be in a room with this many people who even know what Huntington's disease is. I've met so few doctors. They would say, oh, yes, Huntington's, and run to a shelf for a book, and come back and read me the medical definition of the disease but never having really seen it. I have only met about three or four doctors in Montana who have ever treated anyone with Huntington's.

They are "treating" my mother right now. They give her Valium. Now I don't know one treatment from the other, but I know that is the extent to which they have been able to help her. She was diagnosed with Huntington's about 3 years ago, 4 years ago now I guess, and that's the only thing that's been done for her. There are no social services of any kind that are available. She, of course, has not been able to work for the last few years and lives totally on her Social Security benefit.

I can't really discuss her financial needs with you because she won't discuss them with me. She's much too proud to ever tell me that she needs anything, which is typical of her side of the family. On her side, there are six children. The lady who brought my lunch was my mother's brother's wife. He disappeared a few years ago and has never been heard from since. My aunt, my mother's sister, has Huntington's, has had it now for almost 15 years, and I was never allowed to see her until I was 28 years old and had to fly to Boise, Idaho for a meeting and threatened my aunt at gunpoint to take me out to the house so that I could see my Aunt Irene, whom I hadn't seen for many, many years, the first person that I had ever seen who had had Huntington's for an extended period of time--it was a shock to say the very least. Her mind was intact; she still had that sparkle in her eye.

My mother is doing very well, as far as I can see. The generation before that, there were seven children, and four of those died of Huntington's; I think two died of the disease, and two of suicide. My mother has three boys, myself and my two brothers; and I'm almost 30 now, and haven't contracted the disease yet and am very hopeful that I won't. My mother said to me on the phone last night when I told her that I was coming here to testify that she can look at a person and tell whether or not they have the disease. She said there is a look in their face and in their eyes that tells her, that she can see it. She very seldom will discuss the disease with any of us, any of her children, only if we bring her an article or try to get her to go to another doctor.

She sees one doctor, who doesn't know anything about Huntington's, and we've tried to send her to the finest medical clinics in this country; she won't go. That, I guess, is really what I have to say, that there's so much about the disease that my family didn't know, and the reactions that they had because of that ignorance were very stifling. The reactions that I have because of Huntington's are extremely stifling, too. I thank you for this opportunity to testify.

GUTHRIE: Lynn, it was wonderful of you to drive all that way, and I just want to ask you something. Where are your other two brothers now?

HUFFMAN: They are both still in Montana. One is 3 years younger than I, and one is 11 years younger than I. The youngest attends the University, and the other is a carpenter.

GUTHRIE: Living at home?

HUFFMAN: The one who is a carpenter lives with my mother. He has just recently been having some kind of attacks, pulsations of the heart, feeling faint and dizzy. I don't know what that is. I don't know if it has anything to do with Huntington's, but he's been to several physicians and neurosurgeons and so forth in Billings, none of whom can diagnose it; it's just been within the last 6 months.

GUTHRIE: I just wondered, have you boys amongst yourselves ever discussed your family problem?

HUFFMAN: No, and that's not because we don't want to discuss it; it's simply that we can't. I don't know how to explain it to you.

GUTHRIE: No, I understand, and that's why I'm suggesting that in a sense you're perpetuating what the past generations did, and maybe now that you know more, it would be appropriate to seek professional counseling where the whole family sits down with a professional person and has a chance to really talk things out.

HUFFMAN: From the articles that you sent me and the things that I have been able to read, I assume that what you're talking about, something like this would be the best course of action; and I can't find anybody in Montana who can offer the kind of assistance that you're talking about, that kind of a little genetic counseling.

GUTHRIE: Maybe we can establish some kind of outreach program, starting right here, and we'll talk about that as a possibility.

VOICE: How far are you from Spokane?

HUFFMAN: It takes about 3-½ hours from Missoula. I'm the closest to Spokane. My mother lives in Billings, which is another 4-hour drive.

VOICE: There are outreach clinics from Seattle, and Spokane is one of the places where there is a service.

GUTHRIE: This is the kind of thing that we should really try to establish, and there are other families other than yours that we know of who are in touch with the Committee to Combat Huntington's Disease. So it would be important that we try to get some of you together and-- I'm so sorry that you weren't here earlier today to see Mr. Thiessen, who's sitting in the back, with Huntington's, who gave us the most beautiful demonstration of how he's occupied himself.

He calls himself retired because he has Huntington's and he's having a ball with the miniature train which he presented to us on the screen. Mr. Thiessen, would you please just stand up so that Lynn could have a chance to go over and say hello to you. I want him to see another patient with Huntington's who's functioning, and is occupying his time in a positive, happy way. Lynn, after we're over, you may go over and speak to him.

HUFFMAN: Thank you. I will.

GUTHRIE: Thank you. There is one more who wishes to speak, and that is Kathy Bergeson, unless there is someone else who's not on our registry

here who would like to speak. Is there anyone else who would like to
say something, comments of any kind? Kathy. There is another one? Do
come forward and give us your name when you come forward.

TESTIMONY OF
KATHY BERGESON
STUDENT
CENTRAL WASHINGTON STATE COLLEGE

BERGESON: Well, I was really excited to find out that this Commission even existed. It was referred to me by a genetics professor at
Central Washington State College. I'm a student there. My father died
in 1966 at home. He was 45, and he died from HD, and he had been disabled for about 5 years, which, from listening to the rest of the people
today, seems to be a rather short period of time when I hear about these
15- and 20-year cases. His performance just became poorer and poorer
until he was laid off, and consultations with doctors just turned up
nothing. One doctor suggested that his deterioration in performance was
due to yellow fever during the war, and another one suggested it was due
to a concussion from an automobile accident 5 years earlier. Finally,
it was diagnosed by a neurologist as HD, and my father was not told.
He was only told that he was sick, and he would not be getting any better.
Finally, he saw a letter that had been written to my mother from his
sister that said, "Perhaps Virgil has what his father had," and he didn't
know a name for that. All he knew was that it was a terrible disease.

He immediately withdrew for a period of about 6 months, and just
really would sit around just staring blankly and wouldn't get dressed
or speak with his children and such. After that period of withdrawal,
he became really belligerent, and his coordination became poorer, and
he wasn't able to drive a car; and also there was danger when he would
smoke in bed and somehow these privileges had to be taken away from him;
and he became really, really belligerent during that time.

My brother and I were never told. We were just told that Daddy
was sick. This went on for years. It was something that we grew up
with--a sick daddy. The day he died, I heard the words Huntington's
chorea spoken over the telephone to the doctor, and that didn't really
mean anything to me in the fifth or sixth grade, but the words stuck with
me, and I didn't really find out about my personal involvement with HD
until my first year in college. I picked up a paperback book called The
Women in White. It was just a cheap paperback book, and in it was a
character who had Huntington's disease, a fictitious character, but I
just really delved into that book, and I discovered that it was a pretty
awful thing, and I also read of my 50-50 chance.

I became really paranoid at that time, and I was about to be
married, but I just kind of let everything go. I broke the engagement,

and I just started just being really paranoid about everything, not
caring about my studies and about real strong friendships. I was really
paranoid. I was a cheerleader at the time, and every time I couldn't
do a movement right, I just cringed. I was just very, very pessimistic
about this, and I looked around libraries for information, and on occasion I could find a paragraph. With school performance going down and
my performance on the job, it was just kind of an all-time null, and so
finally I just confessed all of this to my fiance, and he boosted my
spirits, and then my mother came onto the scene and decided this was
the time that I ought to know.

She explained, but by that time, I knew even more than she did, and
so I went ahead and was married. But even now there is something that's
really on my mind. My husband doesn't really realize the seriousness of
HD, and I'm here today to educate him to pass on materials; and the subject of having children, I feel guilty possibly of denying him children.
I feel that I could live with it, but I think that it's a decision that
will be put off until perhaps a test can be rendered to find out whether
or not I have the gene. I'll still by that time be maybe 30 or 35,
and we could still have a family.

Another thing that has spurred me on by finding out about this
national group is to get in touch with my father's side of the family,
all of whom I've never met, and they all live back east, but I think
that there are cousins that I don't even know of that perhaps do
or do not know about this, but I think everyone should know.

My mother's never really quite recovered. She took care of my
father at home all those years. When he found out that he was very
sick and getting worse, the one thing that he said to here, the only discussion between the two of them was, "Eileen, please don't send me away
to a home." That's all he said, and she promised she wouldn't, and
she didn't. But she's never quite recovered from the strain of trying
to raise two children and take care of a severe case of HD.

My brother is 26 now, and he won't really think about it
or talk about it. He's still single, but I also want to get him involved.
I think it's so important to talk about it. Sometimes, when I talk about
it for a long time, and then for periods of months, I'll get kind of
paranoid. So then I'll need just some reassurance that I really
shouldn't worry about that right now because you can't worry about
something you can't do anything about anyhow. When I get paranoid
about temper flares, or poor job performance or school performance,
then I should just search and see what the real reason is--maybe it's
just that I'm overworking myself or I'm not getting enough sleep. Mr.
Thiessen was just really, it was just so great to see him, so unlike
my father, who was kept right in the house, and didn't have any outside
interests and that has just really given me inspiration that if I do
contract this disease, there will be something I can do to fill up
those years. Thank you.

TESTIMONY OF
RANDY KARSTETTER
SEATTLE, WASHINGTON

KARSTETTER: I want to take this opportunity to thank you for this opportunity to speak. My name is Randy Karstetter; I am 25 years old, and will be 26 next week. I'm a medical technologist. I work in the laboratory at the Swedish Hospital here in Seattle. I am genetically at risk for Huntington's. My father now is in the VA hospital in Waco, Texas. He is in the later stages of the disease, and he has been diagnosed as having the disease for the last 15 or 16 years.

In our situation, my father knew his mother had the disease. He watched her slowly die from the disease. When he married, they knew that there was a possibility of passing it on in the gene. But at the time, one of my folks' close personal friends was a physician and his wife; and through a great deal of counseling (even though not much was known of the disease), it was decided that they would have children. So, I was born, and my sister, who is almost 2 years younger than I, was born. I was also not told of having the disease or even having the possibility of the disease or my father even having the disease until I was 16. I'd like to reiterate for all those people who said that before, that it is a very hard blow to find out later on in life that your father is dying of a disease when you thought that he was just uncoordinated. That is a very hard way to accept it. As it turned out, he was very productive. He progressed rather slowly, and it was only until the last 5 years or so he retired. We were originally in Alaska, and they moved to Texas, where our relatives are located. It was in the last year, year and a half that he has become institutionalized, with my mother taking care of him until that time.

Something I find amazing is that until this day I have never seen another patient with Huntington's disease; and I have not been around anyone who has even known much of the disease, and I find it difficult talking to anyone. Even being in the medical field, little is known, and it is difficult to discuss it. It's something kind of funny, that I went to Central Western State College, and I may know who you've been talking about. Very little is known to communicate with other people, but it's also difficult meeting other people with the disease, or even at risk. I've really been amazed at the people who testified here today to know that a lot of things that they're experiencing, I'm experiencing also, especially the young man back there who is married and going through the agonizing decisions. I am to be married next month, and I can identify the same decisions with him. I'd like to say that I'm really happy that this day has occurred, and that I hope that this happens much more and that much comes of it.

I'd like to take issue with Dr. Swanson, I think it was, when he said that money doesn't accomplish everything. I'd like to say that

it's my personal opinion, from what little I know, that the technology
does exist; that we could find a diagnostic tool; if not, a maintenance
program, if the funding were there. I think that it is truly amazing
to see what funding does, and I think that from the progress that they've
made so far, from the progress they've made in other diseases that are
very similar to this disease, I think that it will not be that long
if the funding is there.

    So I hope that the funding will be there for research, and most
importantly, the funding will be there for the maintenance of those
people who have it at this time. I hope that, as Mrs. Guthrie says,
that we will all become more aware of each other now and support legislation and funding for this.

    GUTHRIE: Let me just say to all of you how pleased we are that we
could, and I say "we" meaning I am a member of a family, as you know.
It is helpful to share. It is helpful to share our sorrow and our
anguish and our fears. It's equally important that we learn from each
other and share the hopes and the possibilities of what good research
will or will not do. I'm just thinking as you spoke, when I started in
1967 there were 12 genetic disorders that could be diagnosed by examining
the fluid around the fetus in the mother through amniocentesis. Today,
there are 80. Huntington's is not one of these, but from 12 to 80 in 9
years, to me, is progress; and if we can support, I want to say not just
research, I want to say meritorious research, because it isn't a question
of just raising the money and spending it in the way that's going to
bring hopeful results. So we must be very careful to say meritorious,
and I know that you're shaking your heads, that you agree with me.

    I do know that this community has an opportunity to do its share.
From the meetings last night and today, I know that there are people
here in this community, first, who are very concerned and active from
that scientific research point of view, from the social management point
of view. Some of you have commented so beautifully on what's going on
at the University of Washington in the Medical Genetics Program. It
came about and it happened because a few people cared, and those people
have stuck with it.

    I've known Amelia for a long, long time. Those of you who men-
tioned her name know what a supportive person she's been. For those of
you who don't know Amelia, there are other Amelias in your city. If
you will help them to understand who you are, and join with us and
work with us and participate and let Amelia help you, it goes on like
a river. It flows, and it gets stronger and stronger as more people
put into the river what they have to offer. For the people 100 years
ago were hiding because they didn't know what to do; we are in a way
paying the price today, and I sometimes have to say to myself and to
you, in a sense, our young people of today are in some ways suffering

what people long ago didn't suffer, because they know. Knowledge isn't
always helpful or hopeful when you first get started. But once you're
done, and we have, you can only point to the future and say to the future
generation, "It may have been tough for me to come here today and testify,
but I sure do feel good because I did it maybe 5 years ago or 10 years
ago," depending on when we get answers. You should really be proud that
you were part of doing something for the future generation that people
in the past could not do for us. Maybe it was because they weren't
ready. Maybe it's because science wasn't ready; but we are ready today,
and we are sharing hope; and I just want to thank you all for helping
me as well, and all of us who are sitting here are grateful for sharing
with you.

Please work with us; please participate; don't go home and say,
"Well, I'm glad they're doing something." That's not enough. You're not
going to be satisfied, and I know you're not. So take it upon yourselves
and say, "I can help, too." See Mrs. Denney and speak to her. She's
planning a statewide coalition for families with Huntington's disease,
and she wants your name if you haven't given it to her, and she wants
you to get involved in whatever level of interest you may have. Don't
just go home and say, "Thank goodness somebody else is doing it," because
it'll happen sooner and better if you participate.

That's all I wanted to say. Nancy, would you like to say something?

WEXLER: Well, why don't I share with you a sort of peculiar experience that I had the day before yesterday. I'll give you a little
background on this experience. About 9 years ago, when my mother was
diagnosed with HD, it was the first that I had ever heard about it,
much less learned about it in my family. I called the Genetics Clinic
where I was a graduate student in psychology. This clinic is actually
quite an excellent clinic so I'll let it go nameless for the time being,
but I spoke with someone on the telephone and said, "Hi, my mother has
HD, what can you tell me?" This voice came over the telephone, "Gee,"
she said, "I don't know. You have a 50-50 chance. There isn't any research going on anywhere in the world." I said, "My God," and luckily
for me, I knew that that wasn't so because my family had gotten in touch
immediately with Marjorie, and I knew in fact that there was just the
beginning of research that was going on in many places in the world.
Well, I had occasion to think of this experience the day before yesterday because a very superb investigator called me up from Duke, and he
said, "I have a difficult problem. I'm doing some tremendously exciting
research with Huntington's disease. I have something going, which to
me is revolutionary; it's very fragile; I can't publish it; but this
idea is so exciting that I'm afraid to put in the grant application
because I think they'll steal it." I thought, what a radical difference
in 9 years from saying that absolutely nothing was going on, to the
fact that now it's difficult to fund research because all these investigators are being so protective of their ideas; he said, "If anybody

finds this out, they're going to get a Nobel Prize on my idea, and I don't want that to happen. Can't you go out and can't you get somebody in some other discipline to please review this grant?"

I spent 2 hours on the telephone with him on this problem. It's getting to be more of a problem. I would rather we have these kinds of problems where we have to protect our researchers who are out there, than going with a pick and shovel to go and get somebody who will do the research.

I also agree with you. I think that research cannot buy cure. We don't know when the cure's going to come, and when the treatment's going to come, but what we can tell Congress for sure is that without money, there isn't going to be any treatment, and there isn't going to be any cure. So at least we have to give science a chance. That's really what this Commission is all about, that's what you are all about. I think this Commission is much more than nine Commissioners and staff. This Commission has to be every single individual who is involved with Huntington's disease in any way, shape or form. The real test of the Commission is going to be after September, because on August 31, we will deliver a massive report like that to the President of the Congress with very specific recommendations, and the only thing which is really going to insure that those recommendations get pushed through is if there is a firm, united constituency behind them.

If every Congressman knows that all of you out there are going to be calling daily and saying, "What's happening to that recommendation, what are you doing about this, what about the funding for the neurology institute, we're out here, we're looking, we're watching, and we're voting." Without you, our Commission is really going to have been for naught. We can do things, but we're only nine people or eleven people; but with all the Huntington families, for every one patient, you have a spouse and maybe two to four children at least, you have cousins, aunts, uncles, relatives, the grocers down the block, you have a tremendous constituency, and that's really what we're counting on. So you're going to hear from us through newsletters, telephone conversations, any way we can get hold of you. Come September, we're counting on you to be the Commission.

GUTHRIE: Before we adjourn, I want to make one announcement. On Sunday, May 15th, at 6:30 in the evening, there is going to be a 30-minute program devoted to Huntington's disease. It was partially filmed here today. Jim Harriet, on KIRO TV, Channel 7, is preparing that program. I think it would be very exciting if some of you could participate, and see that your friends and neighbors—if you don't ever talk about the Huntington's, at least let them listen to the program. So, I'll repeat it again that on Sunday, May 15th, at 6:30, it's called "Thirty Minutes" and precedes the program called "Sixty Minutes." I hope that you'll be listening. I hope that we'll hear from you.

WEXLER: Tonight, I think it's the 11:00 News, KSTW, Channel 11, 10:00 news on Channel 11.

GUTHRIE: If you can before you leave, do speak to Merle Denney. Stand up. This is the lady you speak to if you can in some way, shape, or form help us out in some organized fashion, and she's going to do this, and she'll help plan out the program. So thank you one and all. It's been a most moving experience, I know, for all of us.

Seattle, Washington   April 14, 1977

MARGUERITE BLUMHAGEN
WENATCHEE, WASHINGTON   MARCH 30, 1977

    I am writing as an interested mother (and wife--husband
deceased 1970 with Huntington's disease) of a living son,
aged 26, who has Huntington's disease.

    My age is 57 and I am a public school teacher. I have
three other living children who show no signs of the disease;
two are married. One has a child but will not have any more
because of the H.D. risk. The spouse of the other does not have
this feeling--but no children yet. The third son has a real
phobia of the disease, having no desire to marry or have children and finds it difficult to talk about it; but it has not
hindered his social life or occupation.

    My husband was a World War II veteran and eventually was
hospitalized in a V.A. Hospital. Under much stress we were
able to hospitalize him in a state mental hospital before space
was available in the V.A. Hospital--necessary because of my job
responsibility and raising of our four children. A very difficult time--had the assistance of relatives and a psychologist.
Could not get medical doctor assistance as to hospitalization
at that time.

    My son who now has the disease was diagnosed at the Uni-
versity of Washington Hospital at age 23--it was not confirmed--
though normal activities and jobs were becoming difficult for
him. It was confirmed at age 24. Since that time he has been
employed at the North Central Washington Supervised Skills Workshop. It has been a wonderful answer to the problem of keeping
him occupied with something besides T.V. We were able to get
Social Security aid as the dependent son of a veteran.

    His brothers are very good about helping with family out-
ings and such which keeps his mental outlook bright. He does
not have any other social life except at the workshop. It
would be extremely difficult without these two sources of concern and occupation.

    Our local neurosurgeon has not been a source of any help.
When I gave him the diagnosis from the University of Washington
Hospital, he said it was their opinion. So my confidence in him
is nil. My personal physician has not seen my son, but will help

when such is necessary. He has given me some counsel as to hospitalization in a local rest home when my son can no longer work at the workshop. As to how this will actually work out, 'tis hard to tell.

I took out a Family Plan Health Insurance with Sunset Life when the children were young, where at age 25 the children can take out their own insurance with no questions asked. My three sons have taken advantage of this.

We have had genetic counseling at the University of Washington Hospital Outpatient Clinic. I paid for this. One son and wife have not attended, but have received all the necessary information.

All in our family have a firm belief and trust in our Creator which holds us together. We were a missionary family before H.D. brought us back to America.

Seattle, Washington   April 14, 1977

CAROLEE J. BUCHER
ARLENE STROWN
SEATTLE, WASHINGTON   APRIL 22, 1977

    The questions you present are very complex and not
easily answered. The only way I can answer them is to express my feelings and the problems I have encountered. I must
simply relate them to you.

    My mother has H.D. She was diagnosed in 1968, but I
think, looking back, that she probably had the disease many
years before that. The neurologist that diagnosed my mother
had seen her for another problem two years before, but because
he was not asked for that particular information, he said or
did nothing even though he noted symptoms at that time.

    There is no family history of this disease. My mother
is an only child and as far as I know has no known living relatives. Her father and mother were first cousins, and she
was born late in life to them.

    But to the present--the neurologist that made the diag-
nosis did just that and nothing more. He simply said my
mother had a year, to a year and a half, to live. The only
other thing he said was that the disease was hereditary.

    Our family then attempted to cope with the situation.
She had been and continued to see a psychiatrist. He knew
nothing of how to cope with or treat H.D. and its related
problems. He only succeeded to confuse and complicate the
situation. My father then became involved with a religious
group of do-gooders. They put a guilt feeling in him, making
him feel as if he couldn't handle my mother's outbursts. They
said he wasn't trying hard enough. My mother is very hateful
and argumentative, making her difficult to live with.

    Only after a minor problem that put my father in the
hospital did we come in contact with a social worker, who then
put us in touch with the University of Washington and Dr.
Amelia Schultz. I had attempted to get information from the
University of Washington in 1968 but to no avail. Through
Dr. Schultz we were able to receive counseling and genetic

guidance. (My sister has two children.) Dr. Schultz also contacted a Dr. Johnson whose wife has H.D. Dr. Johnson has been a big help to my father. He could relate the total feeling of helplessness and frustration.

I think there needs to be more closeness within and openness between H.D. families, so that we can talk out our problems and find ways to cope with them. I felt as though our family was the only one in the world with such monumental problems that only H.D. can bring. Friends and relatives just don't understand and don't seem to want to know. They seem afraid. Just sweep it under the carpet, don't care, and maybe it will go away. They are revolted by my mother's actions and tantrums.

As far as my own feelings and frustration are concerned, when I first learned of H.D., I consulted the University of Washington library for any books or pamphlets. When I wrote for more information none ever came. I felt as though no one felt H.D. was a very important disease, but that if it were heart disease or cancer, all sorts of support and information would be there for the family.

Because of my mother's hatefulness and bitterness towards me, I had a difficult adjustment period. Finally I realized I was expending a lot of energy on a problem I could not con-trol or change. Then I realized that I found I could cope and be around my mother and be supportive of my father.

I did much research into obtaining disability Social Security for my mother and found she could not receive it as she was short one quarter of work. But how could she work? She was having trouble with coordination and her thinking pattern was not functioning normally. But if my father would leave her or divorce her, she could get it in a moment. I don't have an exact dollar amount, but my father has spent thousands of dollars trying to find some answers and the ability to cope. The medications my mother is presently taking are not very effective, but they are expensive.

My father has suffered most:

1. Because of the religious group he feels guilty and
    must keep her at home regardless of how bad it gets.

2. Because of the isolation and inability of friends
    and relatives to understand.

I think it all comes down to informing the public--all
the public. H.D. families must be made to feel they are not
alone or freaks.

I could go on for several pages more in trying to answer
all the questions or presenting the many problems we have had
and continue to have. Nursing homes inability to take H.D.
patients, because they are management problems. The home
therefore "jacks" the prices way up. I wish I had more constructive answers for the multifaceted problems H.D. presents.

Thank you for allowing me to write how I feel and the
problems my family has encountered.

Seattle, Washington   April 14, 1977

MRS. NORMAN BUCKNER
PORTLAND, OREGON   MARCH 20, 1977

    We recently learned that our son's wife, Jerrie Ann
Buckner, of Alameda, California, is afflicted with Huntington's chorea. We, nor our family or friends, had ever heard
of it, much less realizing the awful consequences of it. She
is only 38 years old and the mother of three sons, ages 15,
13, and 7. We are trying to gather information about this
disease, but there is very little written even in doctors'
textbooks. So little is apparently known about this debilitating illness.

    We urge your Commission to make every effort to promote
any program of research to diagnose and treat H.D. There is
need for family counseling, therapy, and some sort of financial insurance, because we can already see that phase is becoming enormous. Mostly, we need more education to be able to
cope a little better with this frightening malady.

Seattle, Washington   April 14, 1977

SHIRLEY R. COOK
STARBUCK, WASHINGTON   SEPTEMBER 16, 1976

        I am sending my testimony on Huntington's disease because
I would like it read at the public hearing in Atlanta on October
21, 1976.

        I am sending it to the South because I was born there and
raised there half of my life, and Huntington's disease started
in my family from there.

        My mother's mother had it and passed away when my mother
was four years old. My grandmother left behind two boys and
three girls. These kids grew up not really knowing what their
mother had died from. Meanwhile, Lizza, the oldest with two
girls, had Huntington's and then each of the others started
getting it, except for one boy, who never showed any signs of
the disease.

        Each one of these children had children that had to be
raised by the other spouse but my mother and my one uncle.

        My mother had it and it progressed slowly on her, until
the last two years and she really went downhill fast. My
father passed away four years ago and Mom has lived in my home
up to last week. One week ago I had to put her in a rest home
or nursing home.

        As to what Huntington's does to your family, let me explain
what I have had to watch all my life.

        When I was a very young girl, Aunt Lizza was taken and
put in a State Hospital. Her girls came to stay with us
a while, and I didn't pay much attention to it at that time
except when we went to visit their mother. She didn't act
the same and I didn't know why.

        Then an uncle started acting funny. He was hard to get
along with. He started shaking and started treating us kids
like he didn't like us anymore. Then he was also put in a
State Hospital.

        Then my parents came to California due to my father's
health. My favorite aunt came to see us five years later and
I couldn't believe my eyes. She shook like the rest of them.

She couldn't hardly walk although she still showed love for us, and she wasn't belligerent. She went back home and it wasn't long until we got a letter that she had also been put into a State Hospital. I cried many nights after us kids went to bed. I also wondered many nights why they all had to be that way, but no one had the answer.

As time went by, I got older and married and divorced right away. But meanwhile I had a daughter. So I took her and myself and went home to Georgia and then went to visit my people; and what I found made my blood run cold. My favorite aunt was all twisted up, her arms and legs. She was so skinny; her eyes were sunk back in her head; and she couldn't even lift her own head. She could not smoke a cigarette or drink coffee. I held cigarettes for her and fed her coffee all the time. I was there, and the nurse informed me they didn't have time to do things like that. They said there were too many patients and not enough help. They said that they couldn't get her to eat and they didn't have time to force her. My favorite aunt did smile though, and that's more than my uncle and other aunt did. When I got to where they were, they were getting the same treatment. These places did not even have time to tie these people in wheelchairs so they could be up for awhile. They didn't have enough help to even feed them. They didn't even have equipment enough to give them the exercise they needed.

I really cried after that and had very bad dreams. I still have these same very bad dreams today. Anyway, I came back home. My mother was starting to yell a lot and she slowly started showing the same things. My father got to where he was very nervous, but he stuck it out and didn't put her in a rest home.

I got married again and my father started making sure he and Mom were very close to us all the time. Mom got worse and worse, so the doctor suggested we put her in the Presbyterian Medical Center in San Francisco. They ran tests on her for two weeks and then called my father and all the kids in for a conference. The doctor then explained all about Huntington's disease to us. He said we should not have kids, but by then it was too late; there are six grandchildren.

Dad got even closer to us, and we watched Mom get a little worse each year.

But the last four years have been the worst. Someone had
to be with her all the time so if my husband and I went somewhere, the girls stayed with her, or we stayed and they went.
We very seldom ever got to go anywhere as a family.

We couldn't go to ball games or sports with our kids, and
when we went to stores, someone had to stay in the car with Mom.
I would take one girl in at a time to get their school clothes.

My girls are teenagers now; I know they feel the same fear
I used to feel when I saw my relatives. They ask questions
all the time--questions I can't answer because I know of no
answer. The oldest one is engaged, and sometimes I find her
saying that she doesn't want to get married and put the husband
through hell. She loves kids, and she can't make up her mind
as to what to do about it. I am of no help, because I can't
make that decision for her.

I love my daughters but I wish to God I had known about
Huntington's disease years ago so I could have had the decision
to make for myself.

I also wish to God they could come up with something to
help the ones that are young, so they could have a bright future
to look forward to, instead of gloom and depression. I am
not very old--35--but I find myself thinking of what the heck
or why try? I find myself very depressed.

I also find that when I let myself get into these moods
that I take it out on my husband and the girls, which really
isn't fair. They have had enough to go through without me
adding to it.

I have even caught myself thinking that I should take my
car, my daughters, and Mom and go off into the hills around here;
but I am not really that weak, and I wouldn't do that.

I have only one brother that moved up here to Washington
about two months ago. He is already showing signs of the
disease. I keep hoping that a scientist will come up with
something that would help. But without the money from Congress
and donations from people who care, my family, my relatives
and other people with Huntington's will be as lost and helpless
and as confused as we were twenty years ago.

Please, won't someone help? Huntington's is worse than
cancer. With cancer you can live a short while and die. With

Seattle, Washington   April 14, 1977

Huntington's, you live longer! With fear and dread you become
helpless and a burden to yourself and to your family. You hate
what you are becoming! But you can't do anything about it.
You pray. Then all that's left is you thank God you have left
what little you do have.

I didn't want to put Mom in a nursing home, but that was
all that was left for me to do, and every time I have been in
there, they have had her tied down in a chair. I did not tie
her at home; she is not an animal.

But they said they are short handed and could not watch
her all the time. They do not have exercise machines for her
to use and they don't have room for her to walk in for exercise.
So I don't figure Mom will be on her feet long. She will become a victim like the rest of her sisters and brothers.

And we don't have the money to put her in a private place.
I wish to God I did. If I could, I would still have her at
home. I also hope the man-made gene will work because that
may open the doors to some of the younger people, and who
knows? Maybe some of the older ones that have already given
up.

The Government helped put a man on the moon. I am now
hoping that they will help the men on earth to look at the
moon. There are more of us on this earth with Huntington's
than they really know of, and a lot of them can't even write
a letter to be read. A lot of them died without even knowing
what they had. A lot of them won't even face what they know
is true.

So I hope my letter will help--not just for my family but
for all the others. I only have one other small thing to speak
about. My mother has a welfare medical card that had to be paid
for each month, which was okay. My only gripe is that they
will pay to keep her in a nursing home, about $500.00 to $600.00
a month, but they won't give me money to take care of her, such
as getting help to watch her, or hospital beds or anything
like that at all.

We were talking of building on a big bedroom with a bathroom with a tub in the middle of the floor so we could get her
in and out, then having someone come in to help with her some,
but they wouldn't even help.

Seattle, Washington   April 14, 1977

     But they have their rules to go by. I just hope they
make the nursing homes and state hospitals more up-to-date,
with the extra help they need and equipment they need to help
these people.

     I hope you can read and understand this letter. I am
really not very good at writing my feelings down on paper. I
am not very good at telling them either.

     The real important thing is, I am not only asking for
help but I am begging for help from Congress.

     All of us need it in more ways than I can put on paper.
I would like to thank you for letting me be heard anyway.

     Thanks a million from all of us.

Seattle, Washington   April 14, 1977

HJORDIS DAHL
JENNIG TAYLOR
BOTHELL, WASHINGTON   MAY 20, 1977

        I am Hjordis Dahl, wife of Edwin H. Iverson. We were
married in 1938. He was 36 years of age. The first symptom
I noticed was eight years later, in 1946, which was the last
year he was able to work. Our son, Ed, Jr., was born in 1941.
He was now five years of age and to raise him and take care of
myself I had to go on Welfare. Mr. Iverson's condition became
steadily worse, to the point that he could hardly walk. He
had meningless motions of his hands, moving them constantly.
He became increasingly out of control and was admitted to Western State Hospital, a mental institution, in 1952. At this
time his illness was diagnosed as Huntington's disease by Dr.
Robert Brown. He was a patient from 1952 to 1956, becoming
practically a vegetable. He died on his birthday, July 8,
1956, at the age of 52 after an illness of ten years.

        My one and only child, a son, Ed, Jr., was born January
30, 1941. He was a brilliant student, had a college degree
in Engineering, and decided to change his course to medicine.
He entered Medical School in New Orleans in 1964. After three
years he was turned down by the Medical School for reentry in
1967. On returning home in 1967 he very definitely showed
signs of Huntington's disease. He inherited the disease from
his father. On August 8, 1972, at the age of 31 years, he took
his own life.

        I am Jennie Iverson Taylor, sister of Edwin H. Iverson.
He was the first male child born to our parents, Julian and
Christine Iverson. Two girls were born before him. My grandfather on my father's side had very bad coordination, was
erratic, and cruel. He had Huntington's disease. My father
had one sister and one brother. The sister had five children,
none of whom were afflicted with the disease. The brother, my
and Edwin H.'s Uncle Iver Iverson, had 12 children, eight of
whom grew to adulthood. Iver was quite elderly when he contracted the disease and died with it. Among the 12 children
one son, born in 1921, died with Huntington's disease at 49
years of age in 1970. He, like my grandfather, father, brother,
and nephew, had a complete change of personality, being irrational and cruel to their closest family members.

Seattle, Washington   April 14, 1977

        I and my brother, Edwin H., were two of eight children
born to our parents--four boys and four girls. Three, two
boys and one girl, died under six years of age, plus Edwin
H. That leaves one brother, 61, two sisters, 77 and 59, and
myself, 66 years of age. None of us are afflicted with the
disease. Of eight children, the first male, namely Edwin H.,
was the only one who inherited the disease, passing it on to
his son, Ed, Jr.

        I will close with the history of my father. His lack of
coordination, change of personality and cruelty to my mother,
was witnessed by me to the age of nine years.

        In closing I hope this information will be of some small
value in your untiring extensive research of Huntington's
disease.

Seattle, Washington   April 14, 1977

ELEANOR DUNCAN
SPOKANE, WASHINGTON   MARCH 3, 1977

RESPONSE TO REQUEST FOR INFORMATION

What are the problems and needs associated with the period
after onset of symptoms prior to diagnosis? Before he went to
nursing home, it was very hard on me and the children. He
would get violent sometimes.

What are the problems and needs associated with the period
during and after diagnosis? Can't find a doctor that knows how
to doctor him. Right now he is in the V.A. Hospital.

What are the problems and needs associated with the period
during which the patient can remain at home but needs increasing
support? Not at home now. Has been in nursing home for four and
one-half years. His condition has been critical three times. Is
in V.A. Hospital just wasting away. He is being fed by tube.
Nothing but skin and bones.

What are the problems and needs associated with the advanced
and terminal stages of the disease? It has been awful for the
children. Kids would tell them he was drunk, retarded. They
would come home crying. My youngest daughter said, "Mom, will
I get the disease?" Marvin would fall, breaking coffee table.
Fell getting out of bath tub. Cut a big gash on his head, had
to rush him to the hospital by ambulance. He fell many times
and has choked on food. Be hard for him to eat.

Your testimony should list the main problems you may have
encountered in the following areas:

I. Medical Care

Did you encounter problems in obtaining referral to a
specialist or medical center? Yes, never did find one.

Did you experience difficulties in obtaining a
correct diagnosis promptly? No.

Was the disease misdiagnosed? No.

Did you receive accurate information about the disease, the prognosis, treatment, inheritance pattern? No.

Did you receive continuing care under general medical supervision? No.

Did either your neurologist or family physician plan and arrange for appropriate care and services? No.

Did either try to explain the special problems and needs of Huntington's disease patients to nurses and other health professionals? No.

Did any single agency or person (e.g., medical social worker, nurse, family physician) take responsibility for arranging for you to get the necessary care and services? No.

II. Care Setting

Were public or private hospitals able and willing to provide suitable care and treatment? Don't understand the disease or what to do.

Were there difficulties in gaining entrance to nursing homes or other similar facilities? No.

In being able to remain? No.

For example, did the facilities attempt to discharge or refuse to allow the patient to remain? No.

What kinds of home health care were available? None.

What about homemaker services, respite care, home health aides? None.

III. Financial Services and Support

Have you been able to qualify for disability insurance under the Social Security Act? Yes.

Are the monthly payments adequate? Yes.

What difficulties have you encountered in being certified eligible for disability payments and in receiving them? What about Supplemental Security Income (S.S.I.)? No.

What about Medicare benefits available to disabled persons? Yes.

What about state vocational rehabilitation benefits? No.

What problems have you encountered in regard to eligibility under Medicaid programs? Getting Medicare, not Medicaid.

What kinds of costs and what portion of them are covered by Medicare or Medicaid payments? Doctors calls and tests.

Does your private or group health insurance plan pay any of the costs? Doesn't have any.

Have you experienced problems in regard to obtaining or continuing health or life insurance coverage? Haven't tried for insurance coverage.

What other financial problems have you encountered, such as a spouse or unaffected parent having to support a family? I don't get any help (financial).

IV. Genetic Counseling

What genetic counseling services have been available? How frequently have they been utilized? Who provided it? There isn't any counseling services.

VI. Psycho-social Problems

Have you been offered vocational rehabilitation, physical rehabilitation or occupational therapy services? No.

What are the problems and experiences associated with the impact of H.D. on the family; on marriage; on family planning; on adoption; on employment; on schooling; on personal and social development and relationships? I couldn't have friends come visit. Would make him nervous. He got where he hated the house we were buying. I couldn't go any place very long. I was seeing somebody. He was always wanting to move. The children and I were nervous wrecks. I had a small heart attack.

Have you received counseling services to aid in coping with the personal and family stresses associated with the disease? No.

Have you been referred for counseling? No.

What has been the impact of H.D. on emotional well-being? For example, has the disease resulted in family breakdown through separation, divorce or abandonment? Has it created problems of emotional disturbance, alcoholism, suicide, crime or delinquency, social ostracism? My son has H.D. also. This is the second time at Eastern State Hospital for setting fires. They don't know how to help him. He is not on any medication. He is 22 years old. He gets so withdrawn.

VI. Other

List any other problems you have experienced as a result of H.D. My husband had a daughter by a previous marriage that died at the age of 18. She also had the disease. His father died also with it. It has really been hard on me, and our two daughters, 18 - 19-1/2 years old, and son. Also his mother. I just hope and pray that the Commission will do all they can to help. Please use my name if you like. It is a terrible disease. Please keep in touch. Thank you.

Seattle, Washington   April 14, 1977

DEANNA GITCHEL
RENTON, WASHINGTON   MARCH 5, 1977

    I first contacted Merle Denny by going to her home in
Everett.

    I was having many problems trying to cope with Hunting-
ton's disease. My husband, Harry Kidder, Jr., had been
diagnosed at the University and was very bitter. He could
not cope with the fact of having Huntington's disease. He
was depressed and became very angry often.

    We had two children that bothered him. He could not
stand noise, crying, arguing and became very rough with them,
even breaking my son's finger and threatening to beat our
little girl beyond the point he already had if I did not leave
the room.

    Problems kept mounting and no one seemed to understand
my despair. Even now it's painful to have to remember all of
this and more.

    I was given Merle's phone and address and went to contact
her. She was very understanding and knew what I was talking
about. When times really got bad and my husband's flare-ups
began getting more frequent and more violent, I didn't know
who to turn to.

    One night Harry got so violent he literally tore the house
apart, throwing chairs, breaking dishes, pulling out drawers
and hitting me. I tried to get help. I called the police,
the county sheriff, the Crisis Clinic. No one would get involved in what they thought was a domestic fight.

    Finally, I called Merle and told her what had happened,
and that no one would help. She came the same evening from
Everett, saw the damage Harry had done and knew how sick he
was becoming. She got on the phone and convinced an ambulance
service to come and take Harry to the hospital. We followed
the ambulance to Harborview where the psychiatrist would not
admit Harry, because Harry said he was sorry. The man did not
know what he was dealing with.

Seattle, Washington   April 14, 1977

        Merle got him to call Dr. Jackson in Bellevue where
we had been counseling, and finally we got him admitted at
Fairfax Hospital for some help.

        I don't know what I would have done without the help of
Merle. Unless someone has lived with a Huntington's disease
patient, they do not understand the problems.

        I have remarried. Henry is in the Veterans Hospital
in Tacoma but my problems are not over. My son, now 13 years
old, has a very defeated attitude. He knows he could get the
disease and is having a very rough time. He's now at Caseadia
and has been made a ward of the state. My hope and prayers
are, of course, for a cure, but I thank God for the help Merle
has been.

Seattle, Washington   April 14, 1977

NAN FREDERICK HACKLER
SEATTLE, WASHINGTON   APRIL 1, 1977

    I am very thankful that after so long, national attention
has at last been focused on the problems that affect my family and so many other families. I have high hopes that the
results of this Commission and the forthcoming national plan
will alleviate not only the problems that I and others have
had to deal with but will also do away with the suffering and
dread and grief; that Huntington's disease will be controlla-
ble. I also appreciate the opportunity given me to submit a
statement. Huntington's disease is a very real thing to me
as my mother has it; I am knowingly at risk as are thousands
of others. But what about the many others who are at risk
unknowingly? Your own children could be potential H.D. victims; an adopted child could be at risk. Any child whose
parent died young or whose parent is unknown or out of contact
could be at risk unknowingly. H.D. is so much more common
than we realize. People keep it secret or patients are honestly
not diagnosed simply because doctors are not familiar enough
with H.D. to recognize it.

    In documenting my thoughts I have condensed our family
story and present it as a personal statement rather than
answering the guideline questions individually. I offer
openly our family history with names, but I am attaching
copies of letters from various doctors that I feel are pertinent but the doctors will be anonymous.

    I am a 32-year-old female; I was married for the second
time 9/11/76--six months ago. We have no children. I attended
college for three years, majoring in psychology and drama.
I moved to Seattle 1½ years ago. The two years prior to
that I spent traveling in Europe and the U.S. My husband
has a degree in architecture and is doing graduate work presently. I am working as a receptionist/secretary and spend
my leisure time gardening, biking, hiking, creative sewing,
reading and acting. My husband and I are very happy, we have
a good life; I am active, healthy and content. But I am at
risk for Huntington's disease. There is always that dark
cloud around the corner that could mean the end to my active-
ness, my healthiness and my happiness. We live not thinking
about it. Most of the time I don't think about it at all,
but it is always there. If I am clumsy on occasion--from lack

of sleep, perhaps, and not dropping anything more than the next person--I think of H.D. A 50 percent chance; either I get it or I don't. If you had a 50 percent chance of crossing a highway alive, would you do it? If you cross it twice, you'll get run over. Of course it depends what is on the other side whether you would take that risk. Would you knowingly marry an at-risk partner?

H.D. became known to our family in 1970. My grandparents died young and the great-grandparents on that side were not in contact. We had never heard of it and were certainly not looking for it. (We have since found that children of my grandfather's brothers have passed it on to cousins that we were not close to. They did not want to upset this side of the family needlessly so never passed along the information.)

My mother and my aunt were always "nervous" and we never thought it could be a "disease." Aunty lives in the east and we didn't see her too often. In 1969 she was driving out to see us and the police stopped her and called us to pick her up in the middle of Ohio. We found her her normal cheerful self, shaken by the experience but nothing extraordinary. They had stopped her for drunken driving; her involuntary movements caused the VW to weave. We thought her worse than we'd seen, her tongue was thick, she wasn't finishing sentences and made a lot of little humming noises and had nervous movements--but that was just Aunty. She had been a widow for 15 years and we just attributed her peculiarities to idiosyncrasies. She had a family doctor she saw regularly; he never recognized H.D.

But somehow, her brother read about H.D. in an article and found a knowledgeable doctor and Aunty was tested and put on medication. She is better now than she was before the medication was started. She is not allowed to drive, but lives alone, takes care of her house, cooks for herself, goes to church and is capable of handling a house full of company. She is 63 and still as cheerful as ever. The time will come when she will not be able to care for herself. She is a widow with one daughter. She does not have money; she does not want to move out of the house she has lived in alone for so long. Her H.D. has not progressed rapidly--but no one knows how long she can hold her own. Will she die in her own home? Will she linger for years in a nursing home vegetating? No one could expect my cousin to take her on if she becomes a burden..my cousin is at risk...she may only have a few good years herself. My cousin was married and working on her Ph.D. when H.D. was

diagnosed. Her marriage broke up; she was extremely upset
but has gotten her degree and has not and will not remarry.
She is active on H.D. committees and has better resources
than we found in the midwest.

When Aunty was diagnosed, it was kept from her that she
had H.D. This was the wrong thing to do. She knew she had
a condition; to sense that relatives are lying makes one
think of things like cancer. Now that she knows that her
condition has a name, she is no more upset and she can read
about the works of the CCHD and know there is hope for future
generations.

However, when Aunty was diagnosed, my mother fell apart.
My father had died and Mother had remarried but was having a
great deal of difficulty adjusting. She had a history of mis-
carriages and nervous breakdowns. She had been a nervous
child and this had been attributed to her being born prema-
turely and ner nervous system not growing. Mother was treated
by her family doctor who put her on tranquilizers. We put
her in the psychiatric ward in the hospital. The doctors
all knew about Aunty and H.D. We had a neurologist examine
her. She was treated by several M.D.'s and psychiatrists.
They concurred. "This woman does not have H.D.," they said.
They gave her shock treatments. She got "better" and came
home. So there we were with an aunt who had H.D. and was
doing fine and a mother who did not have H.D.--she was just a
little crazy.

Mother continued to be treated by her M.D.'s and visited
a psychiatrist. We all knew there was something wrong, but
we did not suspect that a whole staff of doctors could be
ignorant. Her psychiatrist told her that she was so close
to her sister and any involuntary movements she had (which
did get worse if she visited her sister) were just empathy
symptoms. I suppose that we did not pursue it further because
Mother's symptoms were really not like what we saw in Aunty.
We did not distrust the medical profession. We did not really
want Mother to have H.D.; we did not want to be at risk--it
was easier just to believe her nervous system hadn't developed
prenatally.

In 1976 Mother and my stepfather went to England for a
vacation with relatives. Her behavior became so bizarre and
uncontrollable that she was taken to a doctor there. I quote
from a letter from the doctor: "There is no serious doubt

that this patient has Huntington's chorea." Mother did not
stay in England but returned home and was put in the psychiatric
ward for the third time. She had been afraid for so long that
she had H.D.; she was afraid that we were lying to her the way
we had to her sister. She had associated H.D. from the beginning with her sister dying that when she herself was at last
diagnosed, she couldn't handle it. When her psychiatrist found
out, it seems that he felt that since her problem was organic
rather than emotional that there was no way to help her. Her
problem is certainly both a result of H.D. and compounded by
her emotional instability--but she is getting no counseling.

We had already seen the local neurologist and he didn't
know anything about H.D. How to find a doctor who did and who
could treat her? We called my cousin on the east coast and
she was able to give us names of local CCHD people. I was at
all times working with Mother's family doctor, but he was no
help in locating a neurologist. It was through the committee.
I called the president and he gave me the names of doctors and
also offered to provide transportation. Mother was seen several
months later and continued on the medication. The letter from
that doctor was not very informative or helpful; the letter
from her local doctor was not very informative or helpful.
Mother is in Michigan; I am in Seattle. When she does get
worse, she can't call for help, either to me or to her doctors.
My stepfather is 78--he has a lot of problems of his own. They
live very much cut off from the world; they can just manage to
nurse each other along. But Mother can get impossible to live
with and my stepfather drinks when he is upset. There is no one
counseling them, providing any referrals. At no time were any
of us three children offered any information about prognosis,
the treatment or inheritance patterns. Mother is not really
receiving continuing care; she is to see the neurologist when
needed but her local doctor doesn't see the need. She is taking
medication; there is nothing more to be done. Anything that
we, the at-risk children, have managed to learn has been from
literature from CCHD and what we could find in libraries. I
have found that I know more about H.D. than any doctor I have
ever talked to; and still knew more on the second visit after
he had read his medical books.

When Mother was diagnosed in 1975, I was there trying to
pull things together, and being largely frustrated because I
really didn't know where to turn for help. Mother was in the
hospital with a nervous breakdown on top of H.D., on top of
emotional problems, saying she wanted a divorce and that my

stepfather shouldn't be allowed to see her; that he was making her sick. He was at home, crying over H.D. and the
hereditary nature of it and being old and crotchety himself
but being very understanding with Mother and not believing
that she wanted a divorce. I frankly didn't know what to
believe. It was a very trying experience for me. I had been
prepared, I suppose, knowing that H.D. was in the family, and
I really wasn't surprised when Mother was diagnosed, but it
was still a shock. That final, undeniable fact that I and my
younger brother, his son, and my little sister were all at risk.
I was just there visiting; I really didn't have close friends
there to turn to and was running into so many dead ends--pro-
fessionally. At that time I had been doing Transcendental
Meditation for six months and it helped me more than I can say;
I have never been under so much stress and I could really feel
the stress leaving after I meditated. There are several types
of meditation "on the market" presently--I would sincerely
like to see the benefits of meditation researched in relation
to H.D. TM is perhaps the most scientifically documented and
I know the medical profession recognizes the benefits in lower-
ing blood pressure, etc.

When Mother was diagnosed, I was engaged. I was in Michigan with the family; my friend was in Seattle. I wrote him
about Mother and sent him literature on H.D. and told him all
the horrors. I said, "I cannot marry you and it would be
better if I just stayed here and you stayed there and went on
with your life." But being the wonderful person he is, and I
was prepared for him to agree and never see him again, he called
and said that he would come and get me if he had to but we were
going to get married. He said it would be the most cowardly
thing he could do to be scared off by a 50 percent chance.
Things weren't partly cloudy. They were partly sunny. Why
throw away our lives if I never was to get it? We are now
married, but there must be so many people whose lives are spent
just waiting for H.D. to happen, who can't find happiness or
who throw it away because of the risks. I was married for the
first time and he saw Aunty and saw my mother having a breakdown
and it upset him terribly. He had a lot of other hang-ups and
had a drinking problem and we were divorced in 1973. If I had
knowingly been at risk then, he would have left sooner.

My brother was married in 1968 and has a son. My brother
tends to internalize things that are upsetting so it's hard to
know what he is feeling. They never received any counseling
or help from any of their doctors. Fortunately his wife is a

strong person and was a big help; she said, "You all have yourselves to worry about, but I have two--a husband and a son."
Their son is now six and they put off having another child
because of H.D.--but their second child will be born next
week. I think they did the right thing. I cannot believe that
sterilization should be used as a "cure." It is, however, a
personal option that each family must consider their own way.
We are not planning to have children until my husband is out
of school; in two years we will have to decide for ourselves.

I also have a little sister who was living with me after
my father's death. When I was divorced, it just wasn't possible for her to live with Mother and her husband. There were
a lot of stepfather problems, but the greatest thing was Mother
was just too sick. We didn't know then that it was H.D. We
just knew that Mother was too crazy to raise a high-school-age
child. Fortunately, my father left enough money that my sister
could go to a private boarding school. She will enter college
next fall. She is an honor student, a very gentle, sensitive
girl; she is active in all phases of school activities. She
is at risk and it breaks my heart. She has known about H.D.
since she was 13. She knows she is at risk. She is doing a
term paper for science on H.D. (she wrote asking for literature
as she was having trouble finding information). I think it is
easier to grow up knowing about it when it doesn't mean so
much. I think it's easier to accept that way than to find out
it was kept secret until the day before you get married or
after you are pregnant.

My brother was living near Mother but he was just transferred to the west coast. My sister will not be going to
Mother's for vacations; Mother has changed too much that it's
very hard for us to be around her. She has gotten very mean,
she has not been able to make a decision for years, but spends
days trying to. She says yes when she means no. She wants
help but rejects it. We also have a stepfather to consider.
He never liked us kids; his daughter was there for the winter
to drive and cook for them (he can't see to drive and Mother
has a restricted license--she can't drive alone or more than
25 miles from home). His daughter was not happy being there.
We're just waiting to see what they decide to do now; they'll
have to move. It should be to a retirement-type home, or close
to one of his or her children. They need increasing support
at home. Mother will need residential care; it's just a question
of how long my stepfather lives and how rapidly Mother gets
worse. We really haven't looked into nursing homes because of

all the uncertainties; but I understand it can be difficult
finding one. And expensive. As far as the problems of the
terminal stages of the disease I read that it is terminal but
I have never read how. And it seems that the whole course of
the disease varies from family to family, that there are so
many unpredictables. It seems that this is an area of great
need: documenting case histories from enough families to be
able to forecast.

So that is basically our story. Despite it all, I'm
sure that our family has a much less tragic history than
many, many other H.D. families. It seems that all cases
have not shown up till later in life--past the age of responsibility and money has not been a hardship. Our greatest problem has been with diagnosis and treatment. The medical profession just doesn't know about H.D. I did ask a Seattle doctor
about it and he admitted that he didn't know anything but he
would give me a referral. He gave me the number of Amelia
Schultz--the first positive contact I ever made. If everyone
could have someone on the other end of the phone at a time of
need...but by that time I had resolved my problems. I did not
want to be tested. I do not want to find out that I will have
it. I would rather live hoping I don't than take the chance of
finding out, even though a finding that I will never get it
would make life easier. Dr. Schultz also found me a referral
in Michigan for Mother. I called Ms. Caskey and told her about
Mother and how isolated she is. I wanted her to establish a
contact before a time of need. Please see the letter I received
from her. She contacted Mother's doctor and he told her she
wasn't needed.

Mother is perhaps past the point of emotional counseling,
but it just isn't right to not help H.D. victims with the
related emotional problems; some may be caused organically by
the disease but many must be just the knowledge of having it:
the sickening and dying. Do doctors only treat the well?
The recoverable? Imagine Mother seeing a psychiatrist for five
years who tried to convince her that she didn't have H.D.--then
to find out that she really did. How could she--or her husband--
ever trust another therapist? If I sound upset with the medical
profession it's true. I believe there is so much more to good
health than drugs. I am seeing a naturalpathic physician now.
He could not find much on H.D., could not find any documented
histories of M.D.'s treating H.D.'s. He advised me that what
I am doing is the best thing I can do. I eat only whole foods,
no junk foods or preservatives or chemicals or meat. I am very

aware of what goes into my body. I still meditate daily and
have started taking yoga classes. Inner peace is inner strength.
I am not doing these things only because of H.D., but I'm sure
that if I do get H.D. that being better to start with I will
get worse slower. If I am emotionally stable before H.D., I
can cope better. If my body is not filled with poisons but
rather with good health and well-being I will fare better.
It is not a disease that can be prevented but I believe it can
be better prepared for than to do nothing. This is true for
everyone--not just at-risk H.D. people. We are all at risk
for something someday--for death. The fuller are our lives day
by day, the easier it is to accept. I would like to give another
dozen pages of personal testimonials for TM and yoga and healthy
eating. I will refrain. I just know how these things have
helped me so far.

Again, I want to thank this Commission. I would like
there to be a treatment that controls H.D. before I or my
brother or sister or cousin develop it. I am sure there will
be treatment before the next generation grows up.

I want to thank also Marjorie Guthrie who is responsible
for all of this. Any help that our family received--all facts--
came from the CCHD and literature sent by them. Arlo is also
my hero. I will be seeing him April 2 from about halfway back
at the Paramont. Sterilization as a cure? What if Woody had
known and hadn't had Arlo? So many, many people are at risk;
that's a lot of people not to be born.

I will certainly do anything I can to aid in research;
my whole family is willing. Mother has willed her body; we
have sent money; but the more we can be involved in research,
the better we will feel--that something is being done and that
we are helping. It's largely a problem of awareness, having
the medical profession informed and able to recognize H.D.;
to have referrals; to know where to send patients for care, treatment and financial support, and genetic counseling. To have
the public aware that H.D. is and what it is; that the aunt or
uncle you vaguely remember who had the shakes and was put away
could be a threat to next generations. That H.D. is not a
hush-hush thing...that if we are all open about it, facts can
be gathered. Having more public attention focused on finding
a treatment will stimulate researchers. I myself need support;
I can tell people that I have an aunt with H.D.--but I cannot say,
"My mother has it. I am at risk." I don't want an uneducated
public to judge me, reject me, or pity me. I will stand up to

this Commission and say, "Help me. Help my brother and sister and our children. Help the many, many of us who are at
risk to at least have the knowledge that as much as possible
is being done."

I believe that this is the beginning of great advancements
and we thank you.

Seattle, Washington   April 14, 1977

MARY R. JACKSON
SOAP LAKE, WASHINGTON   FEBRUARY 23, 1977

    Being a nurse I intrested in knowing all about this dread
disease which I seem to know I have though keep under control.
I mix mineral oil and Lanacane and wash my bladder. This disease start from acid in blood from their get worse to it become
a cancer by eating linen out of bladder tube letting out pee,
soiling clothes carry a small. Some times I mix a little car
oil to keep feet from swelling. I did carry a cancer smell tho
it gone by washing my bladder once in while.

    God help those that worse I pray.

    I am 63 years old.

    Acid food bad.

    Every morning I drink boiling water, mix milk, honey,
and 1 teaspoon ice cream vanilla for breakfast. Then at nite
no curried meat or barbecue:

    Apple sauce
    corn meal mush mix white and yellow
    vegetables carrots especially
    meat beef

    I keep from child sperm by mixing mineral oil quart
Mississippi caroil here kerosene 1/4 in.

    I'm a retired Government nurse I'd like to go to convention
in Seattle when it come up. So I get my name in.

    I have five children, pretty twins grown.
    1 girl all children took after their dadie.
    2 boys all grown begging to know how to keep childbearing
       from
drunk Indian run over one twin and her oldest baby
parlizing her hand won't grow off with other gash a hole in
her skull. 8 years old. won't heal. she smart. needs good
milk.

    I need a good paying job somewhere.

Seattle, Washington   April 14, 1977

MILTON G. KLEIN
DIRECTOR, STATE OF IDAHO
DEPT. OF HEALTH AND WELFARE
BOISE, IDAHO   MARCH 18, 1977

Despite the assurances contained in textbook material that diagnosis of
this disease is readily evident if certain diagnostic criteria are met,
such as "the typical triad of choreiform movements, dementia in adult life,
and documentation of similar symptoms in family members", it would appear
that patients continue to be misdiagnosed. Often, this is by no means the
fault of the physician, but rests on the tendency of afflicted families to
repress information. Criteria for diagnosis include at least a pedigree
showing that the disease was present, or could have been present, in one
parent and other members of the family. Since psychiatric symptoms may
long precede the neurologic ones, there is further hesitancy on the part
of families to give accurate histories.

Diagnosis is, in my opinion, often impeded by the lack of a sound working
relationship between neurologists and psychiatrists. The behavioral abnormalities in this disease are often too cumbersome to be handled by the
neurologist, who then refers the patient to a state institution wherein the
patient is "lost" to diagnosis and/or treatment. The psychiatrist, in turn,
is often not entirely comfortable with the neurological aspects of the illness, and the patient is again institutionalized. Thus, many patients are
not adequately diagnosed for several years. It is clear that such instances
deprive the patient, and the family, of genetic counseling and the often
much needed supportive psychotherapy.

Physicians should be made more aware of the usefulness and availability of
Computerized Axial Tomography as a means to diagnose appropriately. If further testing is indicated, more funds or grants from the federal government
should be made available to the Neurology Departments in major university
hospitals or private clinics to conduct more exhaustive testing (example:
Creedmor Institute for Psychobiologic Studies, Queens Village, N.Y.). If
these efforts help to weed out the more benign forms of extrapyramidal disorders, so much the better.

It is beyond the scope of these few lines to delineate what happens to a
victim of this disease (and his family) once the diagnosis has been firmly
established. If a diagnosis can be established at a point where little
brain atrophy has occurred, there is a myriad of treatment modalities which
then can be applied to make life more tolerable for these unfortunate victims.

Seattle, Washington   April 14, 1977

ROY F. KOKENGE, M.D.
YAKIMA, WASHINGTON   MARCH 2, 1977

As a practicing neurologist, the major problem with patients with Huntington's disease is the correct and early diagnosis of the disease.

Families are understandably distraught when the diagnosis is made in some one in their family. A reliable biochemical test given to other members of the family would aide in the reassurance of the non-affected members and identification of the affected members. Hopefully, a form of treatment will result so that possible early detection and early treatment will prevent the progressive nature of the disease.

Further medical research is needed inthe areas of diagnosis and detection of the disease and treatment of the disease.

Seattle, Washington   April 14, 1977

HELEN KREUCHER
EVERETT, WASHINGTON   APRIL 13, 1977

    I would like to submit my testimony regarding my hus-
band's illness with Huntington's disease, which he had for
14 years, ending with his death on January 1 of this year.

    It was a long, hard road which I, with my children, had
to bear alone. All the decisions, the work, and caring for him
was my job, until I could no longer do it as it was getting my
health. Not knowing which way to turn, I happened to hear about
Merle Denney whose husband had the same illness. She was so
helpful to me in getting him into a good nursing home, and helping me get the financial assistance which we had to have. She
went with me to the welfare office and assisted me with the many
details of obtaining help. However, the Welfare Department only
allowed me $200 a month to live on. Any money I might earn I
was to give half of it to them for my husband's care. Every
time he received an increase from Social Security, it would
have to be paid to the nursing home. I never was allowed to
keep more than $200. He was there for over three and a half
years and during that time there was a steady rise in the cost
of living, which made it hard for me.

    I cannot begin to mention all the heartache, the loneliness
and despair which I went through during those long years. It
is too painful to write about it and it would take too long.
It is so necessary for families to have someone who can help
them--for counseling and helping with financial problems when
a member of the family has this illness. It is too much to
bear alone.

Seattle, Washington   April 14, 1977

MARTI LEWIS, R.N.
BREMERTON, WASHINGTON   MARCH 14, 1977

    I am an instructor at Olympic College in Health Occupations and am concerned about the lack of textbook coverage of Huntington's disease.

    As the result of becoming personally acquainted with a person who has Huntington's disease (at risk), I started reviewing our textbooks to see what information was available to me and our students regarding Huntington's disease. I was shocked to find such limited, almost nonexistent information in our textbooks! I had to search through physician's reference books to find the disease described in enough detail to grasp what it is!

    Perhaps because of this lack of information in the basic anatomy and physiology textbooks as well as medical-surgical textbooks, supplementary information could be made available to all educators in health occupations.

    In addition, a bibliography would be helpful on Huntington's disease concerning the disease process, nursing care of a patient with Huntington's disease, immediate and advanced stages, and anticipatory guidance to the health practitioner in the care of an H.D. patient.

    Again, our textbooks have very little, if no information concerning Huntington's disease. Our students would know nothing about the disease if they did not have access to physicians' reference books.

Seattle, Washington   April 14, 1977

ARNO G. MOTULSKY, M.D.
SEATTLE, WASHINGTON   APRIL 5, 1977

Thank you for notifying me about the hearings of the Huntington's Disease
Commission in Seattle. I have transmitted the material to several of my
colleagues in Seattle who will respond as requested by you. As you know,
I am on a sabbatical leave at Stanford.

I continue to be worried about the proliferation of efforts for specific
diseases in the HEW/NIH. Special campaigns against a named disease (i.e.,
diabetes, Huntington's disease, etc.) are not necessarily accompanied by
the granting of new funds. Consequently, funds will be siphoned off general
research allotments with counterproductive results in the long run. Success
in creating special status for some diseases, which is not synonymous with
conquest of the disease, will encourage other disease-oriented groups to
establish more and more such fragmented efforts - a move which may have
serious consequences for a productive biomedical research enterprise in the
long run. I hope that this point of view will get some discussion as part
of the final report.

I realize very well the impatience of those who are afflicted with Huntington's
disease and particularly of those who are at risk, with our current inability
to come up with answers. I have spent many agonizing hours during and
following heart-rending interviews with Huntington's disease families in my
capacity as a genetic counselor.

Yet, our well-meaning efforts to do something for this disease should be
viewed against the totality of the biomedical research enterprise and the
historical precedents of possible research leads coming from unexpected
quarters. My involvement with the biomedical research policy committee of
the Institute of Medicine of the National Academy of Sciences has made me
particularly sensitive to this issue.

Seattle, Washington   April 14, 1977

IRMA NORTHUP
VANCOUVER, WASHINGTON   MARCH 13, 1977

        I cared for my son at home as long as possible, then
placed him in Columbia View Manor, a rest home in Vancouver,
Washington. He left his room one evening to get something
to help him sleep. The nurses put him back in his room and
locked it with a coat hanger from the outside. He fell to the
floor and after a time, managed to crawl to his bed and pull
himself on it. One of the nurses told me that she and two of
the other nurses watched him through an outside window. She
said she didn't know how he ever managed it by himself. He told
me about it the next day and asked me to come check on him
about 11:00 o'clock as he had a fear of being locked in. I did
this for him but he was all right.

        They told him that Western State Hospital had a new set-
up for therapy for H.D. patients and he asked me to take him
up there. Told me he would try anything if he could just be
well again. I took him. Again, he was locked in behind iron
doors this time; not like a human being but a criminal. Two
weeks later, my sister and I visited him. When I took him up
there, he walked in. When I saw him two weeks later, he was
in a wheelchair, face black and blue, broken finger, in a
splint. A sight I try to forget. The next week we went back
to take him home, which we did. He complained of his arm hurting him. I entered him in the Highland Terrace Nursing Home
in Camas, Washington. I told the doctor (Dr. Stefan) about his
arm, so he x-rayed it the next day; it, too, was broken. Dr.
Stefan put it in a splint. The nurses asked me what in the
world they had done to that poor boy up at Western State.

        He was content there until John P. Jones, the manager,
wanted me to move him. Said he needed the room for someone
else. My son was on Social Security and wasn't paying too much
as he has a son who was a dependent. I tried several places,
trying to get him in when I got a call from Mr. Jones telling
me they had sent my son to the St. Joseph's Hospital in Vancouver. I went right to the hospital and was told they wouldn't
accept him there as he had torn up the inside of the ambulance
and he was sent to the mental part of Columbia View Manor.
I went down there but they wouldn't let me see him for 72 hours.
He told me then that he didn't know what they were going to do
with him, that they wouldn't tell him anything. Had they told

Seattle, Washington   April 14, 1977

him, they wouldn't have had this trouble, as he was so happy
when he found out he was nearer home than before. He was
there for 60 days, then they had a court hearing and Judge Reid
sent him back to Western State.

In the meantime, I got busy and wrote to Senator Henry
Jackson and Governor Dan Evans about the treatment he had
received while there before. Each of these men had the place
investigated. When my son arrived there, he had a room on
the second floor by himself and the door was always open. Judge
Reid told me he would find a place for my son closer to home so
I could visit him more often and to call him (Judge Reid) at any
time. To this day, I have never been able to get in touch with
him.

My son passed away four months later from bronchial
pneumonia, they said. That has been almost three years ago.

I took Floyd's son when his wife left him when he was
only 1-1/2 years old. The impact of his father's illness has
left him a very disturbed young man. He is now 18 years old
and is taking mental therapy. The pressure on those left is
unbelievable. Lack of understanding by doctors as well as
nurses and staff. Lack of knowledge of H.D. patients. Lack of
proper places available. If you have money, they will take
anyone. Most important is the lack of compassion for these
poor unfortunate people.

I hope this letter helps you in your research. I won't
be around when my grandson reaches the age when he needs help
but I pray to God by that time, things will have changed for
those with H.D. Better yet, I ask God to let it pass him by.

God bless and help you all.

Seattle, Washington   April 14, 1977

DENSLEY H. PALMER
EVERETT, WASHINGTON   APRIL 21, 1977

    My purpose in writing is to lend my support to efforts
to develop centers for the study and treatment of people with
Huntington's disease.

    As a psychologist, I regularly counsel with people about
life planning. We discuss educational and vocational programs
and touch upon such considerations as marriage and family. It
is one thing to impose a relatively stable, chronic condition,
such as a spinal cord injury or an amputation, on a person's
thinking about the future. It is a far different matter to
raise the specter of a serious debilitating process which one
may or may not display at mid-career. How does one plan mean-
ingfully or optimistically?

    The development of centers for the treatment and research
into Huntington's disease will, hopefully, produce resources
and information for people who, like myself, are called upon
for help. I need this. Those who turn to me need this even
more. Thank you for your help.

Seattle, Washington   April 14, 1977

GRETCHEN PEDERSON
McKINLEY PARK, ALASKA   MARCH 5, 1977

        I am writing to urge your Commission to do whatever pos-
sible to combat and find a cure for Huntington's disease.

        I am twenty-seven years old, married but without children,
and am "at risk." My brother and three sisters are also "at
risk," each of us waiting to see whether one, two, three or
all of us might develop the symptoms of Huntington's disease.

        No one had known that Huntington's disease was the
reason that my grandfather had committed suicide. His health
problem had been misdiagnosed by uninformed doctors.

        My mother grew up without ever having heard of Hunting-
ton's disease. She graduated with top honors from her university, married, and eventually had four children, never realizing
that she might be passing on a gene that could have a profound
effect on the lives of those she loved so dearly. She died
three weeks ago from this dreadful disease, approximately fifteen
years after showing the first symptoms.

        Those years were painful for both family and friends.
We were at least fortunate in knowing what it was. Not at
first, but after many tests, the cause of the fidgeting and
jerky movements was determined. It was hard to accept the
fact that her physical abilities and mental acuity would
slowly deteriorate until death, and that the same fate might
exist for me and my siblings.

        As the years passed, my mother's personality changed
and her movements became more awkward. But she still maintained her dignity and her pride in the family that she loved
so much. It was not until the last few years that she was
unable to leave the hospital bed that had been placed in my
father's living room. It became necessary to hire someone to
stay and watch her whenever a friend or family member was not
at home. Just prior to death, my mother had reached a stage
in which her speaking was so slurred that it was practically
incomprehensible. The bed was padded to prevent her from
becoming injured by her flailing limbs and thrashing movements.
She was still able to chew small amounts of food, but was otherwise completely unable to care for herself.

My family's tragedy is not unique. Many others throughout the world are also suffering from Huntington's disease.
It is my hope that your Commission can help to combat some of
the problems caused by Huntington's disease.

Help is needed in patient care. My family learned mostly
from experience about the best techniques in caring for my
mother. Friends helped us in devising new ways of feeding and
transporting her. This type of knowledge should be shared.
Even trained personnel are sometimes not informed or experienced
enough to handle H.D. patients. I will relate one example.
My mother was hospitalized during the week preceding her death.
My father gave detailed instructions to the nurses about how
and what to feed her. Yet when my sister returned later in the
day, the nurses had not fed my mother. They said that she
turned away when offered food. The nurses just hadn't understood, or perhaps hadn't cared, to take the time (often thirty
minutes to an hour) to place each small piece of food deftly
into the moving target of my mother's mouth. They didn't
know that one hand, or even another person, had to steady her
head while the other hand held the fork.

Doctors and the general public should also be more
informed of H.D. Victims have enough problems without having
to deal with doctors misdiagnosing the disease, or with policemen picking them up under the suspicion that they are drunk.

Involved families often need counseling and/or financial
support. Hospital beds, hydraulic lifters, medication, and
other expenses all add up.

Patient care, sharing of ideas between involved families,
education, and counseling and financial assistance for families
are all badly needed, but even more important, is research.
Hopefully your Commission can promote research towards finding
a cure and treatment for Huntington's disease. It would also
be of tremendous value to have a test to determine whether or
not "at-risk" individuals will later develop H.D. symptoms.
Deciding whether or not to marry, have children, or follow
certain pursuits in life would be so much easier if those at
risk knew what to expect. Research for H.D. could help individual victims, their families, and future generations. It might
also have repercussions for other genetic disorders.

Seattle, Washington   April 14, 1977

      Again, I urge you to do your best to help cure Hunting-
ton's disease and solve the many problems associated with it.
The futures of many, like my brother and sister, and my husband
and me, depend on your assistance.

Seattle, Washington   April 14, 1977

LEONA G. ROACH
STRATFORD, WASHINGTON   MARCH 26, 1977

        Thank Heavens! There is something started to aid vic-
tims and their families of the disease called Huntington's.

        My position in this one case is as a friend and part of
a "Team of Friends" to aid a lovely young mother whose name
is Faye Kuch (pronounced cook). The "Team" was organized by
Mrs. Harvey Henke who was a neighbor during Faye's childhood
and whom Faye loves and "adopted" as her mother.

        Three years ago when I first knew Faye, she was able to
walk unaided but was losing some control. A year later she
needed help to walk and her husband put her into a hospital
and subsequently a nursing home. He had said that she was constantly hurting herself in trying to do things when no one was
around to help her. He also said her condition had gradually
worsened over a period of five years, starting not long after
the birth of their third child, following which she had an operation to eliminate any future chance of pregnancy.

        My personal feelings toward nursing homes (my mother had
been in one for a short time until I brought her home) motivated me to conspire, with the "Team's" help, to have her
taken care of at home. We had knowledge of a strong and
healthy spinster lady in her sixties who did that kind of
work. We wrote to various Social Services heads and other
officials to enlist their interest and help in having her
permitted a living allowance to be able to support "live-in"
care. She was only 34 and the nursing homes are so under-
staffed that patients often smell of urine and their hair is
in unkempt condition and dandruffy. A pitiful existence for
a lovely girl.

        On her husband's property were several houses and she
lived in one until he divorced her and put her off the place.
He was apparently fearful of losing his property to the state
for reimbursement if he did not do this. And there are three
boys to support and educate: Rick, now 15, Bill is 13, and
Dan who is 10. Also, apparently her highly nervous condition
was a rather constant source of irritation among the family.

                            5—572

Seattle, Washington   April 14, 1977

        We took her to the University of Washington Research
Center at their invitation to have them diagnose her condition
definitely as Huntington's, with no recommended treatment for
cure.

        This story cannot be told without some background added
to it. You will be appalled, as I was, to learn that this
young lady was a victim of child abuse of the worst kind,
around the age of 12 from a stepmother who threatened her,
her two older brothers, two sisters and a baby brother, with
death if they told their father who worked away from home.
They all had to watch while her stepmother forced the baby
brother to eat and when he cried so hard that he vomitted, he
was forced to eat the vomit. She had so many bruises from
things like a broom being broken over her back that her
teachers became suspicious and caused an inquiry.

        Prior to all of this and soon after the birth of the
baby brother, her real mother developed Huntington's and was
eventually committed to a mental hospital. The children and
father took care of the baby brother until their father divorced their mother and remarried. Her mother died within a
very few years.

        After an investigation of his home situation, the father
was ordered by Court to separate the children from the step-
mother. He died at an early age from a heart attack.

        Two of Faye's brothers developed Huntington's. One has
died. Another, Don, is cared for at the Veterans Hospital
near Seattle, since he spent time in military service.

        It is plain to see the disease created nothing less than
havoc for this family during two generations. Now, in this
generation there are five children, the offspring of these
two, Faye and Don, who have only a 50-50 chance to escape
having it.

        In closing, I wish to say that we of the "Team of Friends
of Faye Kuch" wish to nominate our beautiful Faye as Poster
Girl if you contemplate having one. There is nothing more
heartrending than a little crippled child, unless it is a
lovely young mother who is stricken this way.

Seattle, Washington   April 14, 1977

MRS. ALEX SOLIS
SEATTLE, WASHINGTON   APRIL 12, 1977

        Huntington's has changed our lives completely. My hus-
band's case was not an abrupt one. He did not suddenly find
he could not do things he does every day. His was gradual,
like erosion. During the time he was having his big trouble
I was in the middle of learning to cope with a change of life
baby. I was so nervous that I thought all his problems were
a result of him trying to deal with me and his job. Of course,
he went to doctors but his health was excellent. We had never
heard of Huntington's, and neither had the doctors. Finally
GTE stepped in and sent him to two neurologists before there
was a diagnosis. This process took about <u>six years</u>. Meantime
we lived under an unbelievable strain. Our social life became
almost nil. I made enemies instead of friends because they
would knock my husband, as to his ability. We had enjoyed a
rather nice relationship with the people on the staff and this
went to "pot." The men he worked with had all they could do to
tolerate him at work; much less after work. If we could have
stayed in one place, perhaps we could have survived better, but
he transferred hoping to get a job he could do better, perhaps
not.

        Frankly I have not dealt well with our predicament. My
nerves are in very bad condition. I have tried to get training.
That is out; we make too much money. My husband is still working
which is a miracle. I thank God for every day. Even with this
miracle, we are above the poverty line only enough to be denied
any sort of assistance. Gentlemen, I do not want a <u>handout</u>, now
or later, especially later; what I wanted was a chance to learn
and do a job. Thus far I have made baby-sitting pay the extra
expenses.

        The future to me is so gross that I can not force myself
to even face it, which is the reason I'm sending this letter.
I'm aware that it is full of half-thought, misspelled words
and the works, but I promised to write it. At the time I volun-
teered this letter, I had no idea how much I depend on living
24 hours at a time. Actually I find myself in the position of
being a widow with two children, instead of a husband and a
daughter, but as long as I live only today we have a semblance
of normal, and God knows I long for normal. If this is the
coward's way out, it's still the code I live by.

Seattle, Washington   April 14, 1977

        As to what we want of you, I'm not sure--certainly more
research. I have a daughter who will spend her life in a
dilemma of, "Do I or don't I?" In the future I am sure that
I would wish for anyone to help with medical expenses. To
date most of those are taken care of by our company insurance.
When that expires, only God knows. The ideal thing would be
to have Huntington's under the "Birth Defect" Foundation.
Whatever, the result we need is an opportunity to hold our
head up and be useful citizens. If we were low income, that's
okay, but the way it is we can take welfare or divorce. We
are too young for Medicare and we're too old for Medicaid.
Personally, I have a child of 8 and I do not look forward to
raising her on welfare. I see no alternate route at the moment.

        Gentlemen, I will pray that this jumble of words will
help you realize there is a need.

Seattle, Washington   April 14, 1977

ERNEST H. SPRENGER
RITZVILLE, WASHINGTON   MARCH 14, 1977

     NAME: Mrs. Elizabeth M. (Strobel) Sprenger, known as
"Betty" in this testimony. Born: May 16, 1927; Died: April
26, 1973; the "immediate cause of death--myocardial infarction"
but we know that the real "culprit" cause was Huntington's
disease!

     To those individuals and persons who have experienced the
devastating effects of this disease the stories and testimonies
like this one must sound like sad repeats. And so they are.

     During the years when my wife and family were going through
this tragedy I made the statement many, many times: "If I were
the exponent of evil and intended to design a disease which was
the incarnation of everything that wasn't good...Huntington's
disease would positively have to be my first choice. As a
pastor for almost thirty years I had observed the impact of
many different diseases...none appeared as diabolical to me
as Huntington's disease."

     Before our marriage in 1947 I was first introduced to
the disease when Betty and I visited her grandfather in Eureka,
South Dakota. Her mother had died in 1945 from the ravages of
this disease. The grandfather was 74 years of age at the time.
He was bedfast, his face distorted, his limbs jerking; a slobber-
ing, pitiful sight. He was being cared for by a daughter who
was about 53 years of age at the time. She herself was just in
the early stages of the onset of this disease. Grandfather
Strobel lived to be 81 years of age, the daughter died some
four or five years thereafter.

     Since Betty's mother had died from the illness, Betty's
father was deeply concerned about our marriage and the possibility of transmitting this illness to children if we should
have any. He insisted that she go through the best medical
clinic in Billings, Montana (they lived in Laurel, Montana at
the time). The diagnosis: "Don't worry about inheriting this
illness...if it appears again it will probably be in your brother's lifetime, not yours." This, as we now know, was totally
and thoroughly incorrect information.

The manifestations of this disease first appeared during the pregnancy with our third and last child. Betty suffered from what the doctor at Yankton, South Dakota called more than "normal" depression, nervousness, etc. She had fits of anger during which she threw pictures against the walls, ripped drawers from the kitchen cabinets, etc. I was not convinced that these were manifestations of the disease because I believed the medical advice of the doctors in Billings, Montana. I did have a vasectomy operation--something which, in my case, I believe has affected my sexual performance negatively.

During a visit by her brother in the summer of 1964 he told me that he observed manifestations which were the same as those the family had experienced with their mother, and that we should not waste any time in having it diagnosed. Betty was suffering from uncontrollable muscle spasms and movements in the area of her stomach. Our local doctor (we were living in California where I was engaged in graduate studies), Dr. Heintz A. Von Hungen, Modesto, California, made a preliminary diagnosis on the basis of family history, etc. He scheduled a neurological and psychological examination with Dr. E. E. Lamond in Stockton, California. On September 28, 1964, Dr. Lamond's diagnosis was made and he definitely determined that it was Huntington's disease. Nothing further was said in terms of counseling--just, "You will have to learn to live with it!"

Desiring further professional verification and perhaps some kind of counseling guidelines, we scheduled an appointment with Dr. Donald Macrae, M.D., M.R.C.P., F.R.F.P.S., who was recommended as the one best resource on genetic disorders in the Bay area. This examination was at University Hospital in San Francisco, California on February 25, 1965. The interview lasted twenty minutes (I was never given an opportunity to talk to the man!) and his bill arrived with the morning mail the day we got home! This was cold-blooded professionalism at its worst! Dr. Macrae simply confirmed Dr. Lamond's diagnosis.

In July, 1965 we arrived here in Ritzville, Washington where I have been serving as pastor of the Philadelphia Congregational Church. This employment has offered me the opportunity to take care of Betty in our home until October, 1972 when my own health began to break down. She was in and out of hospitals in Spokane and here in Ritzville many, many times. From October, 1972 until she died she was cared for in our local nursing home. She was mentally alert and able to talk until death came to her.

Major Frustrations and Problems

1. The pathetic lack of up-to-date knowledge regarding
    the disease. Though I realize that 1947 is not
    1977, I have often wondered what the average course
    covers in medical training regarding this disease.

    In twelve years of seeking help and treatment for
    this illness, there has been a good deal of what I
    call "cold-blooded professionalism." I suspect that
    a good many doctors aren't very helpful simply because
    they don't know how to be.

    Through those dozen years of her illness, Betty was
    given many, many different kinds of medication. We
    do have an incomplete history of these but the side
    effects, like illusions and disorientation, were some-
    times as awful and disastrous as the illness might
    have been. Who is to know?

2. Nothing is as devastating as the personal feelings of
    inadequacy. How does one cope with irrational/erratic
    behavior and consequent responses? How does one help
    to alleviate guilt feeling--i.e., after she ripped out
    her children's hair in a fit of anger, or cut up her
    daughter's newly purchased winter coat "because it
    wasn't high-priced enough!" Or how do you cope with
    the attempts and threats of suicide? Which hell is
    worse--to permit her carrying out her attempt, or live
    with a future which has the seal of a lingering death
    upon it?

    Where do you go for help? No "professional" who hasn't
    had experience with this particular illness can possi-
    bly know how to deal with cases like this.

3. The financial strain, with no possibility of Social
    Security disability, or any other kind of resource to
    turn to when the financial burden becomes frightening.
    Without the backing of a loving congregation and a
    fraternal organization (Masonic Lodge) we could still
    be in debt.

Fortunately, also, our group health insurance plan through Travelers was very, very excellent and helpful.

4. What about the future for my three children? Mark, born in 1956, is in the Air Force; Scott, born in 1959, is a senior in high school. Cynthia, born in 1960, is a junior in high school.

Can they be put on a mailing list so they can keep up with the latest research, etc.?

What kind of counseling is available to them? Should they choose sterilization?

I am tremendously grateful to Marjorie Guthrie and all of those marvelous people she has enlisted through the years towards the eradication of this terrible disease. I want to do everything I possibly can to see that the Commission created by the U.S. Congress gets all the necessary information and data to deal with this problem.

Seattle, Washington   April 14, 1977

TEAM OF FRIENDS
STRATFORD, WASHINGTON   MAY 7, 1977

    We heartily applaud the very significant developments in
research on behalf of Huntington's disease victims in the
fields of diagnosis, new techniques for treatment, etc., but
our special interest is in social management which will improve
the lot of those who suffer such physical pain and mental anxiety from this insidious disease.

    We are a "Team of Friends" who aid a young woman, a divorced
mother of 3 sons, who is the victim of this cruel disease.
This task we have been taking on for 2-1/2 years now--so we
are interested.

    We especially desire to have <u>special</u> facilities developed
for the exclusive care of H.D. patients and/or victims of all
neuromuscular ailments, but as above-mentioned, our interest
is specifically in H.D.

    To have such a facility <u>anywhere</u> would be wonderful pro-
gress, however, we respectfully suggest Eastern Washington
State, particularly in the Grand Coulee area as a location
for it. We are adjacent to that area. More importantly,
there is a young and active group there who are working very
effectively to aid H.D. patients, and they are great organizers.

    The one who inspired renewed research in H.D., Woodie
Guthrie, is much loved and remembered there because he wrote
the beautiful Grand Coulee Dam song. Also there are four other
victims of this ailment who come from that area, so it really
"hits home" there.

    We desire that the need for special facilities for the
care of these patients be brought to the attention of Congress
and/or before those various special committees that could help
the cause. For those unfortunate people to be doomed to being
placed in mental institutions, when they are not mentally ill,
OR to be kept in nursing homes when they are yet young and
nothing is known about really helping or arresting their condition, is so unjust.

Seattle, Washington   April 14, 1977

We sincerely want to add our plea for the development of such facilities to the many who are now asking you to exert your powers and good influence toward the fulfillment of this petition.

Thank you for your time and attention to our request.

Seattle, Washington   April 14, 1977

H. C. THULINE, M.D.
SUPERVISOR, BIRTH DEFECTS
STUDY & COUNSELING PROGRAM
DEPT. OF SOCIAL AND HEALTH SERVICES
STATE OF WASHINGTON   APRIL 14, 1977

     The Commission for the Control of Huntington's Disease and
Its Consequences is to be commended for providing the opportunity of testimony from those with a wide range of relationships
to this disorder. The interest I wish to present is, in the
narrow sense, that of genetic counseling, and, in a broader
sense, that of public health.

     The material forwarded by the Commission to those interested
in preparing testimony is very helpful in that it outlines the
concerns identified by the Commission. Examination of this
material confirms to me the deep concern felt over the plight
of affected individuals and their families. The need to assist
them is evident and many individuals will be heard on those
matters.

     An area for which testimony was not directly requested,
although implied in the questions for genetic counselors, is
that of the ethics of dealing with people at risk who do not
know the risk. It would seem that if the Commission can provide firm guidance for at least three matters related to this,
it would be most helpful, whether or not individual counselors
agreed with such guidance in all respects. Some of these issues
are raised in the following situation:

     A few years ago a husband and father committed suicide
when he learned that he indeed had Huntington's disease. He
knew his mother had died with it but had not discussed this
with his wife until his own diagnosis was established. In a
counseling session after the suicide, the widow, mother of
four minor children, was asked if she had preferences as to
the counseling of her children about Huntington's disease. Her
reply was, "I won't tell them and I don't want anyone else to
tell them."

     By her statement she defined the following issues:

     1. The right of ownership over the knowledge that the
children are at risk.

      a.   Do the children have the right to know they are
          at risk? If so, when?

      b.   Does a mother have the right to withhold such
          knowledge from her children while minors or after
          their age of majority?

2. Does the counselor (who has the knowledge) have a
legal duty, a legal responsibility or no obligation to inform
the children of their being at risk? Is this related in any
way to the age of a child?

3. Do this mother's grandchildren have the right not to
be born if they would be affected?

In such a situation an individual counselor will probably
act in accord with one of the following models and the assump-
tions on which they are based.

The "Medical Model":

As to the first issue, ownership of the knowledge that
the children are at risk, the relationship in the medical model
is between the counselor and his client, in this case the
mother, with protection of the perceived rights of the client.
Usually the mother of minor children is perceived to have the
right for decisions regarding her children up to the age of
majority. This perception has recently been breached in the
matter of contraceptive information and methods and abortion.
This now raises the second issue in the medical model as to
whether the counselor has obligations to a sexually active
minor against or without the mother's knowledge.

It has been suggested by Margery Shaw that the counselor
may be able to act in what is considered the best interest of
the children against the wishes of the mother. Laws intended
to control infectious diseases may then afford protection of
the counselor against suit by the mother for disclosure of
their risk to the children. That is, the counselor has knowledge of a risk to the children for development of a disease
and therefore has a duty to inform those children of such risk.
This is an interesting concept and perhaps it should be explored further. It does not, however, speak to the mother's
motive in denying her children the knowledge of their risk.

Her intent was to spare them the uncertainty, anxiety and emotional pain of living and making decisions about vocation, marriage and reproduction while knowing that they had a 50 percent risk of developing a disabling disease for which there is no cure. She is saying they have the right "not to know" that they are at risk as long as nothing definitive can be offered them as a solution to the problem.

The "Socially Coercive Model":

In this model it is assumed that not only the client but society has certain rights in relation to the disease. The rights of society are assumed to be to avoid continuing or increasing economic costs related to the disease and to avoid continuing or increasing economic costs related to the disease and to avoid an increase in the proportion of the population incapacitated by the disease. If the counselor accepts as socially desirable a decrease in the reproductive rate of those at risk, but who do not know of their risk, he may consider this as adequate reason to inform them of such a fact. This would constitute abrogation of their right "not to know" mentioned above. The right "not to know" has come to the fore also in respect to a test which would identify a person as carrying the mutant gene for Huntington's disease prior to the onset of signs and symptoms adequate to make a clear diagnosis. Not only the use but the development of such a test involves the issue of a person's right not to know he is at risk in that suggestion that the test be used destroys the innocence of the situation.

Implicit in this "socially coercive model" is the assumption that the "right to know" overrides the "right not to know" because only for those who are aware of their risk can we apply the social pressure inherent in counseling them about the course of the disease and the choices they have about marriage and reproduction. This appears to be the model being followed at present by most counselors and by those planning programs for the future.

The "Legally Coercive Model":

The rights of individuals to be protected from infectious diseases by legal systems that restrict the exercise of some of the rights of individuals who are or may be infective to others are well established in law. In these cases there is usually no question as to the disease involved, the infectivity

of the disease or of the potential for infection of others
from the person whose rights are restricted. Tuberculosis
is such a disease for which legal systems exist that may remove
a person from his family, vocation and ordinary social contact
until proved non-infective. Although there have been laws in
the past designed for eugenic reasons, they have dealt with a
potpourri of "mental illness" or "mental retardation." Because
of the inappropriate use of such laws they have fallen into dis-
repute and disuse. Also a large factor in such disuse has been
the issue of individual rights. Evolution in our viewpoint
toward individual rights has now brought up a concept which may
be of particular significance in Huntington's disease. This
is the right to a life with normal expectancy for health. The
issue has been couched in terms of "wrongful life" and is a
concept that appears to be pertinent to the offspring of persons known to be at risk or to be affected by Huntington's disease.

Perhaps the Commission could give consideration to the
effect this concept would have, in addition to the societal
concerns of economic costs and increasing prevalence, on reaching a reasonable balance between the rights of living individuals
in affected families and the rights of other individuals and
society. In the event that guidelines are developed, it will
then be more reasonable for a program designed along the lines
of other successful public health programs to be developed.
Programs that provide support and care for those known to be
affected can be successful in controlling the prevalence of
this disease but it would seem from past history that strong
socially or legally coercive approaches may be required. The
question of considering the use of laws designed to control
infectious diseases as precedents is raised.

In summary, the suggestion is made that the Commission
could materially assist in providing more consistent counseling
in relation to the disease by developing guidelines which deal
with the ethical problems faced by counselors, many times without their realization of the issues involved. The initial concerns expressed are in relation to Huntington's disease and:

1. Ownership of the information about given individuals
at risk.

   a. The individual's right to know versus the indi-
       vidual's right not to know.

   b. The boundaries of parents' rights to make deci-
    sions affecting their children at risk without
    the children's knowledge.

  2. The obligation of counselors toward persons <u>not</u> aware
they are at risk.

  3. The possibility that a public health approach modeled
on the precedent of control for infectious diseases may be
developed taking into deliberate consideration of the rights of
living individuals, societal rights, and the rights of the unborn to a life of health.

  Guidelines on such matters would make decisions on proced-
ural matters, such as a Registry and development of identifying
tests, more ordered.

JANICE R. WALKER
BREMERTON, WASHINGTON

FEBRUARY 28, 1977

I can remember when I was in the first grade and my mother was bad enough that my two brothers and I would have to help her walk to the bathroom. That same year, they took her to the hospital and we didn't live with her again.

She was then transferred to Resthaven Nursing Home in Bremerton where she battled Huntington's disease for 11 more years. She had very few visitors except for the immediate members of the family. I visited her every Sunday for 11 years, watching her dribble away to a pitiful sight. While she was sitting in the home, my two brothers and I went from foster home to foster home trying to keep the family together.

In the Resthaven Nursing Home, the help was terrible. The food was usually burnt or would taste terrible. About six months before my mother died, the doctor, along with the nursing home staff, took away her cigarettes and started her on some kind of medicine to relax her. She had previously been up and about, before they decided to give her this medicine; so much so that it was even hard for them to get her to take a nap. All of a sudden, after this medication, she didn't have the strength to get up and go to the bathroom.

My mother told me that she was upset with herself because she just didn't have the strength to do anything. Along with not having any strength she noticed that she started to fall out of bed. At this point, the home started tying her into her bed. Everytime I went to see her and she had to go to the bathroom, she would turn on her light and wait for about 15 minutes and then I would go down the hall and look for someone to help. Usually there was no one to help and I would have to help her go, using a bedpan.

My mother began to yell a lot. I think that she was going through the change of life, but the doctors didn't treat her for anyting. The home started a court order to send my mother to Western State Hospital because of yelling, which was approved. She was taken to the hospital that day after they washed her hair. They didn't take her temperature or give her a required check-up before taking her to the hospital. When she entered

Western State, the doctors checked her temperature and found that she had pneumonia. They started treatment for that when they discovered it. We got a call two days later that she died an unnecessary death.

For me, I worry mostly about becoming like my mother and seeing my children growing up and visiting me in a home. This is why I decided to have a tubal ligation performed on me at the Naval Regional Medical Center in Bremerton. My doctor at the Naval Hospital doesn't know very much about this disease and I was referred to the University of Washington Hospital for research.

I believe if there were any suggestions that I could bring up, one would be to send all doctors a monthly report on what research is being done. I also would like to say that the research for Huntington's disease is much more important than sending men to the moon or selling grain to Russia. I think we should concentrate mainly on finding a cure for this terribly debilitating disease.

Seattle, Washington   April 14, 1977

JAMES G. WILSON
OTHELLO, WASHINGTON   MARCH 23, 1977

I am writing this letter with the hope of promoting financial help and other considerations for victims of the Huntington Chorea disease.

My daughter, Jerrie Ann Buckner, has been diagnosed as having the disease by the Stanford Medical Center in Berkley, California. Jerrie Ann is 38 years old, married and the mother of three boys. Their ages are 15, 12 and 7. Her husband earns an average income but they are quite concerned as to their future both financially and physically. In the past year she has deteriorated physically to a point where she must depend on a walker to attain mobility. They forecast that in another year she will require a wheel chair. In a very few years she will become bedridden and require a nurse at home or be placed in a nursing home. It is not hard to visualize the financial burden this will mean to this family and I am sure it is not unlike many others who find themselves in the same position.

For this reason I highly recommend that money be appropriated or in some way be raised to assist people and families who are victims of this disease. Money is needed for research, therapy and financial assistance.

As I understand it, the present Federal laws will not support any of these needs. So for this reason I am asking your office to do everything possible to bring the victims of this terrible disease into future consideration by those charged with the direction and appropriation of money for such needs.

Thank you for anything you can do.

Seattle, Washington   April 14, 1977

MRS. THEODORE WILSON
VANCOUVER, WASHINGTON   MARCH 30, 1977

    I'm not sure that I can provide the material you want
but I will submit such information to the best of my ability.
I do not care to appear as a witness but you may feel free
to use my name.

    I am a bystander for the Huntington's chorea investiga-
tion, since it was my husband and his mother who had Huntington's
and our children who are "at-risk" H.D. patients.

    Since we were not told what disease my mother-in-law had
we did not realize that the problem existed in our family.

    My mother-in-law, Dorothy Preston, came to Washington from
Galveston, Texas in 1918. She left behind a sister and two
brothers. In 1937 we did hear that the sister was institutionalized at Texas State Hospital. If my mother-in-law knew why--she
never passed the information on. As far as I know the sister
was about 23 years old then and spent her life there. My
mother-in-law was committed to Oregon State Hospital at age 50.
She spent the next nine years there until her death in 1965.
Doctors there did diagnose it as a disease, said it was not
hereditary, but did not name the disease to my husband's half-
sisters. They in turn did not mention it was a disease to us
until four years later when my husband entered a psychiatric
hospital with what was diagnosed as depression. Then they said
the death certificate said the mother's death was from Huntington's.

    In 1957, when I wrote to my husband's grandmother in Texas
to tell her of her daughter's commitment, she told me in a return
letter that another son of hers was also in Texas State Hospital.
So this made three of the grandmother's children hospitalized.
I would assume it was all related.

    Since we did not realize that we were at-risk for H.D.
we did not understand many things that were to occur, and if
I had not been a Christian with the Lord's help to fall back
on, I certainly could not have coped with the problem as long
as I did until my husband was hospitalized.

The main problem we had was "an about-face" conduct of my husband's. During the last few years before my husband's entering a psychiatric hospital, we were raising three teen-age daughters. Every one who has ever raised youngsters understands they can drive you to distraction but my husband had always been a quiet, very sensible person and it seemed that overnight he became enraged at the smallest thing. On one occasion which I later reported to my doctor, my husband completely lost control, flew at one girl and pulled her hair so severely that she hemorrhaged and developed a large lump on her forehead.

We had several such incidents, which the girls and I were at a loss to explain. My husband was a valuable employee at a local warehouse, a respected member of a hiking club in Oregon and had been an A-1 soldier in the U.S. Army for four years.

During the last three years before he entered the psychiatric hospital he complained of his back, his feet and his knees. The family doctor and a bone man found nothing but he did start going to a chiropractor and felt he had some relief. During these years when we would sit reading in the evening his foot would jerk but we didn't realize what the problem was. Also during this time my husband must have felt something in his calf muscles or the lack of something because he would sit and feel his muscles as though he were worried. Since he had been an avid backpacker, having hiked completely across Washington State and also across most of Oregon on the Pacific Crest Trail, I felt he was just a worry wort over his legs.

After we were aware of what my mother-in-law had had, our family doctor of 25 years and the psychiatrist at Columbia View Manor in Vancouver consulted, and it was decided to call in a consultant in Lovejoy Medical Clinic, who was Dr. Larson, a neurologist and psychiatrist. He had previously doctored one of our girls for encephalitis, and another who became epileptic at 18. He diagnosed my husband's problem as H.D. and said he had probably had it for ten years. After this diagnosis my husband was put on medication which was quite effective and was released from the hospital.

For the next five years he steadily saw Dr. Robert McElhoney in Vancouver. Dr. Larson said about all we could do would be to doctor the inner man so we set to work.

Seattle, Washington   April 14, 1977

    My husband was a very disciplined and health-conscious
person who never smoked, drank or overate. He retired on a
disability from his job as a warehouseman. After retirement
he and I set us a schedule of exercising and walking to help
fill his free time. At first we walked as much as five miles
daily. With the medication and the burden of work gone we did
quite well for a couple of years. As time went by the walks
became shorter but he still did quite well though he became
more and more fearful. Every little thing worried him. Where
he had just a few years before hiked cross country from Cougar,
Washington to Spirit Lake all alone through dense woods, he now
became fearful we would become lost in our own area of town.
It was sad to see him go downhill.

    During the last four months of his life he began to have
uncontrollable rages where he would fly at me, hitting and
kicking me. After one such affair I had to call the police
for help. Three policemen had a very hard time and they in
turn called an ambulance, and he was taken to Columbia View
Manor. This was exactly five years after he had been there
when his problem was diagnosed. He was a patient for a month,
then he was released for three weeks until another rage came
upon him and he was a patient again for a month. During the
last two weekends he came home on a pass and did very well.
After he went back on a pass at 7:00 p.m. he suffered chest
pains at 10:00 p.m. and died en route to the hospital. Though
it was a shock I felt this was the Lord's best for him because
the family doctor and psychiatrist had said he couldn't be kept
at home much longer.

    Now that I have given you the main problems I should state
some of the other problems. My husband started receiving Social
Security disability payments and his Teamsters' pension, on
which we managed quite well. The Teamsters' health insurance
was _wonderful_ to help. Though medicine ran up to $40 - $50
monthly for most of five years, they paid 75 percent of cost
after the $100 deductible was satisfied. Medicare and Teamsters'
paid _all_ hospital and ambulance costs.

    The psychiatrist in Vancouver provided our girls and their
husbands with a very good story of the disease and Dr. Larson
of the neurological clinic in Portland had us all come at
once and talked to us. Though we already had three daughters
and two grandchildren we decided to play the hand we had been
dealt with as much common sense as possible. My girls did

worry <u>much</u> at first, but as they saw my husband work at it and
continue to make a life for himself, the fear of the disease
lessened. Though it's been seven and a half years since the
family realized what we had, there have been no more children.
One girl had a tubal ligation. The other two have contemplated
this but so far have not done so.

My husband has one full brother, who had what was diagnosed as an aneurysm at age 50. He is still living, but without
use of one leg and arm. My husband has two half-sisters who
each have three children. His brother has two boys. So all
in all, there are ten children and three grandchildren who are
at-risk H.D. patients. The ages are from 34 down to age 15 in
the children. The three grandchildren are 13, 10, and 10.

Thank you so much for your inquiry.

Seattle, Washington   April 14, 1977

ANONYMOUS
MOUNT VERNON, WASHINGTON   MARCH 25, 1977

The following comments are submitted in response to your request for
information from Huntington's Disease families. Please note that while
I do not want my name published, I am most anxious to be included on
any mailing list for purposes of communicating results of the investigation.

Two years ago, when she was 7½, my daughter was diagnosed with Huntington's
Disease. Symptoms first appeared when she was about six years old, but
pediatricians attributed her coordination difficulties to minor brain damage
as a result of a premature birth. The H.D. diagnoses was made at the Children's
Orthopedic Hospital in Seattle after continued progressively worsening
coordination and after she developed speech problems. She remains emotionally
well-balanced.

Joycie is an only child who attends special education classes in the public
schools. She is the first Huntington's child this school system has had,
so the teachers are not sure how much can be expected of her. I have given
them all the literature I can find, but most of it deals with childhood H.D.
only in passing. It would be helpful if Joycie's teachers could draw on the
experiences of other teachers who have worked with Huntington's children.

Though Joycie is followed very closely by her doctors, there is no treatment
nor medication. There has been no severe financial hardship. Though I
cannot bear to think about the future and what it means for Joycie, I do
know that I will always be able to provide for her.

Joycie's father, who is now 32 years old, is also afflicted with H.D. We
were divorced several years before diagnoses was made for either of them.
I understand now that the cause of the divorce was H.D. manifesting in
mental and emotional aberations, but at the time I could not account for
the radical change in my husband's personality. Knowing now that he is
ill, I still consider the divorce essential to the emotional well-being of
my child.

His condition has progressed to the point that it is impossible to hold a
rational conversation with him. He has become fanatically religious and
seems to have lost all common sense. He is not able to exercise good
judgment, and so is frequently involved in a hassle with landlords, police,
and employers. He is no longer able to function productively - he holds
three college degrees, but is unable to hold a job more than a few months.
His life has become so increasingly unstable that he has lost all personal
possessions and he moves several times a year, living off unemployment and
handouts. He is gradually alienating all relatives and friends who would
like to help him, but cannot deal with his emotional excesses.

Seattle, Washington   April 14, 1977

He harrasses me constantly (almost daily) and I have had to rescue him from
many binds of one kind or another, but so far have been able to shield my
daughter from the most unpleasant of these situations. He is allowed to
visit her in my home only. I cannot let her be alone with him.

His daughter and his identical twin brother have been diagnosed and he is
well aware of the implications. He knows the genetic nature and the
symptoms of the disease, but he has not accepted that he is afflicted. He
has avoided any medical examination, but I have received confirmation from
doctors who observed him while he accompanied his brother for consultation.

He needs help – he needs someone to take care of him. I have had to chose
between him and my daughter. If there were not a child involved, perhaps
I could take him into my home. But his behavior cannot be controlled, and
I know that what respite I could give him would be only temporary, and the
emotional strain on myself and my daughter would be unbearable. I would
not want even a healthy child to live under such conditions.

I have looked everywhere I know to try to find some help for him. It seems
that neither the medical profession nor the state can help him until he
asks for aid or until his situation becomes more dramatically desperate.
I don't want to see him committed to an institution at this point. If
only there were some sort of "outreach" program or if he could get involved in some sort of halfway house that would not deny his freedom, but
would provide some stability and guidance and give him some place to turn
when he is out on the streets with no money and no home. But, I cannot
realistically see him getting along with anyone for any period of time.

His twin brother is living much the same kind of life, but I do not see
enough of him to know his situation. His exwife is physically afraid
of him. There is also an older sister who may be afflicted. She has
been living a borderline life for many years, and if not directly
suffering from HD, she certainly has suffered mentally and emotionally
from experiencing HD in her mother. There are no other siblings. Their
father is remarried and living in another state, and though he does what
he can, he is at a loss on how to help his children. He is living on
social security now, and cannot give them much more financial aid. He
put his sons through college, partially supported his daughter for many
years and is simply exhausted with the worry and effort.

H. D. has totally destroyed this family.

For your statistical information: I am 32 years old, employed as a bookkeeper,
divorced, and college-education (social sciences).

☆U.S. GOVERNMENT PRINTING OFFICE:1978 734-821/648 1-3